SECOND EDITION

Ophthalmic Leadership

A Practical Guide for Physicians, Administrators, and Teams

AF692205

SECOND EDITION

Ophthalmic Leadership

A Practical Guide for Physicians, Administrators, and Teams

John B. Pinto

SLACK
INCORPORATED

SLACK
INCORPORATED

SLACK Incorporated
6900 Grove Road
Thorofare, NJ 08086 USA
856-848-1000 Fax: 856-848-6091
www.slackbooks.com
ISBN: 978-1-63091-980-1
© 2022 SLACK Incorporated with the kind permission of the author, John B. Pinto. All rights reserved.

Senior Vice President: Stephanie Arasim Portnoy
Vice President, Editorial: Jennifer Kilpatrick
Vice President, Marketing: Mary Sasso
Acquisitions Editor: Tony Schiavo
Director of Editorial Operations: Jennifer Cahill
Vice President/Creative Director: Thomas Cavallaro
Cover Artist: Lori Shields

All rights reserved. No part of this book may be reproduced, stored in a retrieval system or transmitted in any form or by any means, electronic, mechanical, photocopying, recording or otherwise, without written permission from the publisher, except for brief quotations embodied in critical articles and reviews.

The procedures and practices described in this publication should be implemented in a manner consistent with the professional standards set for the circumstances that apply in each specific situation. Every effort has been made to confirm the accuracy of the information presented and to correctly relate generally accepted practices. The authors, editors, and publisher cannot accept responsibility for errors or exclusions or for the outcome of the material presented herein. There is no expressed or implied warranty of this book or information imparted by it. Care has been taken to ensure that drug selection and dosages are in accordance with currently accepted/recommended practice. Off-label uses of drugs may be discussed. Due to continuing research, changes in government policy and regulations, and various effects of drug reactions and interactions, it is recommended that the reader carefully review all materials and literature provided for each drug, especially those that are new or not frequently used. Some drugs or devices in this publication have clearance for use in a restricted research setting by the Food and Drug and Administration or FDA. Each professional should determine the FDA status of any drug or device prior to use in their practice.

Any review or mention of specific companies or products is not intended as an endorsement by the author or publisher.

SLACK Incorporated uses a review process to evaluate submitted material. Prior to publication, educators or clinicians provide important feedback on the content that we publish. We welcome feedback on this work.

Library of Congress Control Number: 2021945894

For permission to reprint material in another publication, contact SLACK Incorporated. Authorization to photocopy items for internal, personal, or academic use is granted by SLACK Incorporated provided that the appropriate fee is paid directly to Copyright Clearance Center. Prior to photocopying items, please contact the Copyright Clearance Center at 222 Rosewood Drive, Danvers, MA 01923 USA; phone: 978-750-8400; website: www.copyright.com; email: info@copyright.com

Printed in the United States of America.

Last digit is print number: 10 9 8 7 6 5 4 3 2 1

Dedication

To my son Graham, who at age 15 collaborated with me on the concept for the first edition of this book. Many years have passed. He's a finance wizard now, casting spells in Silicon Valley. Like most of us, he learned more about leadership by living with roommates than going to graduate school.

Aut Viam Inveniam Aut Faciam

This is not my room. This is definitely not my room.
And I don't have my tapioca pudding.
—Dustin Hoffman, as Raymond in *Rain Man*

John is a member of the editorial board of *Ocular Surgery News* and a regular contributor to other eye care publications. He is available for individual physician and practice consulting services to supplement this book. Please contact him at:

J. Pinto & Associates, Inc.
2926 Kellogg Street
Suite B18
San Diego, CA 92106
619-223-2233
pintoinc@aol.com
www.pintoinc.com

Contributing Authors

Amir Arbisser, MD (Chapter 3) graduated from Princeton University (AB) and Baylor College of Medicine (MD). He completed a National Institutes of Health fellowship in genetic/metabolic disease and his ophthalmology residency at the University of Texas Houston Health Science Center. Formal training concluded with pediatric ophthalmology fellowship in Iowa City. He is board certified and practices pediatric and comprehensive ophthalmology. He co-founded Eye Surgeons Associates (20 doctors, 5 locations) and serves as contributing editor for *Ophthalmology Management.* Dr. Arbisser served 6 years on Iowa's public universities' governing Board of Regents, which includes the University of Iowa Carver College of Medicine. He chairs the See Life Clearly Foundation and Minute Suites, LLC. He shares four children and two grandchildren with his wife, Lisa Brothers Arbisser, MD.

Paul N. Arnold, MD (Chapter 30) has served on the executive committees of the American Society of Cataract and Refractive Surgery (ASCRS) and the Outpatient Ophthalmic Surgery Society. He has been chairman of the ASCRS Film Festival and Government Relations committee, as well as serving as an advisor to the American Medical Association Relative Value Update committee and the American Academy of Ophthalmology (AAO) Practice Management committee. He is presently retired and living in Ashland, Oregon.

Priscilla Arnold, MD (Chapter 50) served as the chair of Government Relations for ASCRS from 2000 to 2010. She has also held the position of president of ASCRS from 2004 to 2005, as well as the American Board of Eye Surgery. Dr. Arnold has twice received the Secretariat Award from the AAO. She has been given the Honor Award and Senior Honor Award for service to AAO. She is retired and living in Ashland, Oregon.

Hayley Boling, MBA, COE (Chapter 48) is the chief executive officer for Boling Vision Center & INSIGHT Surgery Center in Northern Indiana. Coming from a long line of medical entrepreneurs, she brings a unique perspective to ophthalmic leadership. She is passionate about developing and redefining practice culture, maximizing practice efficiencies by modernizing practice processes and patient flow, and enhancing the guest experience by consistently exceeding expectations. These passions, combined with the ongoing cultivation of an amazing support team, have been the driving force behind the inspired expansion of Boling Vision Center's practice infrastructure over the past 10 years. In addition to being named an industry "game changer" three times in her career thus far, as well as being an award-winning author, Ms. Boling is an active board member for OWL (Ophthalmic World Leaders, formerly Ophthalmic Women Leaders) as well as the American Society of Ophthalmic Administrators (ASOA), a committee member for ASCRS' Government Relations and Health Information Technology committees, an advisory board member and task force/committee member for several industry organizations, a past chairman of the Board for *AE Magazine,* and actively participates as an Indiana Representative for the Alliance of Specialty Medicine's Fly-In on Capitol Hill. She is a contributing author in various industry magazines, books, and publications and serves as a presenter and panel member at various conferences and meetings across the world.

Let's enumerate 20 of the other attributes of the best practice leaders working today:

1. *Direct job knowledge.* It's not absolutely necessary that a practice administrator or MP know how to post a charge or work up a basic patient, but your staff will respect you much more if these are things that you at least try to do.
2. *Delegation.* Almost all administrators are brought up from the ranks. They know the job. And as working managers they still spend most of their time *doing* the job. But they need to balance this with the ability to delegate. One of the most common complaints leveled at otherwise excellent administrators is that they have difficulty delegating. If you're an excellent leader, you are probably continuously struggling to find the right balance between doing and delegating.
3. *Action oriented.* While every practice executive needs to keep one eye on the future, and work to draw out from your owners their desires, you should not be spending excess time pondering the long-term destiny of the practice. Instead, you should be biased toward operations and drive a process of relentless polishing.
4. *Grace under pressure.* Administrators and the MP they work with most closely are squeezed in a four-way vise, pressured by patients, doctors, staff, and myriad external forces. Great leaders are understated, upbeat, and calm.
5. *Accountability.* Too often, the pressure of pleasing so many parties at the same time can lead to over-promising. Great leaders are able to gauge the needs of the job at hand against their resources and be realistic about what they need in terms of time and staff and dollars to get the job done right.
6. *Communication.* It should go without saying that superior leaders are great communicators, starting with being very good listeners. Although most supervision puts a premium on verbal communication, you must also be able to write clearly. Any practice with more than a handful of staff needs to transition from being a purely verbal culture to writing down agreed protocols and procedures and using frequent memos to keep everyone on the same page.
7. *Discipline.* As a leader you develop and uphold the operational standards of your practice. If these standards are wobbly because of an undisciplined administrator, the practice itself starts to spin out of control.
8. *Tough love.* Holding staff members to the operational standards of the practice takes more than discipline. It requires the ability to be tough with the people you manage. If a staff member arrives inappropriately dressed, that person still gets sent home—even if it means driving 40 miles round trip and the clinic running behind for the rest of the morning.
9. *Fairness.* Staff, when they're being led well, will always tell me something like, "Susan, my manager, is great. She's the toughest boss I've ever had to work for, but she's also the fairest." People do their very best work when they are supervised by someone who's inordinately tough, but combines that with inordinate fairness.
10. *Openness.* People love working for leaders who are open to their ideas. People hate working for a boss who will only take their own counsel … or worse, will twist things around and take all the credit for the ideas of their staff.
11. *Forgiveness.* All staff make mistakes, they're human. They need to be redeemed after every mistake. Nobody likes to work under someone who holds a grudge

for an error made last week. Unless an error has been made that deserves frank termination, every staff should be able to erase their personal error scoreboard by at least the end of the month and start out again with a clean slate.

12. *Adaptability.* Superior leaders may as well wear a button that says, "I Love Change!" Rather than being rigid and bristling at the thought of policy changes or alterations in the routine, they welcome every change for the better and get their more resistant staff to support unpopular changes.
13. *Organization.* The very best practice leaders I've ever met, in more than 3 decades of field work observing thousands of practices firsthand, are engaged parents in their personal life. I'm convinced that if you can properly lead a few kids you can just as easily organize the world.
14. *Guardianship.* Even the most robust practices are relatively fragile as business organizations … especially today, as profits are falling and the economic punishment for making a mistake is rising. A trait you must possess as a leader is being a fierce protector of the enterprise. If you think the practice is heading down the wrong path, speak up—even if it may mean you'll put your career in jeopardy.
15. *Mentoring.* Administrators and practice owners are coaches, cheerleaders, and mentors. Staff protégés are well served if their administrators have the patience and knack for passing along their knowledge, while creating a hunger for career development.
16. *Team playing.* Beyond technical skill, a practice leader should be able to defer to and sacrifice for the needs of the group. This sacrifice takes many forms. Managers have to be open to early and late hours, open to criticism, and open to the adverse consequences of making the occasional crummy decision.
17. *Maturity and respect.* Every leader has the right to their opinion. But sometimes, your board's position—wisely or foolishly—runs counter to your own. The mature department head, administrator, or board chairman publicly respects the decisions of the board, even when they may privately disagree.
18. *Humility.* In a world where you're generating dozens of decisions and requests a day, you're going to make mistakes. Administrators and doctors should readily own up to their mistakes, which will only lead to a virtuous feedback loop of even more respect and responsibility in the future.
19. *Personal reserves.* Ask department heads, administrators, and MPs how much they're giving of themselves to the practice and most will answer, "Why, 110% of course!" This is the wrong answer. Wise leaders only give about 90% so they consistently have some gas left in the tank during crisis periods.
20. *Balanced skill set.* It's unusual to find great people leadership skills (which obliges a large measure of sensitivity, intuition, and emotional intelligence) in people who possess what is arguably the most critical professional skill set in today's health care executives: finance, accounting, and economics. In my experience, financial wizards, for all their ability to read numbers, commonly lack the ability to read people. And vice-versa. Those with innate people skills are commonly "mathophobic." Since you are probably stronger in one area than another, your career advancement requires that you backfill for your weakest areas.

• • •

Obviously, no one ever measures up to all of these ideals. And even if they did, the most appropriate leader for any one organization changes over time, which each year increases the odds of an eventual mismatch between the leader and the practice.

Even at the outset, most practice leaders are at least slightly less capable than the needs of their organization. Certainly in today's bumptious, challenging world few leaders are up to the task, whether they are an ophthalmic practice leader, a Fortune 500 CEO, or the nation's president.

Even the momentarily "perfect" leader soon falls from their pedestal. All organizations (and countries) go through the same amusing cycle: selecting a leader and projecting on that person talents they don't possess. Time passes. The hero-leader inevitably falls short ... the honeymoon ends and the leader's satisfaction ratings goes down.

The common result is a shorter tenure than most leaders deserve. According to *Fortune Magazine,* the average tenure of a Fortune 500 company CEO is under 4 years. The average practice administrator or MP doesn't last much longer. It's sobering to remember that whomever you select for your new leader has probably been deemed a greater or lesser disappointment in another setting.

A few leaders are born. Most are made. But "making" a business leader is quite unlike the fact-cramming process of making a retinologist. Unfortunately, the genetic endowments that make a great microsurgeon do not reside on the same chromosome with the genes for leadership genius.

Business leadership, unlike law or accounting, is not a "learned" profession, but rather largely the slow, personal accumulation of on-the-job case histories. This book is organized loosely into topical sections, each presenting in longer or shorter chapters each author's experience and perspectives. It's an opportunity to add their case histories to your own. Feel free to skip around if some topics attract you more than others.

The contributing authors and I hope that by the time you complete this book a few of ***our*** personal cases, warts and all, will seep in and accelerate your own development as a leader.

—John B. Pinto
San Diego, California

Section I

Leadership Perspectives

CHAPTER 1

Managing Your Effectiveness

Accountability 101

Keith Casebolt

We don't learn from experience.
We learn only as we reflect on our experience.
—Peter Drucker

Just for fun, let's assume that you are the primary factor in your own success. I know, it is so tempting to blame those unreasonable, clueless, and demanding doctors you work for; the stiff competition across town; Medicare rates; the Great Recession; and the lack of motivated and qualified staff. But that would be thinking like a victim. And what do victims do? ***Nothing,*** pretty much, other than whine, justify, and blame others. Since this passes for normal, you'll be in good company in almost any bar and many professional meetings. But you won't get much done.

And getting things done requires change. Change is usually difficult, both in recognizing the need for it and in implementation. Consider these statements:

"If you like the results you are getting then don't change anything."

and

"Your system is perfectly designed to create the results you are getting."

Pinto JB. *Ophthalmic Leadership: A Practical Guide for Physicians, Administrators, and Teams, Second Edition* (pp 3-9).
© 2022 SLACK Incorporated.

Besides blaming others, whining, and denying the need for change, the other possibility is to accept the premise—you are accountable for your own success, much of which will necessitate change. Ouch! If that is so, then what do you do when you don't like the results you are getting? It sounds like a recipe for depression, but it is not. Accountability is the path to personal power, results, and effectiveness. Why? Because once you understand that your attitude and behavior are the only things you can control, then there is a clear path to improving future results. No one can prevent you from improving except you. You don't have to spend a lot of time manipulating others.

So, simply master yourself, make some changes, and your problems are over! (Phone me when you've got that one handled.) Unfortunately, improving your effectiveness is not easy or instant. Here are some strategies gleaned from others that will help you improve your effectiveness:

- There is a difference between reflecting and beating yourself up for past mistakes. Reflecting results in insight: "I see how I could have done that differently, and if faced with a similar situation in the future, I will apply what I've learned." Beating yourself up tends to be repetitive and circular and doesn't result in insight: "How could I have been so stupid? Why do I always do that? When will I ever learn? I am so bad at this!" Once you start in on yourself, you feel worse and worse. Nothing changes and nothing is likely to change in the future.
- Humans have this amazing ability for self-sabotage. You probably won't make a lot of progress with any change until you understand what you are getting out of things being exactly the way they are now. You helped create the current situation by actions you took, or (more likely) failed to take. Why? Here's a hint. Shop for fears. What are you afraid will happen if you make a change? Most of us remain paralyzed by fears of what could happen. But there are other possibilities as well. Let's say you have helped create a dependent relationship with one of your direct reports. You know you need to coach this person to be more sufficient. If you are honest with yourself, you might notice that you enjoy being the expert. You enjoy getting the phone calls asking for your advice. And you fear what would happen to the relationship if you started expecting the person to function more on their own. Until you are clear what your payoff for the status quo is in this or any situation, you will likely subvert your own attempts to make a change. Not to mention handling any resistance you may get from the other party.
- If you make any change that affects others, you can expect these two contradictory responses, often from the same people:
    - "It's about time"
    - "Change back now!"

  If you are not prepared for the "change back" messages, it will be easy to abandon the effort. Remember that most of us agree with this: "There are two things I can't stand. One is the way things are, and the other is change."
- We all hate feeling incompetent. Change will necessarily put you into the zone of learning something new—a new habit, a new skill, or something. And therein lies a trap. By definition, you will be temporarily incompetent and have the feeling that goes with it. High-control leaders tend to avoid that feeling, but if you allow that

to derail you, you will be stuck where you are. Make a choice to be ok with that feeling. It will subside as you acquire a new skill.

- Here's what gets in your way—your ego. Your ego is not about problem solving, it is about looking good. It is about image management. It is about winning. And when your ego is running you and you bump up against someone else's ego, expect a long day. Conflict. Turf wars. We all have egos and they aren't going to suddenly start behaving the way we'd like. So get very clear. You can either be right, or get what you want. The ego wants the former. Effectiveness comes from the latter. So, when one of your doctors suggests a solution that you've been recommending for years, if you want to be right you point out how many times you've already suggested that. You might even complain that no one seems to take you seriously. Or, you could simply agree with the suggestion and be happy that now you can move forward.
- Stop trying to make people feel comfortable. Stop trying to be comfortable. How many times have you heard or said this sentence? "I'm just not comfortable with that." I understand that's usually code for "I disagree." But it is an amazing statement. I think you have to pick one:
    - Learn to tolerate being uncomfortable, or
    - Stay stuck, never change, be safe

  I have a prediction about which one of those will be more effective over time. It's not the second one.
- How do the people you work with see you and does that have consequences? Yes, it does and sometimes it is hard to know what those are. This is a perfectly awful concept. Other people have formed judgments about you. They can't help it, our brains are wired to arrive at conclusions based on limited data. It is pattern recognition software, and unfortunately there are some bugs. Some conclusions are based on total misinformation, stereotypes, and projections. Others have a lot of accuracy. Either way, these judgments profoundly affect how they respond to you. And if you are unaware of their opinions of you, you will be in the dark. How to dispel this darkness? Ask. Ask them to tell you in great detail how you are to work with. What do they like and not like? Specifically, what do they recommend you *start* doing, *stop* doing, and *continue* doing? That pretty much covers the bases. Most people will never sign up for a dose of hearing other people's opinions of them. They are afraid their egos will pop and they will cease to exist. But here's the reality—that has never happened and it won't happen to you either. What does happen:
    - People respect the courage this takes
    - People love to be asked their opinion
    - You will learn many things about how you are perceived
    - You will glean many specific ideas for improving your effectiveness
    - You will have set an example of leadership
    - People with negative judgments of you will stop talking about you behind your back once they've told you directly

 - People's negative judgments of you tend to soften once they feel heard by you
 - You will be teaching everyone that adults talk directly to adults. Children have other ways, like gossip or anonymous surveys. If you want to grow adults, do it directly.
- It gets even worse. I want you to get this feedback in a group setting! And, I don't want you to have any response to the feedback. Just listen. If you want to follow up later on a particular comment or issue, that's fine. In fact, there may be quite a bit you want to follow up on. But in the session, just pay close attention to what they are saying without debate or comment. Ask questions only if you don't understand what they are saying. For instance it is common to hear "continue supporting me." This could mean any number of things, and it would be good to know specifically how they want you to support them. Here is why to do this in a group setting:
 - Counter intuitively, it is safer. If someone is out to get you, it will be obvious to the entire group and no one will like that. And it won't stick to you, but to them.
 - It is efficient. You can get feedback from 10 or more people in less than 1 hour.
 - You can see trends very quickly. If 7 out of 10 people want you to start running meetings more effectively, it will be clearer to you to hear that all at once.
- Take responsibility for reducing your defensive behaviors. What is defensiveness? Anything other than problem solving. A defensive behavior occurs when you feel threatened or attacked in some way, either internally by your inner critic or externally. To avoid feeling this feeling, you employ any one of a number of strategies, such as (this list, and many of these concepts, is courtesy of consultant Thompson Barton):
 - Trivializing with humor
 - Taking offense
 - Poker face
 - High charge in the body
 - Sudden drop in IQ
 - Wanting the last word
 - Denial
 - Playing the victim—"poor me"
 - Terminally unique—"that's just how I am"
 - Loss of humor
 - Retreat into deadly silence
 - Addictions—drugs, shopping, sex
 - Suddenly tired or sleepy
 - Flooding with information to prove a point
 - Becoming cynical
 - Pretending

- Rigidity
- Selective deafness
- Being too nice
- Sarcasm
- Attack
- Holding a grudge
- Endless explaining and rationalizing
- Intellectualizing
- "I'm aware of that; leave me alone" (the defense of awareness)

In the unlikely event you're not aware of doing any of these behaviors, first ask yourself what the defense of denial might look like. You might also ask your spouse or significant other for some input. Pull up a chair and get comfortable. This may take a while.

If you pay attention, you'll probably observe yourself doing these behaviors in sequences. Such as, at first you laugh off the unwanted feedback. When that doesn't work, you start flooding with information, then get a little sarcastic. After that, you retreat into deadly silence. Then you continue on to other topics, pretending you are not upset. When you get home, if you are still feeling bad, you hit the mall and buy something you don't need in the hope of feeling better.

Defensive behaviors are pretty much what we don't like in others and it's easy to see why. They don't solve problems. How would you like to be on the receiving end of the sequence described previously? When you engage in defensiveness, you might feel better in the moment; but nothing changes, except that time goes away. (Oh, and the other person makes a judgment that you're highly threatened and difficult to work with.) So your task is to reduce the amount of time and energy you put into being defensive. The best way to do this is "with a little help from my friends." By definition, defensiveness starts with unawareness, so you need some support. Make a new deal with the people you work most closely with. The deal is: "When you see me doing these behaviors, would you point that out? I'd really like to spend less time and energy being defensive." Ask them to tell you what defenses they see you doing most, and in what situations. Check in with them once or twice a year on this subject.

- Improve your listening. This may be the simplest and often most difficult way to improve your effectiveness. Most of us, and therefore most of your staff, suffer from the hurt feelings of not being heard. One author said, "Being heard is so similar to the feeling of being loved that most people can't tell the difference." Truly listening has that profound an impact. Listening, contrary to what we've often been taught, is not a technique, it is an intention. If it is your intention to listen, your behaviors will look like this:
  - "Tell me more"
  - "What I think you are saying is…"
  - "What I think you are feeling is…"

Core Strength

Another metaphor for understanding core strength is the oak tree. The stronger, more deeply, and firmly rooted it becomes at its base, the more secure it will be when adverse weather strikes. A healthy oak can withstand hurricane-force winds. Limber branches bend nearly to the breaking point while the deeply rooted trunk barely strains.

Do you have the same deep roots for your practice? Do you have the flexibility required to bend rather than break when challenged by crisis? One of your main jobs as a practice leader is to foster both the core strength and flexibility of the organization.

Group practices must establish "roots." Think infrastructure, here ... the kind of grounding that comes with authentic vision, mission, and values statements; written rules that are followed and that have real consequences; boards and administrators who are both competent and aligned. All of this creates an organizational structure that thought leader Stephen Covey calls a "corporate immune system," enabling resistance to virulent threats.

These threats are now endemic in our environment. Pending fee adjustments. Higher operating costs. Greater competition from peers and institutions. And a regulatory storm that obliges every practice to have a de facto compliance officer.

Organizations with mature, stable cores can flex under pressure and simultaneously pursue entrepreneurship. Conversely, practices with unstable, weak cores most often demonstrate surface-level rigidity. Such practices commonly retreat toward the status quo in the face of uncertainty.

A Simple Key to Success: The Leadership Dyad

How can ophthalmic group practices develop the security that flows from core, corporate strength, and set the stage for more nimble growth and development? The answer lies in a simple, familiar concept with a funny Greek name—"dyad"—which in this context refers to a pair of leaders, the administrator and elected MP of the practice.

As Nathaniel Williams wrote in *The Affordability Factor: The 4 Cs of Change*, "One of the hardest things to do in life is to suppress our individuality and work as part of a team." There is no more important structural catalyst for your practice's purposeful growth than the MP and administrator working productively in tandem.

Think of how this works in a familiar, personal context. Children at home and adults in the workplace need a foundation that secures and empowers them. The most functional two-parent families enjoy relative stability and peace while nurturing the growth and development that embraces change as the kids grow up.

Misaligned parents can ruin young lives, just as misaligned practice leaders can ruin their businesses. We've witnessed numerous practice settings where a disengaged physician-leader or defensive manager can lead to perpetual crisis rather than forward movement.

In both family and business settings, the "offspring" (ie, the real kids, or the adults working in your practice) invariably play, divide, and conquer when they recognize that the "parents" are not aligned. In such cases, authority ultimately shifts away from the nominal leaders, and an unstable and chaotic core results.

The highly effective practice dyad mirrors an appropriately stern-but-benevolent, parent-like authority and responsibility within group practices. A unified, mutually respectful, and complimentary relationship between lead doctor and practice manager looks just like the effective co-parenting dyad.

In practices with this kind of dyadic core strength, today's rampant changes are seen as exciting opportunities, not as a source of paralyzing dread.

It may seem paradoxical, but setting up your MP and administrator in this model—having them provide limits, boundaries, and consequences to the rest of the "family"—ultimately creates more freedom for everyone in the practice to grow and adapt to change.

Although your organizational chart probably casts the administrator as subordinate to the MP, in the most effective settings these two become peers, creating a palpably unified quasi-parental dynamic. This builds respect and confidence in the practice work force at all levels, and especially among owner-physicians. Such doctors (even if once quite at odds with each other) will commonly settle down once they respect the authority they have formally granted to the dyad.

Core-Building Leadership Principles

Once the MP and administrator are annealed (and your practice may, as you read this, be missing one or the other or both halves of the team), the dyad's effectiveness begins with a clear understanding of three well-recognized leadership skills:

1. Humility with resolve
2. Emotional intelligence
3. Inspiring others to find their voice (after you have found your own, of course)

Humility With Resolve

As Jim Collins describes in his classic text *Good to Great,* leaders channel their ego needs away from themselves and into the larger goal of building a great company. "It's not that leaders have no ego or self-interest," Collins writes. "Indeed, they are incredibly ambitious—but their ambition is first and foremost for the institution, not themselves."

Inspiring leaders credit their people for successes while taking personal responsibility for failures. Trust is multiplied when the dyad functions as an advocate for, rather than a competitor or obstacle to, success. Great leaders are more like "plow horses" than "show horses." They have a humble, unpretentious nature. Their strengths are not worn

Competition is not uniformly bad, however we must maintain constant vigilance to prevent suboptimal patient care driven by business or other nonmedical metrics. Some of us are old enough to remember prerobotic surgical competition within a specialty cohort: "Through how small an incision can I deliver that baby, that tumor, that cataractous lens, or that lens nucleus? How fast? How many can I perform in an hour/day/month, etc?" At the beginning of our clinical practice it seemed amusing when nurses compared surgical procedure durations—especially since we "beat" the competition. When nurses pitted my wife Lisa's times with mine—in the words of the B. B. King song: "The thrill is gone." The humor evaporated. We reconsidered whether patients benefitted from this competition. We insisted our nurses seek more beneficial pursuits immediately.

Mixing competitiveness with economic drive can yield counter-productive partner behavior and dysfunctional groups. When the partner compensation methodology depends primarily upon an "eat what you kill" jungle mentality, it's not surprising that partners compete with each other for big-ticket services. For example, in some groups, many surgeons (including vitreoretinologists) perform refractive procedures instead of directing patients to a smaller cohort of procedural masters. The result? Individual docs performing more procedures certainly feather their own nests, however their group could suffer a flattened procedure growth curve or, worse, a decline in cases due to more mediocre results.

During my tenure as the founder and past MP, it was important to me to both redirect individuals' competitiveness away from each other ***and*** to cast myself as a noncompetitor. My compensation formula de-emphasized but did not eliminate the cash register incentive. The distribution calculation rewarded desired behavior appropriate to the enlarging group. We redistributed a significant portion of the group's income to incent physicians to examine patients to find pathology to refer to our most masterful subspecialists. We reassigned postoperative visits ***with*** compensation to our more medically oriented doctors to further free the master surgeons for more procedural opportunities. Directing pathology resulted in more efficient and effective use of ancillary income producing resources like our optical and our ASC. Since income distribution ultimately depends upon the bottom line, we all worked together to grow the pot to distribute. We recognized a large increase in new pathology resulting from patients' word of mouth. Our doctors ultimately prospered by successful group growth more than they might have by diverting an extra procedure or two away from their colleague. Most important, our patients benefitted from the alignment of physician compensation with outstanding clinical outcomes.

I wasn't always this kind of leader. My evolution into more selfless leadership ultimately depended upon my recognizing and implementing goals that obviously benefitted others first.

Let's start with cataract procedures. During the late 1980s and a period of egalitarian philosophy (thanks for that liberal arts education, Mom and Dad!), I consciously rotated new cataract evaluation/procedures among ***all*** the surgeons within our group. On subsequent retrospective analysis, I noted our previously robust procedure growth curve flattened apparently because one surgeon failed to produce positive outcomes as predictably as his colleagues.

Word of mouth is a double-edged sword. It moves quickly within a relatively small population base like ours to either benefit or harm the practice. In July 1990 we attended Dr. Howard Gimbel's meeting, where my wife Lisa became intrigued by technically advanced anterior segment procedures that obviously surpassed our training. Within months her passionate commitment improved her techniques beyond mine. Since I enjoyed a thriving strabismus practice, I elected to cease performing cataract surgery. Our group's commitment to procedures most benefitting patients helped to restore our growth curve quickly.

Even as a pediatric ophthalmologist, I soon applied the same philosophy to pediatric cataracts—Lisa performed the best technical procedure and I managed the patients medically. We experienced outstanding visual results with fewer complications than were typical.

The next opportunity for selfless choices presented when two subspecialists (in corneal refractive and orbit/oculoplastics) left the military and joined our team. Lisa stopped offering corneal procedures (remember this was the era of widespread AC lens aftermath), and I discontinued a moderately busy plastics practice. These doctors offered opportunities for enhanced patient care rather than competition for our established pathology referrals. The four of us enjoyed predictable success. A huge added benefit? The practice's focus on optimal patient care attracted an outstanding and stable lay staff.

With experience I instinctively started leading by example and understood ***not*** to ask colleagues to undertake tasks I might refuse. When the technical staff occasionally failed to stay ahead of me, I'd grab charts to perform workups to help the staff catch up. We were massively busy in our main offices. When I proposed new locations, I volunteered to serve as part of the initial staff—with some predictable loss of personal income while benefitting the group strategically. All new locations grew as a consequence, but not all grew adequately to warrant their retention. When I proposed Saturday morning hours I was first on the schedule. (Fortunately, that scheduling "experiment" failed.)

Several years later a new opportunity presented itself. At a national pediatric ophthalmology conference I discovered a nearby competitor's ad for a pediatric ophthalmologist! Once my visceral response calmed, I concluded the threat to my group's long-term success overshadowed any personal affront. Despite my relative youth at the time and a successful and satisfying strabismus practice, I recruited my own wonderful successor—a few decades ahead of my life's theoretical timetable. It definitely sweetened the offer that our new colleague transitioned almost directly from fellowship into a mature practice complete with the orthoptist who co-authored the field's textbook. I seldom performed another squint, and my new colleague hit the ground running instead of competing with an active, established, relatively young, senior associate. ***Plus*** the presence now of two pediatric ophthalmologists within a relatively small territory effectively terminated any outside applicant's interest.

Over time other less obvious patient care-oriented opportunities presented. These require a leader to brave risks first for group benefit. Lisa and I once purchased a prime piece of commercial real estate across from an announced future hospital location. This proved too bold for our partner's temperaments or wallets. Years later we sold it to our land-locked and frustrated neighbor specialists—*after* the hospital was constructed. By then it was much too small for our needs. We banked substantial profit on that investment, but did not replicate similar success with another large project in a neighboring expansion community. In business and medicine, entrepreneurial behavior yields wins and losses but requires risk-taking.

Though employee/owners in the boardroom still typically wear a "Me" hat instead of a "We" hat, examples of selfless behavior occur more frequently than they used to. Some years ago we were negotiating with an excellent, seasoned specialist. Their expected minimum salary guarantee exceeded most equity owners' economic tolerance. Recognizing the opportunity, our group's senior owners personally guaranteed the substantial spread between the offer approved by our general membership and the needs of the doctor being recruited. Fortunately that bet paid off!

The selfless leader respects the group's needs. A selfless leader requires adequate insight to appreciate and accept that not *every* idea they propose deserves action. I'm pretty sure the majority of our ideas never gain traction; however, enough enjoyed the light of day that I've been very satisfied with my role.

As an optimist I occasionally erred in recruiting associates by rationalizing how they might fit in instead of focusing upon why they might not. I transferred that recruiting role to another partner to better benefit the group. On the other hand, I initiated a recruiting strategy we still employ—partner site visits to seriously interested final-stage recruits.

Recruits historically display impeccable manners and behavior on site visits to practices like ours—they "Ooh" and "Aah" over facilities and laugh at partners' dinner table jokes. Other than great phone and cocktail chats, our practice had few tools with which to "look under the hood." And references were typically shallow and unduly glowing. I proposed that a partner spend a day or two with the applicant in their current location. We'd see how they treated their own patients in both the clinic and the OR. Obviously we didn't expect a trainee to perform procedures like a senior partner, but we were fascinated how they handled tissue and responded to intraoperative surprises. More important—we'd see how the staff interacted with our applicant. Were nurses and techs eager to interact with our proposed doc—or did they avoid eye contact with our potential newbie? I bet you can figure out who volunteered to make those first visits—me.

While my interest was chiefly in practice share growth within our regional market, our younger cadre sought a more economic, profit-biased practice model. The appropriate response meant hiring an excellent nuts and bolts administrator and implementing a separate finance committee populated with partners with an affinity for calculators.

Selfless leaders must actively embrace succession planning. The transition plan initially meant engaging equals into our practice. Instead of my retaining decision control, equity and governance travelled together. From the moment we were a foursome we created an annually rotating fifth vote to break any potential ties. It has never been invoked in more than 20 years, and during that time no equity owner has ever departed our clinical practice. Today we have 10 equal partners.

Our compensation formula predictably assigned significant fixed overhead equally to all 10 owners. That provision's intent was to economically insulate younger partners from additional shifted overhead as senior members elected more leisure time later in their careers. Seniors' leisure time off becomes increasingly expensive.

More recently I suspected that filling Lisa's and my increasing leisure time schedule with production by surrogates might reverse the equation and spread the group's overhead while increasing production and the group's profit pool available for distribution. Lisa and I were not ready to retire, but blocks of time off were desired. We were lucky enough to find another late-career surgeon-couple to job-share with, cycling one month on and one month off. This, of course, represented another of my "experimental economic adventures" for the group. No model existed for comparison or analysis. When I presented my job-sharing concept to the group, I walked in the boardroom door proposing that Lisa and I would assume the entire economic risk for this venture. Our risk assumption substantially shortened board discussion and expedited implementation. I'm delighted to report the success of this venture.

• • •

I adore the nexus of ophthalmology and strategic planning, however as the balance began to change between my personal and my practice schedule, I groomed a successor MP within the practice before my personal needs harmed the practice. In the corporate world, the immediate past leader quietly disappears. I still actively practice, but I made a very conscious effort to be less visible and I generally participate now only when I'm invited.

Whether a doctor leads, votes on the board as an equity owner, or is a nonequity associate physician, I'm convinced that a bias toward "Me-ness" over "We-ness" counts. If you consider your patients, your colleagues, and your staff before yourself, you'll enjoy a better and more satisfying practice.

CHAPTER 4

What Do You Believe In?

Developing a List of Core Values for Your Practice

John B. Pinto

The 20th century advertising legend David Ogilvy, an Oxford University dropout, door-to-door salesman, and farmer, was one of the most revered marketing minds in the world before his death in 1999. Among thousands of brilliant client campaigns, he launched the most famous automobile advertisement of all time:

At 60 Miles an Hour the Loudest Noise in This
New Rolls Royce Comes From the Electric Clock.

Was his inner secret to success mere hard work and a fluent typewriter? No. As odd as it may seem to say about a man from the rascal-filled world of advertising, I believe Ogilvy's fame—and his customers' victories—came from a few core philosophies and values about what worked in his particular profession.

Pinto JB. *Ophthalmic Leadership: A Practical Guide for Physicians, Administrators, and Teams, Second Edition* (pp 23-25).
© 2022 SLACK Incorporated.

CHAPTER 5

The Thermodynamics of Practice Leadership

John B. Pinto

Thermodynamics is built on the study of energy transfers that can be strictly resolved into two distinct components, heat and work, specified by macroscopic variables.
—P. W. Bridgman
The Nature of Thermodynamics

Despite the title, you'll be relieved to know we're not going to discuss a lot of higher-order math here, but rather the central, applicable take-home lessons from what might have been one of your least favorite pre-med courses in college.

Getting your practice's positive "chemical reaction" going takes loads of human energy. Keeping the resulting, inherently unstable "business compound" from flying apart at the seams takes even more energy and careful handling.

Your practice is a complex, day-by-day laboratory experiment. Although you may not have thought of your business in these terms, you are adding energy (in this case, human time, financial capital, and expertise) to grow something unique,

Pinto JB. *Ophthalmic Leadership: A Practical Guide for Physicians, Administrators, and Teams, Second Edition* (pp 27-30).
© 2022 SLACK Incorporated.

profitable, and enduring. Along the way, you have to overcome operational entropy and friction, and sustain an economically favorable chain reaction. Business, chemistry … they're all the same, really … with a bit of physics thrown in for good measure.

Conducting a business chemistry experiment successfully always starts at the top. Just one or two alpha leaders in every practice are the critical source of energy.

Here's a thermodynamic metaphor: a summertime campfire. If you were a Boy or Girl Scout who won your camping merit badge, you'll recall that you can't light a big log with a little match. You have to nurture a campfire by degrees. First the kindling. Then twigs. Branches next. And, finally, the log.

Until that first log is burning, you have to sit right next to the new fire and keep feeding it. After you have a blaze started, you have to keep it going by adding more logs hour after hour. If you neglect the fire, it runs out of sufficient heat to ignite the fuel and goes out.

Your practice is just like that campfire. It once started small, most likely with a single doctor and a couple of staff. In the early years, the founder's long hours, daily attentions, and highly directive leadership were essential. In a few years, less energy and attention were needed. The workdays shortened a bit. The practice had finally "caught fire," and there could be fewer meetings. With time and mastery, operational details perpetuated with little oversight from the top.

But like the fire, even the most modest practice needs a critical continued energy input. When that energy is withheld, the fire dims and eventually goes out.

Here's a case in point. I've just returned home to San Diego from a visit with a middle-aged ophthalmologist with a slowly dimming practice. Let's call him Dr. Brown. The light is going out and his practice is faltering for one clear reason: Dr. Brown, himself, is faltering.

Brown was once, himself, on fire to succeed. He would arrive an hour before the first patient to tidy up paperwork and rally the troops. Dr. Brown would take lunch with his staff weekly. At night, he'd go over the books, and the next day tweak revenue and expenses. He would stoke the fire, both his own personal one and that of the practice.

But that was more than 20 years ago. Today Dr. Brown is in his early 60s. The fires don't burn as hot as they once did. Dr. Brown commonly arrives an hour after his first patient arrives. He rarely meets with staff anymore. And evenings are spent watching sports instead of the bottom line. A once-energized staff and doctor cohort have now settled into a much more relaxed pace, too. "If Dr. Brown doesn't seem to care or exert any extra energy, why should we?"

I've seen this "energy withdrawal disorder" (or EWD) play out in numerous settings, most commonly in larger, closely held practices owned by just one or two older providers who have delayed the admission of partners. EWD is compounded when both the owners ***and*** the key staff members are at a stage of life and practice where energy levels decline. EWD is less often seen in widely held group practices with a healthy age distribution of doctors and lay leaders.

• • •

For the doctor and manager, energy contributions take several forms. Raw, observable intensity prominently frames the gulf between great and mediocre practice leaders. A lot of this intensity is innate. Intense doctors and managers can't help themselves; that's just who they are inside.

Those who are not naturally intense—but who have leadership roles obliging at least the appearance of energy and enthusiasm—need to summon the inner equivalent of a high school pep rally. This can be personally engineered in a number of practical ways:

- Listening to recordings of motivational speakers ... Tony Robbins and the like. Some leaders I know who would not be very motivating on their own, have gathered a large library of these recordings and start each day on the commute to work with a pep talk.
- Selecting an administrative assistant or similar aid with a cheerleader personality ... or at the very least, NOT working with a dispiriting sourpuss.
- Reading the biographies or watching the video documentaries of great leaders, or inspiring narratives from those who have overcome adversity. You can't read *Between a Rock and a Hard Place* or the derivative movie *127 Hours* about Aron Lee Ralston, the hiker who had to self-amputate his arm to save his life in the wilderness, without bringing some of Ralston's do-or-die intensity into your practice.
- Holding the business equivalent of pep rallies. Practice life and high school life are not really all that different as it turns out. Enthusiasm is infectious. Instead of pompoms, football heroes and cross-town team rivalries, your practice will thrive if it has the grown-up equivalents: spirited department heads, surgical heroes, and economic points on a publicly viewed scoreboard.

To what end should one apply the resulting intensity? The most effective application is a sustained drive to continuously improve clinical processes, business operating standards, and ultimately the customer's experience during a visit to your practice. As an MP or administrator you should be intensely (but kindly, patiently) interrogating everyone, up and down the ranks, about what they are doing and why they are doing it. The questions you ask are as critical as the urgency in your voice. "What's one thing we could do differently here on the clinic floor allowing us to see one more patient per hour?" "Are we making patients just as comfortable and relaxed as possible?" "Could we have seen today's patients with one less receptionist and one less tech?"

In order to continuously improve, one has to have the energy and courage to listen to and act on staff and customer feedback. Short comment cards and half-hearted exit surveys fall short of the necessary quality feedback process. Office managers should casually query dilating patients. Opticians have a perfect opportunity to follow up with a patient who says, "I didn't really understand what the doctor said." Someone in your practice should be calling about five random patients per provider per month and reporting the results to all hands.

If successful, the owner can readily find a buyer, either a private party or even the jackpot of an initial public offering. If the owner is young, they can readily start all over again at the beginning and invent a new concept, this time with a much larger personal capital base.

This pathway is rarely followed by ophthalmic entrepreneurs for numerous reasons:

- Eye surgeons by their nature are more risk adverse than the average business entrepreneur. (This is paradoxical, of course—when an eye surgeon's business fails, they can typically secure a six-figure job offer in a few weeks.)
- Eye surgeons are raised up in a culture of perfection. Inasmuch as growth necessarily begets imperfection, growth can be restrained because "we're not perfect yet."
- Restaurants need managers, chefs, wait staff, and bookkeepers ... all of whom are readily available at modest cost on the open market. Practices need surgeons, specialist-managers, experienced techs, billing and coding experts, etc.
- Restaurants have a relatively low level of enterprise complexity: a few dozen products, modest regulatory oversight, at-will pricing, simple accounting systems. Practices have a profoundly high level of enterprise complexity at all levels.
- With the right manager and chief chef, a restaurant owner can drop back from daily involvement and still collect a paycheck. It's far more difficult for an ophthalmologist-owner to run their practice passively—most qualified fellow surgeons are unwilling to generate passive incomes for owner-employers beyond a brief partner-track associate period.
- Practice succession is harder and less leveraged than ordinary business succession. Successful restaurants have a ready buyer pool, paying many multiples of annual earnings. Ophthalmic practices sell today for their net tangible asset value plus a modest goodwill value, and the latter is slowly eroding.
- The new restaurateur can hold onto the dream that they'll have a winning franchise concept and go public one day, netting tens or hundreds of millions of dollars. Few eye surgeons harbor such dreams.
- When a restaurant chain gets larger, its variable costs for food (which are high as a percentage of revenue) come down in percentile terms. In ophthalmology, most costs are fixed, not variable ... so economies of scale are difficult to achieve.
- Most practices secure a customer base through the consistent excellence of their celebrity doctors. The ***doctor*** is the product. Restaurant chains secure a customer base by serving consistently "great" food. The ***food*** is the product. And with thousands upon thousands of new chefs graduating from culinary school every year, the product is more dependent on the recipe than the maestro in an apron and tall, white hat. You don't walk into an Applebee's and ask the hostess, "Who's in the kitchen tonight?"

That having been said, the motivations for buoyant practice growth to a larger scale include:

- Theoretically better access to contracts in the future
- A large cohort of owners, making the buy-out of any one owner easier
- With more owners, the odds increase that at least one person will be able and interested in leadership
- With more owners, decisions are slowed, but can be more rational ... rash, outlier opinions are dampened by a thoughtful majority
- Large practices have the capital base to venture into riskier opportunities to drive passive income (eg, optical, ASC, optometrists)
- The practice is less susceptible to the loss of any one key-man provider
- The practice can afford a stronger management team, including in-house IT, marketing, and other specialists
- There can be marketing economies of scale (a $10 million practice would have to spend 9% of cash flow to have the same visibility in the market of a $30 million practice spending just 3%)
- Modest optical, medical supplies, and technology economies of scale
- Coverage of a wider span of professional services and duplicate coverage for critical subspecialty areas (eg, two retinologists)
- The pride of saying, "We are the largest practice in the area"

To balance out this list of growth drivers, there are nearly as many motivations for relative stasis or even downsizing your practice from where it stands today. There are well-recognized difficulties seen with large-scale practices, both economically and interpersonally. There is better proportionality between practice scale and doctor leadership resources ... there are low odds of finding an engaged partner with free time to be the serious executive needed in a large practice. With fewer owners, decisions are faster. Both large practices and small have ready access to money for worthy business ideas in today's capital markets, so you do not need to get bigger to fund new projects. Importantly, practice problems are largely caused by people. Odds are that a practice with twice the number of doctors, staff and patients will have twice the problems of smaller practices. Finally, most eye surgeons are pretty individualistic, control-oriented people. Bankers and sales executives and lawyers who used to play football may inherently love being part of a large corporate team. But as a general observation, ophthalmologists tend to be happy in their businesses in inverse proportion to practice size.

Errors and misfits takes different forms in different settings:

- The soloist who builds a 15,000 square foot building (because they so loved the process of design and construction, and assumed that their practice would bloom) but who doesn't have the energy or risk tolerance to build a practice of comparable scale.
- The large-practice surgeon who feels lost in a crowd of partners, when they would really prefer to call the shots all by themselves.
- The doctor with real leadership talent who works in a market that's so competitive that building a larger group is almost impossible.

The Paradox of Practice Size

Remember that except for a few unusual, very large settings, practice scale has little influence on the profits flowing to a given doctor-owner. Indeed, because of the commonly observed diseconomies and inefficiencies that can attend scale, I get lots of calls from surgeons in 8- to 12-doctor practices who start the phone discussion by saying, "We were doing so well with five doctors. Profit margins were high, and managers could understand and control all of the moving parts. Now, profits are down, confusion is up, and one hand doesn't know what the other is doing. What happened to us?"

The answer to the doctors' lament, *"What happened?"* is best visualized by this simple two-line graph. How can you know your own boundaries? Your own just-right-practice sweet spot? Here is a discussion of eight simple determinants that may help you decide if you're better suited for large or small practice.

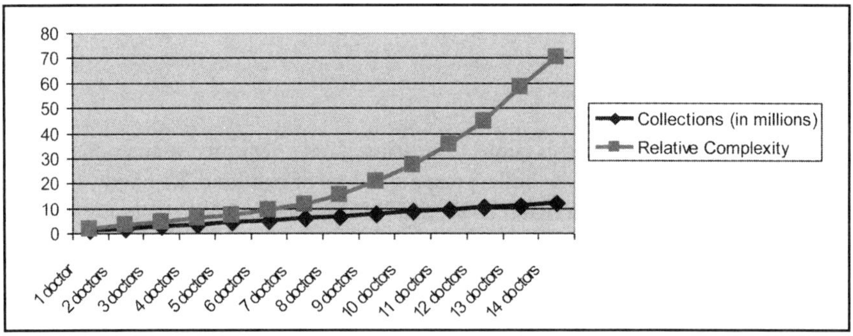

As you'll read, some surgeons committed to developing or joining a large practice may be better suited to stay small. While others who are attracted to work in a modest, boutique practice would do better to overlook the challenges of scale, get out of their personal comfort zone, and gravitate toward building or joining a large practice.

- What size practice team makes you most comfortable? The answer to this may be obvious from your personal history. If you played large-scale team sports back in school (eg, football, baseball, basketball) you're probably going to be comfortable jostling in a crowded boardroom or at a meeting with a hundred support staff in attendance. And vice-versa. If, like most ophthalmologists, you revel in a quiet dinner party with two or three couples but can't stand plunging into a raucous New Year's celebration, this may be all you need to know about your happiest practice scale.
- How well can your personal time availability rise to meet the constant baseline commitments—and periodic sky-high demands—of large practice ownership? If you employ 50 staff, you will have 10 times the personnel headaches of a tidy solo practice. Ten times the absenteeism. Ten times the job-site drug abuse. Ten times the exposure to customer service gaps. Some relish the larger playing field, some shrink from it.
- What's the best fit with your personal lifestyle and competing interests? It's no secret that eye surgeons in their 30s and 40s today are a bit less workaholic than doctors from previous generations. Physicians who are simultaneously practicing and raising a young family, or juggling other outside interests (eg, teaching, research, or a budding art career perhaps) would do well to consider the proper practice setting to fit with their other demands. Successful, entrepreneurial private practice of any scale obliges 50- and 60-hour work weeks, more in the early years. Happily, given the significant and growing number of openings, employing practices are more flexible than ever before in granting a creative template.
- What's your risk tolerance? Is the safer bet in these challenging times being part of a larger or a smaller practice? Actually, the answer is more braided than the question suggests. The risk of being an ophthalmic business owner was once negligible. Today, many more practices falter and fail than ever before. While a small, boutique practice may seem more fragile and riskier, such businesses can make faster changes, reducing costs or entering new service lines with little notice. While large group practices may seem less risky, some become ossified and unable to adjust to fast-changing conditions. Bottom line: You have to evaluate every setting differently, and especially examine the second-order variables beyond practice size (eg, local population-to-provider ratios, the age distribution of patients and payers, managed care penetration, and the strength and unity of the owners).
- How do you feel about time off from practice? In a large practice, coverage in your absence is no problem. In fact, in a few large practices partners are encouraged to enjoy larger sabbatical breaks, something that is nearly impossible to accomplish in small-enterprise practices.
- Are your physical and emotional energies, and reserves, in line with the demands of leading a larger or smaller group? As you can see, leadership demands rise at a faster pace than practice scale. To some extent, these higher demands can be passed off to a growing cohort of middle management staff. But at the root, as a large practice leader you simply have to exert yourself more, physically and emotionally, than in a small practice. Meetings run later into the evening, and there

are more of them. Since the stakes are higher, arguments can be more heated and stresses rise, all of which obliges the fortitude to withstand (ideally, even relish) conflict.

- How high is your demand for personal control? Running a solo practice board meeting is pretty simple … all decisions are unanimous and you always get the vote you were looking for. Not so in group practice. A consensual style of practice decision making works with two or three owners, but "kumbaya management" breaks down with scale. Eventually, majority voting is obliged. If you aspire to a jumbo practice scale, your new favorite saying has to be, "I can live with that."
- Are you concerned about getting your investment out when you retire? Selling a practice was relatively easy a generation ago. America was making nearly 3% more ophthalmologists every year, and a flood of new grads were all too happy to pay a premium to buy in. Now, however, we're not graduating enough new eye surgeons to cover the existing retirement pace of baby boomer doctors, much less take care of the roughly 3% annual growth in the number of new American seniors each year. These stark demographics mean that your practice—any practice of any size—will probably be worth a little less in the years ahead. When selling, however, the edge goes to larger practices. A soloist has to find a doctor to take over … a 100% shift in professional labor is needed to accomplish the transaction. A 10-doctor practice has a lot more flexibility with the same succession event: Nine doctors can buy out the retiree painlessly and probably absorb their patient base. Or the large group can simply hire a new grad (who may be easier to coax into a large group in today's environment), splitting the cost and risk nine ways. Without advance planning, an increasing number of peri-retirement soloists in the years ahead will simply be closing their doors, getting little more than salvage value for their tangibles.

CHAPTER 8

Business Pathology

Applying Health Care's Disease Management Model to the Management of Your Practice

John B. Pinto

This somewhat off-handed chapter is derived from an intentionally humorous presentation at the 2011 Hawaiian Eye Meeting. It is offered up only half in jest. Between the laugh lines, I hope you'll discover something essential to the success of your practice, especially as successful business leadership is becoming a greater challenge with every passing year.

It's the "inner game" of practice administration, something I've appreciated ever since the early 1970s when I took a left turn on the way to medical school: The key to better management of your practice is always hiding in plain sight … in the form of medicine's elegant intellectual model for finding and treating disease.

Pinto JB. *Ophthalmic Leadership: A Practical Guide for Physicians, Administrators, and Teams, Second Edition* (pp 41-47).
© 2022 SLACK Incorporated.

If you want to be a great practice owner, you do not need to adopt some unaccustomed mindset. Just prepare yourself with a few underlying facts and concepts … and then keep thinking like a doctor.

Unlike formal business training, which remains pretty nonstandardized in even the most rigorous B-school settings, mastering a body of basic professional expertise is much more uniform in medicine. Medicine, like law, engineering, and the like, is a so-called "learned profession," with relatively little nuance and a high ratio of science to art.

Learn the science, and they make you a doctor. By contrast, business practitioners get very little of what's needed to lead a company from formal schooling, which is why experienced high school drop-outs can sometimes manage circles around younger baccalaureates.

But beyond divergent training regimes, business and medicine converge more than you might imagine as professional disciplines. Medical and business practitioners both hunt for problems. These problems often first present as vague, subjective complaints that become hard facts with tests and measurements. The human patient complains of burry vision, which emerges as nuclear sclerosis and a BCVA of 20/70. Your practice (the "patient" in this case) mysteriously bogs down at 11 o'clock every morning, which emerges as an easily cured 35% technician staffing deficit.

In both cases, a "cure" is applied—surgery for cataracts, hiring for the staffing gap. Weeks and months later, improvements are confirmed, and you keep checking periodically, chasing down the next most important chief complaint, while monitoring for regression and adverse side effects from the last treatment you provided.

Your practice is the patient. As an administrator or MP, you are the patient's doctor. Looked at in this manner, you'll come to appreciate that the intellectual challenge and stakes of great practice "doctoring" are as large as the challenge and stakes of being a great ophthalmologist.

• • •

Here are some of the most common forms of ophthalmic business "pathology."

Adminorrhea

Characterized by bloated management ranks, endless meetings, elaborate feasibility studies, and organization charts in six-point type. This is a slow, progressive practice disease that often commences in times of financial abundance and is only discovered years later when you notice that to talk to Amy at the nurse's station about an unclear chart entry you have to make advance arrangements with Amy's bosses' boss. Resistance to treatment is common. Treat Adminorrhea with combined therapy: peeling back excessive layers of middle management, excising bloated staff hours—sometimes even erasing whole segments of the organization chart.

Servus Redundo

Latin for "excessive staffing," this is less commonly seen today since the advent of modern benchmarking ... but is a persistent condition in primitive settings. Servus Redundo is a routine finding in practices with end-stage Adminorrhea. Signs and symptoms are readily determined and often show up as staff standing around chatting beyond their break periods, more than one hour of tech time for each patient visit, and less than $10,000 per month in collections per lay staffer. The core treatment approach, as with all administrative hygiene, is to gather the data and let the data make the decision about how many people you really need.

Interdepartmentalitis

Presents as larger or smaller frictions between practice workgroups; can be especially great between technical and receptionist staff. This malady is endemic to the profession of eye care. Treatment should be applied directly on the problem, counseling or removing individual bad actors. Interdepartmentalitis generally clears up spontaneously when you excise just one pot-stirring employee, although the experienced management practitioner will need to be vigilant for recurrence.

Metastatic Overhead

The malignant proliferation of practice costs out of all relation to practice collections. Early, subjective findings are subtle ... masked administrator anxiety during each biweekly payroll cycle ... doctors quietly cancelling long-planned vacations. These subtle signs will be rapidly followed up by the capable administrator. In addition to gross external findings (ie, costs in excess of 65% of collections), various practice organ systems must undergo separate exploratory procedures. Staffing costs in excess of 32% of cash flow, facility costs in excess of 6%, or marketing costs over 5% are the most common observations. Unfortunately, most practice expenses are fixed. Aside from rare cases of grossly malignant supervision (in which case radical surgery is always indicated), Metastatic Overhead responds best to dual therapy: a gentle downward traction on costs and a gentle upward traction on revenue. Gifted managers and owners can reduce the largest cost tumors briskly, treating the inevitable residual expense nodes with stern eye contact and progressive spending authority withdrawal therapy.

Hypomedicos

Characterized by an abundance of patients and an insufficiency of doctors. This has, unfortunately, been a very rare administrative condition since the 1960s and the bloom of medical training slots. Studies show that Hypomedicos is now mostly limited to the rural outposts of America. Gross symptoms include provider fatigue and 3-month delays until the next available appointment. If your practice is one of the few now experiencing this condition, early treatment is preferred. If allowed to linger, Hypomedicos can lead to the infiltration of your service area by competing providers and rebound Hypermedicos that could be fatal to your practice. Take steps to add doctors such that local population ratios settle in at 20,000 people per ophthalmologist and 10,000 per optometrist.

PolyEdificium

More Latin, for the creation of excessive, often part-time satellite offices, resulting in low aggregate profitability and excess enterprise complexity. This was once, in the era of $1500 cataract fees, a harmless, even beneficial condition. If you suspect your practice has PolyEdificium, you can screen for this simply by determining the net profit per physician-hour for each location. This exercise may reveal office locations with well under $200 in net profit per hour; such facilities can then either be rehabilitated or amputated from your system.

Officemia

An insufficiency of office space. The key finding is more than 200 patient visits per month per exam room. The only treatment options available are more exam rooms, longer hours, fewer patients, or a new espresso machine in the staff lounge to accelerate throughput. At times, in a zeal to cure Officemia, treatment is carried too far, resulting in Polyedificium and rebound Metastatic Overhead.

Promotional Atrophy

Also known as "Skinny Practice Syndrome" ... The withering away of new patients which can be readily predicted to form whenever marketing budgets fall below 3% of practice collections." The most prominent finding is a persistent year-on-year trend of fewer new visits. Diagnostic caution is obliged when evaluating a practice for suspected Promotional Atrophy. False positives emerge when comparing summers and winters in Miami (or Detroit). Restoring promotional nutrition is the first line of treatment. However, it's critical that these marketing nutrients be well-balanced. The atrophied patient will rally slowly at first, but baseline strength is eventually restored in nearly all cases.

Philanthromania

Giving away too many of your services for free or at an excess discount. This depresses the average revenue yielded per patient visit and sharply reduces profitability. Philanthromania also distresses staff when they see their next hoped-for pay raise handed out in the form of courtesy care to one patient after another. The thoughtful manager will treat this malady by measuring and reporting on the annual cost of excess kindness. In a group practice setting, they'll shift any excess generosity directly to the cost center of the too-generous provider.

Refraction Fee Insufficiency Syndrome

A particularly virulent form of Philanthromania, characterized by fees under $45 charged to fewer than 25% of the practice's total patient visits. The first line of therapy is intensive counseling on the benefits of daily hygienic charging practices. A single anterior segment provider, seeing 6000 visits per year, should be charging out 1500+ refractions for a net revenue yield approaching $68,000 or more. When not charged, this represents a 10% to 20% pay cut for the provider.

Floppy Billing Syndrome

Also termed "Collectionopathy" ... quite common, particularly in practices with inexperienced billing staff and inattentive oversight ... Floppy Billing Syndrome is one of the most consistent comorbidities of Philanthromania." Fortunately for the patient, the lab panel for this disorder is robust and positive findings for the disorder are well-understood, including net collection ratios below 95%, more than 12% of open accounts aged over 90 days, and the absence of a collection agency. Floppy Billing most often results from too few staff. About 18 minutes of clerical time are needed for each practice transaction. Once the contributing factors are corrected, all lab panels typically restore quickly to normal range.

Surgiphobia

The maddening tendency of otherwise well-trained providers to delay needed surgical care. Surgiphobia is easily detected by examining the surgeon's average preoperative BCVA figures. Average BCVA values over 20/60 commonly respond well to peer coaching and ongoing vigilance. Average values over 20/70 suggest highly advanced Surgiphobia. In such cases, the kindest course of treatment may be a surreptitious editing of the doctor's bio on the practice website, and revised patient appointing directives for the front desk.

Numeralgia

Mild to intense pain experienced by practice owners during the monthly finance meeting, leading to an avoidance of all subsequent economic discussions. Numeralgia can be treated effectively by improvement of the underlying performance of the practice, so the numbers are less painful, as well as the application of appropriate analgesic agents during all practice finance meetings. (I find that red wine works best.)

Technophilic Reflux Disease

As the term suggests, Technophilic Reflux Disease results from the excess or overly hasty adoption of new technology, and subsequent disgorgement of same. Signs include closets filled with abandoned gadgetry and providers who run chronically behind in clinic because they are always trying to master the latest time-saving device. Technophilic Reflux Disease is the opposite of the equally disabling "Luddite Syndrome," wherein all things new are rejected. Treatment for Technophilic Reflux Disease often obliges harsh aversion therapy, where the affected doctor is given a retrospective cash-detriment analysis of the last decade's purchases.

Peripheral Business Disease

Most often found in practices owned by highly intelligent and energetic surgeons, who get bored running just one great business at a time. Peripheral Business Disease is characterized by many distracting side projects, juggled at the same time to the detriment of the main business: eye care. Point out to the affected surgeon the trajectory of former, failed projects ... hold up for contrast the comparative brilliance of the core practice. In the most challenging cases, intervention by the surgeon's accountant is required to shock the patient into the needed behavioral changes.

Precocious Sweatophobia

The intractable resistance of many recently graduated eye surgeons to work more than 36 hours per week. Formerly known as GWAS, "Generalized Work Allergy Syndrome. This is always best handled prophylactically. Be sure to undertake a deep review of every candidate's work history.

When Dr. New describes that your practice, "Would be, like dude, my first 'real' job," gently show him the way to your competitor's office. Sadly, Precocious Sweatophobia appears at present to be incurable with even the best tools available to management science. If prophylaxis has been unsuccessful, the only treatment remaining may be a gentle doctorectomy.

Failure to Thrive

Like its human cognate, the failing practice may decline due to any number of causes. If detected early, through regular trend analysis, the prognosis can be excellent. One of the earliest warning signs can be a drop in established patient volumes. In smaller practices, the most common etiology is provider-based: too little attention to the needs and details of the company. As these needs are rising each year, surgeons who are not up to the task should consider consolidation with larger practices. A reversal of this disorder, in practices large and small, can be accomplished with superior management talent. Advanced cases of the disease require time, patience, and sustained capital infusion by the owners.

Accountus Sicca

AKA: "Dry Bank Account"... Generally, an end-stage finding; not so much a disease entity to be treated as it is a terminal sign. Graded from Stage I, when you inadvertently bounce the occasional check, to Stage V, when a van pulls up and two guys named "Joe" start removing the office furniture.

• • •

Business Is Just Like Medicine

1. First, do no harm.
2. The diagnosis is in the history.
3. Start with the subjective complaint ... move on to the objective facts.
4. Know when it's better to treat briskly or rely on the tincture of time.
5. Triage is key ... prioritize your treatment plan.
6. Businesses and bodies both have organ systems.
7. Business diseases can be organ-focused or systemic ... acute, chronic, or episodic.
8. Business is complicated and experimental ... keep up your charting ... be ready for surprises.
9. Adverse side effects are common even with the best treatments ... some cures can kill the patient.
10. Healthy bodies (and businesses) seek homeostasis ... excesses and insufficiencies generally signal a disease state.
11. Prevention is always best.
12. Sometimes, the patient must simply live with the disease.

CHAPTER 9

How Well Will You Adapt to the Future Eye Care Business Environment?

John B. Pinto

Availability, affability, and ability are what young doctors need to build a practice. And, in that order of importance.
—Sir William Osler

Sir William Osler, one of the great teachers of premodern medicine also said, in an 1897 address to the New York Academy of Medicine, "When schemes are laid in advance, it is surprising how often the circumstances fit in with them." In other words, for success, plan your work and work your plan. It sounds like he was time-traveling to the present era, yes?

Had he worked in today's fast-changing environment, Sir Osler probably would have underscored his philosophy of practice success. And I think he would have added a fourth "A" to the familiar medical student's 3-A axiom. He would have added "Adaptability," and put it at the front of the list.

You should, too, in this weird, peri-recessional, breath-holding era.

Pinto JB. *Ophthalmic Leadership: A Practical Guide for Physicians, Administrators, and Teams, Second Edition* (pp 49-52).
© 2022 SLACK Incorporated.

This moment in medical economics should be stimulating your instincts to loosen up and become more adaptable. This month let's discuss some practical things to keep you and your practice light on its feet and nimbly adapting to the world ahead for all of us.

• • •

First things first. The largest operating expense in every practice is lay staffing, so that's the first place to be braced and ready to take action. If against all sound predictions fee cuts do occur in the next few years—or indeed, if fees don't rise, but inflation does—you may have no option but to trim staffing costs. Such cost-cutting can snip in numerous variations, large and small:

- Cutting the number of staff to transit a given volume of patients
- Cutting staff hours across the board to accomplish the same economic result
- Freezing or reducing wages ... this could include eliminating annual cost-of-living allowances (replacing them with spot bonuses) or selective pay cuts
- Labor substitution ... this can take many forms: replacing full-time staff with part-time to save benefits costs, replacing low-level adult clerks with casual labor from the local high school, eliminating tech positions and performing some of your own work-ups, and terminating underperforming associate providers (putting their patients on your own schedule)
- Outsourcing back-office business functions, such as billing, payroll, or human resources, that may be more costly for you to manage than an outside specialist

Most of these changes are painful to one degree or another, which gets to the heart of being "adaptable." You have to be able to personally accommodate to this kind of discomfort, and be willing to confront tough decisions *with the interests of the practice placed ahead of any one individual, including yourself as a leader.* Not to press the survivor analogy too far, but this is no different than a lost hiker adapting to their new situation by fighting back fear, drinking brackish water, and pushing their body to the edge of endurance.

Such unpleasant, even painful changes must of course be in line with the rest of your behavior as an owner. If the day arrives when you have to prescribe bitter medicine for the staff, you can't turn around and order a new luxury car, buy a nonessential clinical tool, or book an island cruise.

The second largest outlay—and a target for adaptation efforts—is for office facilities. There are several ways to increase adaptability in this area.

- Commit to shorter lease periods, and more liberal escape clauses, even if it might cost a bit more ... this is especially the case for any facilities beyond your core location
- Unless growth is highly assured, err on the low side of how much space you will need
- When opening up in a new area, lease office space until success in your own building is more assured (of course, the catch-22 with this more cautious strategy is that by that time, land and building prices may have gone up)

- Rather than owning or leasing your own dedicated office, rent space (and staff) by the day or month from compatible colleagues, who may also be in a position to refer patients to you
- Be more circumspect in examining satellite office opportunities ... having two offices can be four times more complex than a single location, and lead to operational mix-ups in the original office

Of course, enhancing bottom-line performance is more a matter of boosting revenue than containing costs. Remember that adding just one patient per clinic day can generate enough incremental revenue in a year to cover one staff member's salary and benefits.

We are entering an era when the demand for services is rising, while fees are stagnant (and falling in real, inflation-adjusted terms). Now is the time to discover a few new personal "gears." If you have been operating two cases an hour, call the team together and shoot for three. If you have a backlog of patients (increasingly common in some areas) and are topping out at 45 visits per day, take a field trip to a 60-patient-per-day colleague to see how it is done. Remember the words of ophthalmic legend Dr. John Corboy: "If you're not smarter than those other fellows, you may have to work harder than them to keep up and get ahead." The times certainly call for it.

Looking more broadly at adaptability, your practice should have a written disaster plan. This can be a few short pages. Here's a way to get a quick start. As soon as you finish reading this chapter, take 10 minutes to write down the potential disasters you now face: fee cuts, unfriendly moves by the competition or local hospital, loss of an office to natural disaster, and your own disability (or worse). Then take another 10 minutes to write down what you would do in each circumstance.

If you think about it, this informal disaster (read "adaptability") plan is not unlike how you prepare now unconsciously before every surgical session. What if a patient moves or has a health crisis? What if the electricity goes down or you drop a nucleus?

Everyone likes a simple scorecard approach. "Am I ready or not for what lies ahead?" Here's a quiz that will test your own adaptability to the environment we may well be facing. If you can answer "Yes" to a majority of these five questions, you may already be sufficiently armored for the future:

1. Imagine that double-digit fee cuts are a reality. Your personal income will soon also drop by double digits. Are you the kind of person who could probably learn to live with this new reality and shift your source of satisfaction to other spheres?
2. Adapting means changing, and all change (even the good kind) is stressful. Would others say about you that you have always adapted well to stress and change?
3. Do you have a clever, inventive nature that makes you relish the thought of operating an eye clinic in tougher circumstances? (A hint: if you have ever been on an overseas mission, that was a perfect test for this kind of ingenuity and ability to do more with less.)

4. You cannot control the trajectory of fee reform, but you ***can*** control your ability to mitigate softer fees with harder work, seeing more patients every day. Do you possess the health and energy reserves that would allow you to ramp up your output?
5. If you work with partners, are your relationships with each other strong enough to endure any financial or other resource challenge anticipated in the years ahead?

Section II

Awakening Leadership Skills in Yourself and Others

CHAPTER 10

Character and Leadership

Creating a Positive Work Environment for a Highly Successful Practice

Jaci M. Lindstrom

Character is a diamond that scratches every other stone.
—Cyrus Bartol

Trust men and they will be true to you; treat them greatly, and they will show themselves great.
—Ralph Waldo Emerson

The process of building a business culture starts with the integrity of the leader's character and is strengthened day by day in actions, not words.

I have been working for the last decade to bring women leaders in ophthalmology together in a meaningful way that supports their aspirations and motivates them to provide great leadership in their practice areas. Over the years, it has become increasingly evident to me that no matter the size of the medical practice, success hinges on a leader's ability to create a positive work environment. Studies have shown that employees, and business, thrive where there is a positive work environment or culture.

While it is important that an organization's leadership be educated, make good decisions, be emotionally intelligent, and communicate well; it is strength of

Pinto JB. *Ophthalmic Leadership: A Practical Guide for Physicians, Administrators, and Teams, Second Edition* (pp 55-59).
© 2022 SLACK Incorporated.

character that carries a leader. It is from character that a leader leads and creates a positive work environment. As Peter Drucker, the legendary management consultant, once pointed out, "For it is character through which leadership is exercised, it is character that sets the example and is imitated in turn."

This chapter seeks to expose the reader to the idea that a positive work environment can only be achieved with a leader that demonstrates a strong moral character each and every day in the workplace.

Character Matters, Character Leads

One of the greatest business minds of our time, Warren Buffet, was known for selecting leaders based simply on character—before resumes or experience. Buffet was also known to buy companies and keep management in place. If he could trust a person, if they would work hard, and if they truly cared about the people entrusted to them, then he felt he could teach them the rest. The success of a company is intrinsically linked to the behavior of its leaders and the character of those leaders matters.

With the rise of corporate social responsibility, there has been a rise in character education in public schools as well. It has become increasingly important to build the character of our future leaders from childhood, and so recently, a program called Character Counts, from the Josephson Institute's Center for Youth Ethics, became our nation's largest character education program used in our public schools. Character Counts teaches the Six Pillars of Character: ***trustworthiness, respect, responsibility, fairness, caring,*** and ***citizenship.*** Using these as a measuring stick for character in our leaders, let us look more closely at the importance of each one in the context of business leadership and the creation of a positive work environment.

Trust

First and foremost, a leader must be trustworthy and strive to create a culture of trust. Trustworthiness is the obligation and responsibility of someone in whom we place our faith. As a core value, trust underpins almost every other attribute of leadership character, and is an unbreakable bond—that if broken is almost always unrecoverable. When employees trust their leader, that leader can inspire employees to overcome daily work challenges and innovation thrives. Create a workplace where employees feel free to try and fail, rather than keep a low profile, never take initiative, and perpetuate the status quo. This doesn't make for a very exciting company or a highly-performing operation.

Respect

The respect you give comes back. Respect everyone you meet, from the administrative assistant to the leading surgeon in your field. Former Chrysler CEO Lee Iacocca was known to say that when your people begin to respect you, "they'll follow you to the death" (metaphorically speaking of course). Leadership must show respect for the talent and abilities of its workers, and in turn, the employees will believe in themselves and show the same respect for their leaders. The old Biblical proverb of the Golden Rule applies here, "Do unto others as you would have done to you." Leaders who demonstrate a high degree of respect create engagement and commitment.

Responsibility

Strong leaders accept responsibility for their own actions and decisions. When leaders demonstrably hold themselves accountable for their actions, their direct reports are more inclined to do the same. Still, it is the role of the leader to "inspect" not "expect" and pay attention to the outcomes of their teams. Leaders recognize performance accomplishments and coach team members with corrective feedback regularly. This promotes attention to the goals and standards that the leader wishes to reinforce, develop, and achieve, as ultimately it is the leader who is responsible for outcomes. Leaders have a vested interest in helping and improving staff performance.

Fairness

Numerous studies have shown that fair treatment of employees by leadership is critical to developing desirable workplace habits and behaviors. Rewards and benefits include: greater satisfaction with and acceptance of decisions, higher perceived legitimacy of authorities, higher job satisfaction, greater commitment to the organization, higher task performance, and less theft.[1] A leader's effectiveness, or ability to mobilize and motivate a workforce, is directly contingent to staff perception of a leader's ability to "be fair." Fairness is perceived by employees in their day-to-day interactions with leaders, policies and procedures instituted, and the equality or fairness of how a leader handles often similar or different workplace situations over time.

Caring

A leader who cares is probably the most human of the characteristics necessary for strong character leadership. Leadership is foremost responsible for creating a workplace that is safe, clean and free from any kind of abuse; be it physical, emotional, or verbal. Leaders can provide programs, encouragement, and even workplace activities that help employees maintain and increase their health and well-being.

Leaders also care for team members by showing empathy and compassion, which is the counterbalance to discipline. Leaders must be firm, but they must also look at people as individuals with self-esteem, value, and worth. Being empathetic as a leader is to put yourself in the shoes of your subordinates, to see things from their perspective, and to understand their feelings. Empathy is closely related to compassion. If you are empathetic, then you understand another's pain. If you are compassionate, you feel or show sympathy for another. That's taking the empathy one step further. Understanding the pain is critical to being able to behave in a way that is sympathetic or compassionate to another individual. Together, compassion and empathy are key to being a caring individual and leader, to being human.

Citizenship

In recent years, leaders have been coming out of the boardroom and affecting change in their organizations through acts of good citizenship. Organizational citizenship involves behavior that is discretionary, or not recognized by formal reward systems. It involves behavior that effectively promotes the success of the organization. It involves giving of oneself, helping others, and performing in a conscientious way. Effective leaders help their staff by listening to their problems, often affecting change through collaboration, and the sharing of ideas and views. As a practice leader, it is important to do more than is required, go above and beyond the call of duty in a way that demonstrates the quality of service and organizational values important to you as a leader, and inevitably, nurturing the change you wish to affect in the organization as a whole.

Setting an Example … Building Integrity

The greatest way that a leader leads is by setting a good example. It's not enough to possess the qualities enumerated here; character is demonstrated by its integrity each and every day. Given that the substance of character is composed of trustworthiness, respect, responsibility, fairness, caring, and citizenship, then the glue that holds character together is integrity. The integrity, or consistency, of a leader's character sends a powerful message to subordinates and sets the tone and character that is amplified throughout the organization as a whole. The chief characteristics of integrity are sincerity, consistency, substance, and being a good finisher.

Actions Speak Louder Than Words

Be sincere. A story of Gandhi describes a mother who brought her child to him, and asked Gandhi to tell the child to stop eating sugar. Gandhi replied that he cannot tell him that, but to bring him back in a month. The mother was very dissatisfied. She had traveled some distance, and she expected the famous leader's support. So she left, and came back a month later. Gandhi knelt beside the child and said, "Do not eat sugar. It is bad for you." Then he gave him a hug and returned the boy to his mother. Perplexed, the mother asked Gandhi why he didn't say that a month ago. Gandhi explained, "A month ago, I was still eating sugar." Your actions should match your words, or they will hold no water.

Once Is Not Enough

Be consistent, once is not enough. This goes back to fairness and equality. A leader must consistently show integrity and create systems that also show integrity. For example, disciplinary standards must be enforced consistently from person to person, and from incident to incident. Theft by an administrator should be handled with the same degree of seriousness and process as theft by a custodian. Making exceptions to process and rules for the sake of position or friendship creates low morale and threatens employee trust in management.

Be What You Say You Are

Leaders must have substance. Appearances are not everything, as your employees will soon discover. Trying to impress will not build trust. Abraham Lincoln was known to tell the story of a tree and a squirrel. A squirrel ran up a tree and into a hole in the tree. Upon closer examination, Lincoln discovered that the tree he thought was so strong was actually hollow. A storm could have easily blown that tree right over on top of his house. Much like the tree in a storm, leaders who lack integrity will not be able to weather the storms of tough times.

Finish What You Start

Persistence. Determination. No matter the odds, a good leader finishes what is started. This is where you really see what people are made of, who has the heart to complete the task despite the odds or the challenges, perceived or real. Follow-thru. Do what you say you will do. Keep your word. Do the right thing, even when it is difficult.

Creating Positive Work Environment Begins Anew Every Day

The challenge of building character and building integrity is something that leaders must work on every day. The challenge of character is not just to understand its core values, but to live them. It is only by setting an example, one day at a time and one project at a time, that leaders create the positive work environment where people can thrive and business can be successful.

Without character, true leadership is virtually impossible. Character establishes trust, loyalty, respect, and motivates followers. Moral character lifts the team in bad times, carries it through struggles, and points the way to success. A leader's character is the backbone of every company or practice, and its integrity a key source of power.

These are some pretty basic concepts of leadership and life. No doubt you have heard of others, as have I. These, however, have been my basic and fundamental rules of the road. I sincerely hope they can be of benefit to you as they have been to me.

Reference

1. Van Knippenberg D, De Cremer D, Van Knippenberg B. Leadership and fairness: the state of the art. *European Journal of Work and Organizational Psychology.* 2007;16(2);113-140. doi:10.1080/13594320701275833

CHAPTER 11

The Eight Roots of *Healthy Power* in Effective Medical Leadership

Craig N. Piso, PhD

Life ultimately means taking the responsibility to find the right answer to its problems and to fulfill the tasks which it constantly sets for each individual.
—Viktor Frankl

This material is intended to provide a framework for understanding *healthy power* in effective medical leadership and to delineate the eight psychological principles upon which it is built. It is written especially for self-examining physicians who are striving to understand why they usually excel in medicine/surgery but sometimes feel challenged and less competent in handling administrative matters as practice leaders.

Pinto JB. *Ophthalmic Leadership: A Practical Guide for Physicians, Administrators, and Teams, Second Edition* (pp 61-78).
© 2022 SLACK Incorporated.

Power and Effectiveness

He that is good with a hammer tends to think everything is a nail.
—Abraham Maslow

Every effective leader generates the influence to align and motivate others so they strive together toward successful outcomes through their *power.* Accordingly, it cannot be expected, in general, that practice staff will readily follow directions, make adjustments, or embrace even moderately difficult changes without first having respect for the authority of the person to whom they report in the chain of command. Further, it is apparently part of our innate wiring to become most responsive to those people who carry sufficient power to make meaningful differences in our work lives—those who can wield rewards and punishments—and to be especially attuned to those with whom we experience healthy fear ... the precursor to respect.

Daniel Pink makes a convincing case to argue why the traditional "carrots and sticks" model for motivating people often does not work.[1] He asserts that the most important drivers among workers at higher levels of maturity are "autonomy," "mastery," and "purpose." However, the fact remains: People at all levels of maturity become more willing followers in response to stronger, more powerful leaders—those who can impact their lives most meaningfully—regardless of their benevolent or malevolent intentions.

Whether they are working productively with loyalty and commitment for a *servant leader* with whom they have an intimate yet deferential connection, or merely toeing the line because they fear for their very survival under a dictatorial boss, the underlying dynamic is the same: People are emotionally and behaviorally responsive in direct proportion to the magnitude of power they ascribe to their supervisor. Parallel with effective parenting, any supervisor who is perceived as lacking power, and therefore evokes little or no fear in their staff, receives proportionately little or no respect.

The key to creating enduring organizational health and effectiveness that together generate healthy practice results, however, is not simply a matter of growing one's arsenal of power without regard for interpersonal fairness or individual well-being. If it were truly the case that "might makes right," then medical leaders would do well to rule dispassionately with a dictatorial iron fist; however, this is clearly not the case. Not only is the quantity of one's power a prerequisite to leadership effectiveness, but also, and more importantly, the qualitative features of one's power and its perceived expression.

Healthy Versus Unhealthy Power

Perhaps the best way of understanding the contrasting features and dynamics associated with *healthy* and *unhealthy* power is to apply the analogy of a swimming pool and its purification/filtering system. The water is chemically treated to achieve the right balance of PH, alkalinity, and chlorine, and it is filtered each day to remove foreign materials and contaminants that otherwise cloud and pollute the swimming pool. This keeps the water clean and sparkling clear, thereby making for a high-quality swimming experience as well as an attractive sight for observers nearby. Anyone immersed in such a pristine pool at just the right temperature will invariably enjoy a wide array of wonderful aquatic feelings through most of the senses. The water looks, feels, smells, and even tastes inviting.

Now liken this analogous description to an ophthalmic practice that is both operationally functional and culturally wholesome—one in which there is such regular, effective dedication to the appropriate empowerment of staff and patients alike that people enjoy becoming "immersed" within it, time after time. This is a system that is built upon *healthy power.* It develops its healthy core strength, both operationally and culturally, and then it embodies high functioning, attractive features throughout the system and at its surface for all to witness and enjoy transparently.

Returning now to the pool analogy in a sharply contrasting manner, the system undergoes an increasingly dramatic change of both functionality and aesthetics when the water purification/filtering system either stops or becomes operationally ineffective. When pool maintenance duties are performed poorly and/or neglected, one can enjoy relatively clean water and adequate pool viewing for a short while; however, one is soon reminded that continued imbalance compromises performance, thereby producing toxic results. As algae grows green on the pool bottom and sides, the water becomes cloudy and murky over time, and the quality of swimming and observer aesthetics are similarly degraded. Unchanged, the system will inevitably deteriorate into such dysfunction and ugliness that people not only will cease to swim there, they avoid the sight and smell of it altogether in pursuit of a better pool.

Whether the practice leadership as a whole is characterized by *unhealthy power* and its accompanying core weaknesses or merely harbors a small but significant faction of managerial toxicity, such a practice becomes at risk for operational dysfunction and cultural contamination the longer the lack of healthy balance continues. As described in the swimming pool analogy, abuse/neglect of the machine (operations) and/or its people (culture) will, in the short run, enable those in charge to believe falsely that (for example) profit-generating short cuts and abuse of power without accountability make for business success. However, Jim Collins asserts through his recent research that the first three stages of business failure are typified by: "(1) Hubris Born of Success; (2) Undisciplined Pursuit of More; and (3) Denial of Risk and Peril."[2] In the absence of a paradigm shift toward *healthy power,* the longer term results are quite predictable: People (both patients and staff) leave in search of a better pool.

In view of these contrasting, abstract depictions of *healthy* and *unhealthy power,* what is now required is a framework for understanding these dynamic forces in order to apply practice management strategies toward the development of greater organizational health and effectiveness. This framework and suggestions for its implementation are presented in the remaining sections.

The Eight Psychological Roots of Healthy Versus Unhealthy Power

A healthy root system growing deeply downward into fertile soil sustains and nourishes the mighty oak toward mature thriving so that it can branch out, thereby bearing good fruit (acorns) plentifully in its season. By contrast, undeveloped, inadequate roots, or even good roots drawing upon poisonous soil, threaten the tree's very survival, making fruit bearing in maximum quantity and/or quality impossible. In this regard, some might relate well to Gary Cooper's 1941 portrayal of Alvin York in Warner Brothers' *Sergeant York* in which he exclaims amidst his early life struggles, "I reckon I ain't found no roots that'll hold me up. That's why I'm hell-bent to fall!"

The framework depicted below shows the continuum for each of the eight "roots" that nourish either form of power, *healthy* or *unhealthy*, first within individuals, and then as a ripple effect within their sphere of influence systemically. Accordingly, the more influence a person carries within a group practice, for example, the larger and more far reaching will be the ripple effect they generate, positively or negatively. Therefore, this model is an especially important tool for understanding how those at the top of an organization's chain of command influence the culture, staff morale, operational integrity, and, ultimately, the quality of overall patient experiences (ie, patient satisfaction with both customer service and medical/surgical outcomes).

Here is the applicable leadership paradigm for creating ***powerful*** group practices:

Healthy Power*..** ***Unhealthy Power

*P*ersonal Responsibility..*P*ersonal Irresponsibility
*O*ptimistic Expectations..*O*rchestrated Suffering
*W*in-Win Relationships ....*W*in-Lose Relationships
*E*nergizing Joy ....*E*gocentric Pleasure
*R*eality-Based Choices..*R*egressive Choices
*F*ocused Action ....*F*ragmented Activity
*U*nrelenting Courage..*U*nsettling Fear
*L*ifelong Purpose...*L*ifelong Grasping

P: Personal Responsibility Versus Personal Irresponsibility

The first root in this model stems from the following premise: *Power and responsibility develop in direct proportion to each other and are functionally related in healthy individuals and systems (ie, power = responsibility).* That is, any mature, well-developed person working within a predominantly healthy organization will become more powerful as they act more responsibly in handling positional duties. Therefore, the willingness to take complete ownership of and accountability for one's choices is the pathway to self-empowerment within any healthy system. Conversely, such a person predictably becomes more responsible to the degree that they are appropriately empowered and supported. It follows, then, that the fundamental way to help someone with an adequate sense of conscience to become even more responsible is by empowering that person with greater positional authority (eg, supports and tools, staff direct reports to manage).

This, then, becomes a quite useful diagnostic formula to apply in both personnel recruitment and management. For example, it is usually quite illuminating to ask candidates during the interview process about their handling of previous difficult, challenging professional situations. There is a striking and important distinction between those who report having been able to overcome and solve problems and those who point the finger of blame, make excuses for failures, and present their "victim" role in such responses.

Since power and responsibility always travel together in a healthy (eg, mature, competent) recruit, such persons are likely to report a sense of ownership (eg, responsibility) when having faced earlier problems. Whether or not they solved the problems, they will describe their experiences from an internal *locus of contro*l (eg, origin of power) and, therefore, with a strong sense of accountability for their handling of them.

On the other hand are those candidates who deny culpability for their past struggles or failings while attributing responsibility to people and/or forces outside themselves, thus from an external locus of control. The problems that such recruits manifest once hired quite often are the result of clinging to their positional power while shirking and shedding responsibility for their performance when it does not meet expectations. Enabling such behavior is characteristic of relatively unhealthy systems. Recognize that the operating system of dictators and other dysfunctional individuals is one in which one wields authority while holding others accountable, especially for their problems and/or failure. Thus, *unhealthy power* is sought through *personal irresponsibility,* and its arising logically manifests in dysfunction.

According to Jim Collins,[3] "Level 5" great leaders embody "Humility with Resolve," demonstrated in part through "The Window and the Mirror." Looking unselfishly through the "Window" to give full credit to staff when things are going well, while looking courageously in the "Mirror" to take responsibility when things are going poorly. He also found that ineffective leaders, with no surprise, tend to do the opposite, thereby generating tension and resentment as fallout.

Here are three *healthy power* prescriptions for developing *personal responsibility* as a leader:

1. Walk the *power = responsibility* talk. Speak frequently about this dynamic when explaining the rationale for your decisions and actions. For example, "Because of the consistent manner that Jan has made effective choices (ie, exercised her power) to succeed at projects, I recommend her for this promotion with expanded duties (ie, responsibilities)." Conversely, the same principle applies when communicating about negative performance or behavior: "Jane, you are being terminated (ie, being held accountable) as the result of your choice to belittle your supervisor to a vendor after being warned repeatedly and in writing that the next infraction of this sort would result in your loss of employment here."
2. Ask and answer these self-diagnostic questions, including input from trusted staff and peers where feasible:
   a. Am I an accountable *servant leader,* humbly striving to serve a mission greater than myself, or do I impress others as being primarily concerned about my own welfare and prosperity, using my positional authority in self-serving or arrogant ways that could demean, frustrate, or hurt others?

b. Do I demonstrate a democratic leadership style in which others feel empowered, valued/appreciated, and encouraged to find and express their voice, or do I show more of a dictatorial approach (eg, unilateral decision-making, double standard behavior, controlling others without holding myself equally or more accountable for my actions)?
c. When I become frustrated, anxious, irritable, and tired, do I take responsibility for my reactions to others, graciously trying to become part of the solution, or do I focus upon others and expect them to change or adjust in order for them to improve my moods and feeling states?

3. Clarify the performance expectations you have for your staff since, according to practice management consultant Walt Underwood (personal conversation, 2011), "all conflicts are the result of two or more people not sharing the same expectations." You will have fewer such conflicts with your staff and, when necessary, the disciplinary actions through what you hold people accountable to will be logically determined by having first empowered them with clear expectations for their performance.

O: Optimistic Expectations Versus Orchestrated Suffering

Two mid-twentieth century ground-breaking works set the stage for what has become currently exciting research material within several technologically accelerated areas of neuroscience: "psycho-neuroimmunology"—mind-body connection, brain-behavior relationships, brain training, etc; and "positive psychology"—the burgeoning interest in human happiness and well-being. The first, *The Power of Positive Thinking,*[4] provided an inspirational description of the positive power a person develops from within and then attracts toward oneself via faith and optimism. The second, *Pygmalion in the Classroom,*[5] provided empirical findings to support the power of expectations to empower or disempower oneself and/or others via "self-fulfilling prophecy."

The assertions of these pioneering authors/researchers are directly relevant to this broader discussion about *healthy power* in leadership effectiveness. A leader who demonstrates authentically positive attitudes and expectations about both people and circumstances tends to generate hope and confidence among staff, thereby providing psychological fuel (energy) for the team's goal-directed behavior. Since people generally work up or down to the expectations held about them by those deemed to be most important in their lives, these processes in leadership can be a double-edged sword. On the one hand, a staff member might be buoyed up by a manager who sees their greater potential, especially if treated with compassion while struggling to perform well. On the other hand, prejudice (negative self-fulfilling prophecy) can erode that same person's hope, dismantle their confidence, and rob the person of motivation to make their best efforts toward success—the dynamics of *orchestrated suffering.* (*Note:* For those reading this section familiar with placebo effects in medical/surgical outcomes, it becomes clear that setting genuinely positive expectations with patients with a realistic and prevailing overall sense of confidence regarding outcomes is an integral part of any patient-centered and empowering bedside manner.)

Here are three *healthy power* prescriptions for developing *optimistic expectations* as a leader:

1. Instill hope in your people about their goals, their potential, and their long-term success and fulfillment. If you believe genuinely in the unique strengths and untapped potential of your people, then they naturally feel the contagiousness of your positive view of them. For example, when someone says, "I just can't figure this one out," a helpful reply is, "You will, you just haven't figured it out *yet.*"
2. Commit to face-to-face discussion of difficult issues, rather than "splitting" or "triangulating" (ie, complaining to others while avoiding confrontation and/or conflict), and address issues in a timely manner, rather than allowing them to "fester." This courageous commitment to having what some have called "fierce conversations" with everything put on the table in person, ironically, creates a more positive working environment and atmosphere of increased safety/security because the process increases trust, leaves no stone unturned, and most often results in logical resolution of issues for greater stability.
3. Always represent the best interests of the practice and its governance, even when problems are apparent and still unresolved. Just as parents do well to support each other, especially when a complaining child attempts to stir strife at the top of the family pecking order by turning one parent against the other, do not allow anyone to play "divide and conquer" with you and your managers, doctors, partners, etc. Understand and respect the power of words to help or hinder any initiative that you oversee. In this case, never diminish the authority of your staff or supervisors, thereby exposing an "Achilles heel" at which others will predictably shoot more arrows of negativity.

W: Win-Win Relationships Versus Win-Lose Relationships

It takes a mature, confident, humble leader to create a culture in which a "win-win" mentality becomes woven into the fabric of all interpersonal relationships. This type of practice is characterized largely by its people showing consistently cooperative and unselfish dedication to each other for the success of the practice as a whole, even if this means making individual sacrifices to support that success. This also runs directly against the grain of many predominantly western values espoused in business, sports, and otherwise where competition and winning are inextricably linked. Vince Lombardi is well remembered for saying, "Winning isn't everything … it's the only thing!"

The now familiar and increasingly prevalent "win-lose" paradigm had its modern era roots in "social Darwinism" – a socio-economic model that was extrapolated from the early work of Charles Darwin[6] wherein "survival of the fittest" became the mantra for social and business competition. Unfortunately, once this work ethic is embraced, it tends to give license to play by one's own rules because, as they claim, "It's a dog-eat-dog world, and this dog won't be eaten!" Further, then, it's not a big leap for many such individuals to live and work under the belief that "the end justifies the means," leaving others floundering and swamped amidst the hardship created by their one-sided wake of success. In this model, *unhealthy power* in its most extreme forms is seized by sacrificing all others without regard for healthy competition, sportsmanship, or regard for the greater good. One might recognize our current American political in-fighting and nonproductive gridlock as symptoms of this leadership model at its most tragically flawed. It also permeates much of corporate America with comparably toxic side effects.

A "win-lose" leadership style and related culture in group practices tend to propagate systemic mistrust and accompanying in-fighting (eg, "turf wars", resistance to change, silo behavior). A leader's espoused attitude and perspective about winning within one's group practice, therefore, becomes a driver at many important forks in the road. If, for example, the practice leadership operates from a "scarcity mentality," then the culture will become characterized for the most part by staff behavior that is biased toward a "win-lose" orientation toward all relationships. This unfortunately includes those operating between peers and other departments, not simply against outside competitors. Nobody normally likes to lose, thus avoidance of losing becomes a powerful source of negative reinforcement for staff behavior when a more secure, attractive paradigm is not in operation.

Stephen Covey, an organizational development and leadership icon, argues that what is needed to produce a healthy culture of aligned and empowered team effort is a completely opposite perspective: "Think win-win or no deal."[7] While we certainly want to instill a strong sense of competition with outsiders and rise to the highest pinnacle of success that is possible in the larger arena, what's critical here is to recognize two key reference points for any such efforts: (1) the locus of control; and (2) the model through which "winning" is achieved.

Productive, healthy teamwork across departments and disciplines is most frequently fostered by leaders who inculcate staff within an "abundance mentality" so that they will behave in manners that empower and support each other interdependently. A practice model then emerges in which there is room for everyone to share in the resources and become both individually and collectively successful. Accordingly, effective leaders make skillful use of both key reference points in their management efforts:

1. Rather than spending time/energy focused upon the competition and being fearful of outside threat, staff are redirected to pay most careful attention to their own behavior from an internal locus of control, thereby increasing their confidence through their self-initiated, developing competencies.
2. Such a leader will create a "win-win" environment in which people become other-directed. That is, they become primarily oriented toward the organization's mission with a service focus, a servant leadership orientation, altruistic sharing, and the formation of creative synergies among coworkers to become more productive while, at the same time, working more enjoyably.

Here are three *healthy power* prescriptions for developing *win-win relationships* as a leader:

1. Enable every staff member to feel like a "winner" by catching them in the act of doing something of extra great value on behalf of the practice, and then commemorate that incident with a written memo and/or certificate (suitable for framing) that is kept in their personnel file for reference during the next performance review process. If you cannot do this at least once for each person during the year, then you might have the wrong person in that position (or perhaps you need to

adjust your managerial radar in order to notice more of the positives in their performance).

2. In addition to developing individual performance goals for the upcoming 12-month review period, develop team-oriented goals for which the team enjoys a shared sense of pride and tangible rewards both for their attainment. Healthy internal competition is also part of this equation, as long as no "loser" is created in the process (ie, establish tiered rewards for all, rather than a winner-takers-all, all-or-none outcome).
3. Whenever staff become distracted or derailed by being concerned with what others are or might be doing, within or outside of the practice, redirect them to focus exclusively upon the duties of their position. Similarly, assist with making inner comparisons only (eg, comparing today's performance with that of last month), rather than comparing oneself with others.

E: Energizing Joy Versus Egocentric Pleasure

This is one of the most important and yet elusive areas for advancement in leadership effectiveness, largely because many people do not consider nor understand the significant differences between *joy* and *pleasure*. Further, such people do not develop their leadership style to evoke and mobilize the potential *healthy power* that arises spontaneously when workers become joyful. This is in sharp contrast to the popular but temporary (and usually counterproductive) dynamics that are spawned in the workplace in pursuit of predominantly self-serving forms of pleasure, such as *quid pro quo* ("this for that") sexual harassment. Therefore, let us examine those differences and the implications they hold for the development of truly great, empowered leadership.

Joy always arises emotionally from deep within us, being heartfelt and uniquely personal, thus it is under our potential control and it invigorates our lives without creating entrapment or leaving any form of "hangover."[8] Almost universally among people and across cultures, joyfulness is spontaneously derived from other-directed, mission-focused service to others and for causes greater than oneself, thereby coloring one's life with a deeper sense of purpose and meaning. This is not to be confused with "lose-win," self-defeating behavior. To the contrary, joyful sharing within a healthy workplace is reciprocally contagious because it tends to spiral the professional lives of like-minded coworkers upward. Working so among those who understand and appreciate your pursuit of joy will prompt others to connect eagerly with you more fully as "kindred spirits," thereby bringing even more joy through such social connectedness.

Most importantly, joy can last indefinitely, even for a lifetime, since there is none of the "withdrawal" process found in chemical or other forms of overdependency or addiction. The pursuit of joy in a world filled with *hedonism* (ie, the instinctive pursuit of pleasure and avoidance of pain), cynicism, and accompanying misery is part of the exceptional journey described eloquently by M. Scott Peck.[9,10] Applying these precepts to for-profit medical leadership effectiveness might seem to some like an irrelevant generalization. However, let's consider the other side of this enigmatic coin.

Pleasure is most frequently triggered, at least initially, by outside forces, including people and things that stimulate ("turn on") the brain's pleasure center. This process can foster our external dependency upon that pleasure, wherein we unwittingly empower an external locus of control, thereby leading progressively into dependency or addiction. Given that overdependency and addiction are most often perpetuated through the defense mechanism of *denial* (ie, believing what one needs or wants to believe in lieu of factual risks and dangers), any person so inclined falls prey to what Andrew Olendzki describes as the "hedonic treadmill": Striving relentlessly for more and more *egocentric pleasure* while engaged in denial.[11] Engaging denial as the primary means of ignoring warning signs and the deterrents to continued dysfunctional behavior is disempowering because any form of deception, especially self-deception, erodes our *healthy power.* Ignoring or otherwise being unable to recognize the truths regarding their pleasure-seeking behavior is a primary feature of those individuals who unwittingly sacrifice real power for the illusion of control in an unending cycle of driveness that yields only temporary relief from their discomfort, while inviting serious problems.

When the pursuit of pleasure in the workplace is overdone, misguided, and otherwise overshadowing opportunities to generate joy, that workplace and its people become entrapped in their ongoing, unsuccessful attempts to enjoy the *unhealthy power* they've found. Like any addiction, these pursuits are ultimately disempowering because they redirect primary energies toward the self, repeatedly looking for and acquiring doses of pleasure and/or pain avoidance at every opportunity, and yet never being satisfied for more than brief periods. The accompanying roller coaster of such emotional up's and down's usually creates a cadre of coworkers who share in their unhappiness (ie, "misery loves company") and bemoan a sense of victimization, the latter stemming directly from the law of *power = responsibility* described previously. The externalization of *responsibility* by looking outside oneself for pleasure and pain relief (eg, smoking, overeating, alcohol/drug abuse, affairs at work) naturally leads to an externalization of one's *power,* and when a person is unhappy in this scenario, they will feel like a victim: suffering, unable to change things substantively, and not responsible for the inescapable sense of helplessness.

Here are four *healthy power* prescriptions for developing *energizing joy* as a leader:

1. Seek joy through inner transformation, relaxed self-mastery, and autonomous freedom. Minimize cravings for external pleasures and any accompanying self-deception, overdependency, and addiction.
2. Practice being nondefensive with all others by developing realistic self-confidence and self-acceptance in order not to take things personally. Act as your own final judge, holding yourself wholly accountable for your choices with authenticity and public transparency. Model these traits with humility and grace, and coach others to do likewise to create a more joyful atmosphere.
3. Count your blessings with daily appreciation and a joyful focus, comparing yourself and your professional life situation with no one else. Failure to appreciate your blessings is the root of discontent, a sense of want, and painful envy. Instead, as much as possible, inspire others to focus upon and appreciate every aspect of each moment by being mindfully present at work with a positive (ie, "glass half full") outlook.

4. Dare to dream regarding your developing leadership role with zest and passion, a sense of adventure, and excitement about embracing appropriate professional risks. Faith in your meaningful dreams generates hope contagiously throughout the practice, and hope provides you and your team with energy for striving more productively and with greater fulfillment during the journey toward goal attainment.

R: Reality-Based Choices Versus Regressive Choices

Especially as a leader in health care where the stakes are inherently high, become determined to understand and accept the *truth* (eg, facts, reality) in all matters pertaining to the practice, not limited to one's medical/surgical services to patients. This admonition is offered because truth is the basis of *enlightenment* (ie, seeing and understanding lucidly) and, because "information is power," contingent upon such information being accurate. Such discernment and acceptance of any truth, even the most unpleasant of truths, then liberates energy to make more confident, fact-based decisions.

Leaders, by contrast, who tend to make choices based upon incomplete and/or inaccurate data, suffer the painful, energy wasting consequences of rework and repair after lesser quality decisions have been implemented. Relatively ineffective leaders too frequently deny and/or avoid the truth out of fear, insecurity, or simply a lack of resilience—the ability to rebound from a set-back after finding that a mistake has been made—which, ironically, contributes to making more mistakes. This decision-making style is more prevalent among those medical leaders who strive for perfection in all that they do, a not uncommon characteristic among ophthalmologist owners, MPs, and medical directors.[12]

Recognize also that *unhealthy power* always seeks to perpetuate itself through deception and misuse of information with others. Falsehood (eg, lies, distortions, propaganda) is the currency through which immature and/or aberrant persons often acquire and expand their base of power by influencing decisions that are then based upon misinformation (eg, *regressive choices).* Thereby they are manipulating, ensnaring, and controlling others for personal gain.

Here are four *healthy power* prescriptions for developing *reality-based choices* as a leader:

1. Study and develop your *emotional intelligence*[13] in order to reduce or eliminate any "emotional hijacking" that triggers you to become blind to what is factual and real. Recognize your leadership "buttons" that when pushed tend to render you less discerning and poised, and then practice the skills that will disable those buttons (eg, refrain from making impulsive decisions, ask for help from trusted peers, embrace all truths as dispassionately as possible).
2. "Keep the jury out" when you hear reports of interpersonal strife and conflict within the practice. That is, give the benefit of the doubt regarding any negative report you hear about a person, including peers, administration, patients, other providers, etc. Reserve judgment until all of the required facts are understood, thereby restraining the urge to reach closure prematurely, especially under the strain of intense feelings, such as anger/frustration and worry.

3. Allow your more rational thinking and behavior under pressure to flow into edifying calm and personal poise. Show others how to "let cooler heads prevail" amidst the chaos through your silence and dispassionate reflection whenever necessary.
4. Let your word be your bond. Always mean what you say and say what you mean. Without exception, demonstrate an unwavering commitment to truthfulness through your honesty, transparency, and authenticity, thereby causing people to listen to what you say with experience validated trust and confidence. Your impeccable honesty engenders trust, and trust produces followership and loyalty—basic sources of power for any leader. Maintain confidences, keep your promises, take responsibility when appropriate, and apologize when you're mistaken. Follow these prescriptions faithfully and your people will more reliably make *reality-based choices,* too.

F: Focused Action Versus Fragmented Activity

Paraphrasing and highlighting the pearls of a conversation with John Pinto this past year, he likened the power that is generated through focused action to pressing the sharp point of an awl into a plasterboard wall, therein making a deep, penetrating impact quite effectively. By contrast, he went on to describe the relatively futile effort to make a hole in the wall by pressing the palm of one's hand onto the same spot. Laws of physics enable the increased force created by concentrating the point of pressure into a narrower, precise focal area to break through the wall. He drew a parallel to what is required to become most successful in any pursuit that requires making a penetrating impact toward breakthrough. Thus, the focus here pertains to leadership behavior that drives positive growth and change through strategically focused, concentrated team effort.

Jim Collins[3(pp95-96)] has written about the paradigm he uncovered for building and maintaining business greatness through the identification of one's empowering strategic focus: "The Hedgehog Concept." It is comprised of what he called the "intersection of three circles: (1) What you are deeply *passionate about;* (2) What you *can be best in the world at;* and (3) What drives your *economic engine.*" He contends that businesses tend to lose their greatness and sometimes fail when they act "foxy," allowing themselves to become distracted and derailed by drifting away from the primary focus that produced their initial success.

Similarly, Stephen Covey[14] described the positive alignment of effort and results generating dynamic associated with leadership that consistently drives intensely concentrated, focused team behavior toward a prescribed set of business priorities. In doing so, the leader differentiates those tasks that are most important, both urgently so and otherwise, from those that should receive little or no attention. Since, as Wayne Dyer has asserted, "what we focus upon tends to expand" (personal conversation, 2011), it becomes critical in all forms of leadership that we select and maintain the most appropriate and important focus day-to-day, both individually and collectively. What, then, will expand is the developing nucleus of effort to make the penetrating impact required for goal attainment and breakthrough success.

An inspiring act of powerfully focused leadership heroism took place on January 15, 2009 when Chesley Burnett "Sully" Sullenberger, III saved the lives of all 155 people on board US Airways Flight 1549 by successfully ditching the aircraft in the Hudson River off Manhattan, New York City. Speaking afterward with news anchor Katie Couric regarding the focus of his preparation over many years for such an event, Sullenberger said, "One way of looking at this might be that for 42 years, I've been making small, regular deposits in this bank of experience: education and training. And on January 15 the balance was sufficient so that I could make a very large withdrawal."[15]

Here are four *healthy power* prescriptions for developing *focused action* as a leader:

1. Use the power of focus. Recognize that our focus upon people and things tends to expand, either positively or negatively; thereby influencing how we interact with them. For example, a steady focus upon another person's faults only serves to expand our sense of their faults, creating tension as well. Accordingly, we become more effective when we maintain a focus upon those things that contribute most to our goals, rather than letting ourselves become distracted by lesser or counter-productive things. In your communications, therefore, create and maintain a positive outlook and focus. Help your people to shift their focus in ways that support their successful actions and create a more positive work environment. When, for example, a staff member is complaining about their struggles with problems, whether real or imagined, help them by shifting their attention toward what is working, their available resources, potential solutions, and their choices and options; rather than perpetuating the negative focus in which they have become stuck.
2. "Put first things first" each day by first identifying your strategic business priorities and action steps toward their attainment, both as an individual leader and through inspirational guidance and support of your team practice wide. Choose your priorities carefully and remember, "Where your eyes go, your car follows."[16]
3. Develop your "Hedgehog" focus by identifying the intersection of three circles described previously as part of creating the *strategic plan,* both short- and long-term, for the practice. Then develop tactical plans in direct support of the strategic plan that can be applied to all managerial efforts by you in concert with your administrative team.
4. Uphold the chain of command. The organizational chart defines roles and reporting relationships with an explicit structure through which power and control are to be mobilized. Consistent focus upon this chain of command is essential for the support and continued empowerment of every position in the hierarchy. Therefore, ensure in every communication that no manager or supervisor is overlooked or bypassed because doing so renders them less effective, especially in the eyes of the person(s) who succeed in nullifying their authority. For example, if someone complains to you without first having broached their complaint with their immediate supervisor, redirect them to their supervisor with the clear expectation that they will handle their situation competently. Should that not be the case, schedule a meeting of all relevant parties and discuss the matter transparently toward resolution, always supporting the supervisor in question, especially in front of the staff.

U: Unrelenting Courage Versus Unsettling Fear

Courage is often misunderstood as the absence of fear, therein associating a person who experiences fear with being a coward. In truth, courage is not the absence of fear, anxiety, doubt, or discomfort. Instead, courage is demonstrated by taking deliberate, effective action in the *presence* of fear and/or other such unpleasant emotions. Derived from the Latin root *cour,* it has its meaning in the word "heart." Therefore, the emphasis here is placed upon developing effective leadership through the skills of *taking heart* in the presence of fear, etc in order to initiate undeterred, powerful action steps while being fully cognizant of the risks involved.

It is especially important to their success that leaders develop the skills required to confront issues and people courageously, the latter confrontations being more difficult (eg, addressing behavior and performance problems). Yet this is the area in which leaders most commonly fall short, demonstrating and/or enabling such common practices as avoiding conflicts, procrastinating on projects, minimizing issues, and other means of simply not handling the problems found too often in their own and others' performance. Why is this so? Leaders frequently put off doing the very things that are most vital to their success simply because they are afraid of failure, discomfort, or change (eg, *unsettling fear).* Their ripple effects are similarly unsettling to both staff and patients.

As a useful, magical analogy, think of such avoidant and self-defeating behavior to be the equivalent of locking a monster in a closet where "out of sight is out of mind" and where "ignorance is bliss." However, there's a catch: The monster feeds on your inattention (which is how it grew to become a monster in the first place, instead of being handled before it became frightening). Each day that the monster is ignored, it grows bigger, scratching at the door as it tries to reemerge, increasing in its dangerousness as the days continue to pass (akin to the approaching deadline for that "gorilla" project assigned 3 months ago but still not begun)!

Avoidance and denial continue until the haunting, stress-producing noises coming ever more loudly through the door compel the person to peek into the closet to take stock of what now lurks within. While initially shocked to see how big the monster has become during the interim period, one notices that it begins to shrink in size almost immediately now that attention has been directed toward it, reversing the effect that inattention had in inflating its growth. Therefore, mustering the courage not only to open the door, but also to embrace the monster behind it, will speed the rate of making it more manageable. After all, it became monstrously larger than life primarily in the mind, anyway.

The moral: Open your closet door and hug the "monster(s)" that have been growing amidst any neglect, and learn to tackle people and projects with courage in the early going when careful planning and diligent effort thereafter keep things under better control. Remember, what we don't confront, we enable.

Since the greatest common obstacle to leaders confronting major issues in a more direct and timely manner is fear … fear of conflict, fear of failure, fear of repercussion, etc. John Maxwell described "failing forward" as an empowering reframe of fear in order to propel more courageous, perseverant action, especially for embracing more challenging confrontations.[17] Resilience, the ability to bounce back productively following any setback or disheartening experience, therefore, is developed by accepting that feelings of fear, hesitation, etc are normal, rather than indicators of cowardice or being a "failure." A failed attempt is just that—a behavioral trial and learning experience to be factored into the next planned and more seasoned effort—rather than evidence that the *person* is a failure.

Here are four *healthy power* prescriptions for developing *unrelenting courage* as a leader:

1. Become a stronger, more courageous leader by practicing the habit of acting in real time to solve problems and to complete key tasks first, rather than procrastinating about jugular issues (ie, "hug your monster").
2. Reframe challenges and adversity as opportunities to develop resilience while maintaining faith that you and/or your staff will prevail in the end, thereby showing and engendering confidence among your team ... a foundation of core strength.
3. Expect and teach your staff to find the courage to follow your good example in order to meet the challenges that they face, insisting that courage is not the absence of fear but, instead, taking decisive action in the *presence* of fear.
4. Influence open and courageous interpersonal exchanges. Expressing empathy and understanding with staff is the most important communication skill that you can demonstrate in order to influence the courageous communication exchanges you desire. This begins with the willingness to listen to what others have to say and giving genuine respect to their ideas and opinions, even when they are quite different from your own. It means meeting your people where they are before attempting to move them where you want them to go. This has a profound impact upon others because it gives them a sense of being safely valued and understood, two of the most important factors that determine how secure your people will feel working under your direction. By having first validated the other person's right to their opinions and feelings, even if you strongly disagree with them, you have reduced the tension that otherwise would stand in the way of their open communication. By patiently and respectfully understanding the person, you help them to take heart and more openly express their voice with courage.

L: Lifelong Purpose Versus Lifelong Grasping

Purposeful, values-driven leadership is probably the very most important root principle driving *healthy power* of the eight described in total. As Rick Warren has written, "When life has meaning, you can bear almost anything; without it, nothing is bearable."[18] The extrapolation made here is that such perspective infuses positive energy also into one's work life. Obstacles are then transformed into opportunities by a committed team that you lead with an *esprit de corp* and enlivening vibe that patients and others visiting the practice cannot help but feel. What, then, are the qualities of such values-driven leadership that galvanize a practice to form a culture characterized by *lifelong purpose?*

Inspirational healthy leaders (eg, Dr. Martin Luther King, Jr.) always evoke deep, positively transforming emotions in others. Thus, in having such an effect, they enjoy the power of aligned and loyal followership that was described previously. Note, however, that Hitler, Stalin, and other dictators through the present day temporarily enjoy the same empowering dynamic. However, this continues only until loyal constituents discover that they have been deceived and/or ensnared by the carefully hidden true intentions and closely guarded weapons of *unhealthy power.* Such a reign of *lifelong grasping* then inevitably falls apart.

Achieving this pinnacle of leadership success begins with a clear and passionate commitment to one's dreams ... visions that are so transparently benevolent and health promoting that most people who hear them cannot help but identify with their importance and lend their full support. However, there is a caveat: Some who ascribe primarily to a self-serving, primitive agenda either cannot or will not fathom such benevolence, and they will predictably resist and undermine its enactment within the practice. The most effective leaders, therefore, recognize this archetypal conflict between *healthy* and *unhealthy power.* They then intervene to protect and preserve the practice through all necessary and appropriate management efforts. This might require taking the most challenging ultimate step of "getting the wrong people off the bus."[3] However, even this extreme measure is carried out with the leadership values of compassion and goodwill melded with skillful execution, thereby demonstrating the previously described ideal features of strength married with benevolence.

Leadership in every aspect of health care, including both administrative and medical/surgical activities, must embody the intangible qualities of "spirit" in order to create an atmosphere of purposeful excellence. As described by Thomas Moore, when this is the case within a practice, "You are not just doing a job, and you're not just a technician. Your whole being is involved in your work. People see it in the air around you."[19]

Perhaps no one has demonstrated more inspiring *healthy power* in leadership during challenging circumstances and then emerged more triumphantly than Viktor Frankl, who, as an Austrian Jew and psychiatrist, spent almost all of World War II in Nazi concentration camps, 3 years of which were at Auschwitz. Through his prolonged and tortuous trials, including the murder of his entire immediate family, he discovered many of the keys to psychological survival. He not only applied such strategies toward his own survival, but also played the roles of physician and spiritual guide to bolster the spirits and very lives of his fellow prisoners wherever he was held in captivity. Reference is made here because the modern day challenges emerging within economic and health care arenas now require the same fundamental, purpose-driven leadership skills that Frankl applied during his captivity[20]:

> As we said before, any attempt to restore a man's inner strength in the camp had first to succeed in showing him some future goal. Nietzsche's words, 'He who has a *why* to live for can bear with almost any *how,*' could be the guiding motto for almost all psychotherapeutic and psychohygienic efforts regarding prisoners. Whenever there was an opportunity for it, one had to give them a why—an aim—for their lives, in order to strengthen them to bear the terrible *how* of their existence. Woe to him who saw no more sense in his life, no aim, no purpose, and therefore no point in carrying on. He was soon lost.

Here are three *healthy power* prescriptions for developing *lifelong purpose* as a leader:

1. Strengthen your commitment to building meaningful interpersonal and professional relationships toward the achievement of worthy goals. Nurturing healthy interdependence between yourself, your coworkers/staff, and your family/friends/community is important for living with a sense of wholeness, safety, and purpose.
2. Develop and consistently demonstrate your *integrity* (ie, the depth and degree that your values align with your observable actions) so that you embody internal harmony and core strength. Accordingly, lead others with transparency, authenticity, and trustworthiness—the keys to empowerment of others and, thus, to gaining their followership in support of your leadership.
3. In parallel fashion, determine to build a culture of integrity within your practice that is forward thinking, results-oriented, and values-driven. Toward those lofty ends, create meaningful vision, mission, and values statements that are aligned with and supportive of both business and cultural development goals, and then make them palpable in everything you do.

Summary

Healthy power in medical leadership is derived from the eight root psychological principles described here working together in harmonious balance, so that the whole they create is greater than the sum of its parts. They then combine and resonate like the finely tuned instruments of an orchestra to produce a powerful yet beautiful symphony. Accordingly, as the "conductor" leading such a practice, you will manifest those root principles most effectively by:

- Taking complete *personal responsibility* for every choice, decision, and action that you undertake, and then fairly holding your staff accountable in like fashion.
- Developing and expressing your *optimistic expectations* with unwavering confidence and faith that you and your team will ultimately prevail.
- Building *win-win relationships* with everyone as much as possible in an atmosphere of abundance and good spirited competition, comparing yourself and the practice primarily against internal benchmarks.
- Creating a culture of *energizing joy* in which you and your staff experience intrinsic motivation, an internal locus of control, and freedom from self-serving distractions with any related overdependency.
- Making only *reality-based choices* with careful and thorough information gathering, fact-based analyses, and team planning so that decisions foster confident action and minimize the need for any rework or damage control later.
- Initiating and mobilizing intensively *focused action* in order to maximize alignment of prioritized effort and to create sufficient impact toward breakthrough successes as a practice.
- Demonstrating *unrelenting courage* by taking decisive, effective action, even amidst fears, doubts, or other discomfort, and then expecting the same of your staff.

- Envisioning a *lifelong purpose* for your practice that involves service to others through your team's passionate, inspired, and altruistic behavior, trusting that both the journey and the outcomes will be tangibly rewarding and emotionally fulfilling for everyone touched by your leadership legacy.

The combined effect of such *healthy power* described here fosters a seemingly effortless ability to create positive, values-driven results through people. Such results flow from loyal, committed, and enthusiastically engaged staff—people providing the *followership* that empowers your *leadership* in a healthy *quid pro quo* paradigm. As a key part of such, the most effective leaders nimbly play alternating roles: at times the teacher, at other times the student; at times the speaker, at other times the listener; at times the service-oriented leader, at other times the appropriately enabling follower.

Lastly, commit yourself to gaining the confident, undying trust of your professional staff and all others with whom you interact by being both professionally competent and of fine character, for both are necessary but insufficient conditions upon which trust is given. And when people trust you unflinchingly as the result of experiencing both your competence and fine character, they will then entrust you with their most precious assets, tangibly and intangibly, thereby empowering you to influence even greater and more positive changes in their lives.

References

1. Pink DH. *Drive, The Surprising Truth About What Motivates Us.* Riverhead Books; 2009.
2. Collins J. *How the Mighty Fall: And Why Some Companies Never Give In.* Author; 2009.
3. Collins J. *Good to Great.* Harper Business; 2001.
4. Peale NV. *The Power of Positive Thinking.* Prentice Hall; 1952.
5. Rosenthal R, Jacobson L. Pygmalion in the classroom. *Urban Review.* 1968;3:16-20. doi:10.1007/BF02322211
6. Darwin C. *On the Origin of Species.* John Murray; 1859.
7. Covey SR. *The 7 Habits of Highly Effective People.* Simon & Schuster; 1989:204.
8. Noble Heart, Pema Chodron, Sounds True audio recording, 1998.
9. Peck MS. *The Road Less Traveled.* Touchstone; 1978.
10. Peck MS. *People of the Lie.* Arrow; 1983.
11. Olendzki A. *Unlimiting Mind.* Wisdom Publications; 2010:6.
12. Pinto JB, Piso CN. The ophthalmic personality: how to more successfully and happily be, or work among, some of the most talented professionals on earth. *Ocular Surgery News.* 2009:Parts I, II, III, March, April, May.
13. Goleman D. *Emotional Intelligence.* Bantam Books, Inc; 1995.
14. Covey SR, Merrill AR, Merrill RR. *First Things First: To Live, to Love, to Learn, to Leave a Legacy.* Simon & Schuster; 1994.
15. Newcott B. Wisdom of the elders. *AARP Magazine;* 2009:52.
16. Stein G. *The Art of Racing in the Rain.* Harper; 2008.
17. Maxwell J. *Failing Forward: Turning Mistakes Into Stepping Stones for Success.* Thomas Nelson Publishers; 2000.
18. Warren R. *The Purpose Driven Life.* Zondervan; 2002:30.
19. Moore T. *Care of the Soul in Medicine.* Hay House; 2010:56.
20. Frankl VE. *Man's Search for Meaning.* Beacon Press; 1959:84-85.

CHAPTER 12

Grooming and Moving Line Staff Up to Middle Management

Corinne Z. Wohl, MHSA, COE

A blue-ribbon leadership culture includes opportunities for growth and promotion within the organization. Opportunities to advance not only allow but also encourage the best employees to stay. The advantages of retaining and promoting well trained, dedicated, experienced-in-your-culture employees are numerous. But beware—not every wonderful employee is manager material, even if they want to be. Let's discuss ways to assess their future ability and to assist a motivated employee to become a terrific manager. This chapter will review the pathways to grooming line staff to become the middle managers you want running your practice.

Pinto JB. *Ophthalmic Leadership: A Practical Guide for Physicians, Administrators, and Teams, Second Edition* (pp 79-84).
© 2022 SLACK Incorporated.

Identification of a Potential Manager

Let's start by identifying the traits that are needed to succeed as a manager. Unfortunately, company longevity, technical expertise, loyalty, and ambition do not equate to leadership skills. This common promotion pitfall has led to disappointments for both employer and employee, and often leads to the loss of a not-so-great manager who was in all other respects a superstar on the clinic floor or in the front office.

So how can you foretell supervisory success? Look for evidence in their current position. Do their peers look to them for guidance and advice? Are they considered an informal leader within the organization? Have they made productivity suggestions? Have they shown by example how to accomplish more with less? Are they comfortable sharing workload balance, indicating they can be a future delegator, or do they behave as if they are the only one that can do it right? Do they act as if they want to make everyone around them happy all the time or have they taken a stand to do the right thing even if a coworker may not have appreciated their action? Have they ever advocated for staff in an appropriate or inappropriate manner?

Asking yourself some of these questions will help you determine whether or not to encourage the time, energy, and risk it will take to groom a line staff employee to become a middle manager.

Test the Water

If you've got a candidate in mind to promote, but you are still not sure if they are manager material, here are six safe assignments you can try:

1. Ask them to help organize an office fundraiser for a community purpose.
2. Have them help to identify the top three issues in their department that could use retooling.
3. Incorporate them into an assignment that crosses department lines to see how they interact with employees not in their department.
4. Assign them the taks of performing patient satisfaction surveys and have them present the results to a committee of managers.
5. Have them lead a multidepartment task force or committee.
6. During a department or full staff meeting, have them present an educational update on one of the assignments they completed.

Once you evaluate the results of their efforts, see the commitment from the potential candidate, and have the confidence in them to move forward, it will be time to prepare the new path you will both follow.

Develop a Plan

Establish a written plan that includes goals for both yourself and the promotable employee. Based on the person you select, each plan will differ from the last. This plan ideally includes basic orientation for new managers and goals that reflect any immediate skill deficits you want to address. Very few managers are strong in all areas of management skills. Expect this and be prepared to nurture, not browbeat, the weak spots.

Be sure to include the anticipated timelines for each action or goal listed. Here are a few sample goals you can use for a newly promoted mid-level manager:

- Demonstrates an ability to effectively influence and direct employees.
- Projects self-confidence, authority, and enthusiasm.
- Develops fresh and resourceful solutions.
- Makes decisions that consider the possible consequences of change, and then communicates these decisions with confidence and clarity.
- Recognizes the importance of working with the team by demonstrating effective delegation skills.
- Identifies staff development needs and encourages employees to strive for improved skills.
- Clearly establishes performance objectives and evaluation criteria for employees.
- Takes prompt measures to identify behavior problems or performance issues from becoming a pattern; supervises fairly and with consistency.
- Shows appreciation for the contributions and achievements of department members.

A long-term plan that evaluates the first 2 years (ideally quarterly) of being a manager is also a good way to stay current on a new manager's progress. This provides the feedback they need to make any mid-course corrections and avoid developing long-term bad habits. The evaluation should be structured in a measurable format with the understanding that expectations will evolve and change over that period of time. This will be a challenging time for both the new manager and the manager leading the way. Highs and lows are to be expected, and continual support of the new manager is critical to their success and ultimately to the whole process. Remember that other line staff are watching and will decide based on how this internal promotion proceeds if they will throw their hat in the ring when a future opportunity arises.

Commitment to Proceed

You have identified your future manager and are ready to start the process. They are up for the challenge and now you need to put your plan into action. A limited orientation training by a senior person and some "on-the-job" training are often inadequate and fail. Your plan should include a mentor (or two) who acts as a coach, a specific list of managerial responsibilities (in addition to a formal job description), and a time commitment to the transfer of new knowledge. Anticipate both the training time for a new manager and for the anticipated mid-course corrections. Be generous with the time allotted.

Selecting the Mentors

Mentors can be from middle and upper management positions. It works best if they are role models: exhibiting good work ethic, patience, intuition, and people skills with a personality that is inspiring and motivating. If these people are difficult to find in your organization, then at a minimum select the person that will teach by example and is well respected within the organization. Make sure the mentors are fully engaged with your corporate philosophy and will be able to pass this along.

Role of the New Manager

Here is a sample list of 13 leadership abilities. Add your own to coincide with your unique practice culture:

1. *Active listening skills.* Management skill depends as much on listening as it does on directing, if not more. Observing and listening to doctors, patients, employees, and other managers is a key to earning respect and making good decisions.
2. *Setting expectations.* Goal setting is a powerful tool that newer managers may not understand. Written goals are key to success. Developing this great habit from the start will be very helpful. It will save a lot of aimless flailing around and frustration if mentored properly.
3. *Giving and receiving feedback.* Effective managers give feedback every day, both positive and pointing out areas for improvement. They need to catch staff doing something right and acknowledge it. When reviewing a situation that could have been handled better, make the constructive feedback a two-way street, so the correction can start at the core. It is best to end the feedback session on an upbeat note and set goals and expectations for future review.
4. *Decision-making acumen.* New managers can agitate forever over decisions. It is best to learn early on that taking a reasonable, well thought out action at a faster pace is better than delaying a decision while waiting for the perfect solution to evolve. Actions can always be revised, and often need to be, once put into motion. Explain to the new manager that even experienced managers make plenty of lousy decisions. Great managers just know how to identify and fix them quickly.
5. *Effective delegation.* A big transition from line staff to manager is learning how to delegate. It includes being able to "let go" and trust that others will do a good job. It also means you have to develop a way to direct and instruct staff to perform functions they may not prefer to do. The best approach for this is directness and emphasizing that the common goal for all employees in the practice is patient satisfaction.
6. *Time management.* This ties into effective delegation. As one develops as a manager, it is important to continually reassess what you are doing on a regular basis, how long it takes, and is there a better way to accomplish the same task or goal? Many roads lead to the same destination in the land of management. Being flexible and open-minded to new pathways enables managers to view issues and opportunities in new and creative ways.

7. *Developing trusting relationships.* Set this as a goal and remind oneself often that integrity and honesty will lead to developing trust. Encourage new managers to expose, not hide their weeknesses or errors in judgment they have made. Now is the most comfortable time for a new manager to admit a lapse in judgment or knowledge. Later on, they may be embarrassed "because they should have known better" or fear not meeting expectations and may be less likely to come forth. If they can trust in the process of admitting they need help, the years ahead will provide more opportunity for future growth as opposed to hidden or embarrassing professional shortfalls.
8. *Credibility keeping confidences.* Being considered a person who keeps confidences is incredibly important as a manager. Second chances are few in this area and newer managers need to understand that although "information can equate to power," it will be a short-lived power. Better to establish oneself as a trusted confidante and earn the respect and knowledge that follow.
9. *Self-confidence.* A new manager must learn steps to overcome stress and develop a confidence in themselves that can be recognized by others. Being a new manager can be overwhelming and frustrating. Use of mentors as a sounding board for questions and guidance can be useful, productive, and calming. Confidence develops in layers and laying a solid foundation is important.
10. *Confronting difficult situations and standing by your decisions.* Concern about being liked by everyone they supervise or the opposite, to forcibly impose boundaries to avoid the appearance of favoritism is a challenge for new managers. They must find middle ground and stand strong. It is certainly acceptable to re-examine decisions, but in this early stage showing spine and not constantly wavering is also important.
11. *Start fresh and avoid the appearance of favoritism by ignoring former coworker influences to maintain fairness and objectivity.* It is challenging for new managers to supervise people who were previously their peers and who may still be their friends. It may be difficult for their former coworkers and even fellow managers to accept their new role. Avoiding the appearance of favoritism from the very start will earn the new manager immediate respect and quicken the transition in the minds of others.
12. *Strategic thinking.* This area can be developed over time. But initially, it is important for a new manager to develop a more strategic overview of the work being done and to have a greater understanding of the impact their department has on the practice as a whole and on the other departments. It is making the shift from "what is best for me as an employee" to "what is best best for the practice and its patients."
   Rotating a new manager through all the departments during the orientation period is a good way to encourage the new manager to have a fresh perspective of the organization and see from a new vantage point how the pieces fit together. If the new manager performs some of the daily functions side-by-side with the employees, it makes an even stronger impression.
13. *Become a change agent.* The goal to have a smooth running department that is respected by doctors, staff, and even patients is admirable and not to be underrated. But the fact is that daily operations running smoothly is just one part of the job.

In the challenging health care environment we face, managers need to be change agents who are able to continually identify opportunities and take the steps that morph their department and the practice toward future goals. Encouraging newer managers, once their feet are planted, to foster new ideas and be flexible helps everyone in the long run.

Supporting the New Manager

The best way to support and strengthen a brand-new supervisor is to set a good example yourself. The boss's behavior affects morale and productivity in every workplace. Make sure you embody what you are teaching or at least admit that you try and do have your own weaknesses you are working on.

What else can you do? Stand behind their decisions, supporting them, especially when they err. This avoids embarrassment and avoids inadvertent undermining. Afterwards, review the problem together, and make sure they understand and agree that they erred. Allow them to resolve the situation themselves. Do not step in and save the day. They need your support to succeed, not undermining. Long term, this approach benefits everyone involved.

Review successes and failures regularly as a part of continued guidance, support, and a feedback process.

The Results—Management and Leadership Skills

The energy it takes to identify and help a future leader evolve within your organization is worth the effort. Having the opportunity to move up within an organization creates a strong bond between the worker and their practice, and develops a sense of purpose that transforms a job into a career.

The best advice you can impart to a new manager is to clearly define the difference between mere management skills and leadership skills. Managers oversee projects and tasks. Leaders influence and inspire people. Leadership is all about the goals. It takes time, effort, self-discipline, and courage to be a leader. It is a goal that all outstanding managers can strive toward and develop over their career.

CHAPTER 13

Best-of-Class Administrators

The Triumph of the Tortoise Over the Hare

John B. Pinto

... the Tortoise plodded on and plodded on, and when the Hare awoke from his nap, he saw the Tortoise just near the winning-post and could not run up in time to save the race.
—Aesop's Fables

Although you work in eye care, and you probably think that what one ***sees*** is pretty important, appearances can be meaningless when gauging the output and efficiency of doctors and staff, alike. For example, the most laconic-appearing practice managers—those who seem to dawdle through their week—may actually be the ones getting the most accomplished for your board, your practice, and for *you* as a provider.

The first time I understood this was not watching an ophthalmic manager, but watching a carpenter who was working on a Texas client's private residence.

Mike was the slowest moving tradesman I had ever seen. And yet, not a single motion was wasted. Nine hours a day, Mike moved deliberately from task to task. The result—working almost entirely by himself to build a 6,000 square foot house

Pinto JB. *Ophthalmic Leadership: A Practical Guide for Physicians, Administrators, and Teams, Second Edition* (pp 85-88).
© 2022 SLACK Incorporated.

in under a year—was a masterpiece created in less time and at less cost than could be accomplished by the typical five-man crew.

Here's what I saw.

> Mike would walk from his truck when he arrived on the job site, past the building materials staged out front. As he walked past a stack of wooden studs, he would grab an armload and move to the closest place they were needed (where he also had a saw plugged in and ready to go). With a fluid series of motions—but by no means quickly—he would measure, cut, and hammer in place one stud after the other. Observed for just a few minutes, Mike looked like a very slow worker, indeed. But Mike's slow pace camouflaged the fact that he never *stopped* working. He was in constant, purposeful action for the entire day.

Seeing Mike in slow-steady action, compared to other carpenters, brought to mind some of the most effective administrators and office managers I've worked with through the years. These executives are not so much the caffeinated "hare-paced" set; but the ambling tortoise, plowing ahead without wasted motion and little drama.

If you're a practice manager, or manage a manager, here are eight things you can do to relax, know that the job is getting done, and bring more efficiency to the process of running your enterprise.

1. *Judge a manager's performance by outcomes, not just time and motion.* Yes, showing up is important. But a punctual administrator rolling out 20% profit margins isn't doing your practice any favors. Quite often, the manager who stays on hours after the practice has closed down, or who has to take home mounds of unfinished work each night, is not so much dedicated as drowning and inefficient.
2. *Make sure major time is spent on major tasks.* To stretch the construction analogy, a building's foundation, walls, and roof should get most of the attention ... arranging the landscaping so it is "just right" is way, way down the list. In your practice, managers should apply most of their time to buttressing the core assets of the organization: the doctors, the staff, the facility, and the sources of new patients.
3. *Foster and praise delegation to help assure a calm environment.* The hare-like administrator, hopping around in anxious circles with their hair on fire, is a sure sign of underdelegation. Imagine how frantic you as a surgeon would be, too, if you had to room every patient, post every charge, and personally handle credentialing. If your administrator underdelegates, it is unlikely they will change much if all you do is admonish or tease them. It *will* help to walk them through the following exercise:
   a. List, in the greatest possible detail, all of your management job functions (this is going to be a long list ... potentially 100 items or more)
   b. Next to each item, write a number between 1 and 10, with "1" being of little importance to the organization, and "10" being of very high importance
   c. Then, go back to each item and score it on the same 1 to 10 scale, but this time with "1" being very easy to delegate to someone else (inside or outside the practice) and "10" being essentially impossible to delegate.
   d. Multiply the two scores and rank in order all of the resulting composite scores
   e. Commit to delegating everything below a selected composite score

Here's an example of four items:

Job Function	Importance to the Practice *1 = Low importance* *10 = High importance*	Ease of Delegation *1 = Easy to delegate* *10 = Impossible to delegate*	Composite Score
Prepare for board meetings	9	9	81
Screening new hires	8	7	56
Biweekly payroll	7	2	14
Stocking exam rooms	5	1	5

4. *In this example, the first two job functions are very important and difficult to delegate, and they have high composite scores.* They should definitely be retained by the administrator. The last two job functions are much less important, easier to delegate, and should probably be passed on to others.
5. *Be clear about communicating deadline expectations.* If you work with a tortoise manager who is eventually going to get things done quite well—but who, along the way, will generate in you a high level of anxiety about, "How are we coming along with Project X?"—then make sure you've worked out a regular time for your manager to report in to you. And by all means, tell your manager, "When I don't hear from you about Project X, I assume it's not getting done, which makes me uncomfortable … so please keep me in the loop."
6. *Make sure your manager is clear about the outcomes you seek.* I've talked to managers who thought the goal was cutting costs at every turn … and then heard their doctors say, "We're not that interested in cost-cutting. We want to grow the practice at the fastest possible pace and understand that this may require extra outlays and some waste." Ideally, you and your administrator have codeveloped a written plan for the next 3 to 5 years (5 to 10 years for larger institutions) with sequential, measurable hallmarks. (It's like Mike the carpenter having written blueprints for the house he was building.)
7. *Do one thing at a time.* OK, maybe two things. Excessive multitasking leaves lots of unfinished balls up in the air to fall on your head. The most effective ophthalmic executives will delve into one or two projects at a time, resolving each issue intelligently, deeply, and finitely, so that it doesn't rise up again. Less effective managers can have dozens of projects in the works (and appear to be highly accomplished) but only have time to apply temporary, incomplete solutions. This results in the same issues arising over and over again, and never really achieving closure.

8. *The basics are essential.* Communication should be clear and, with increasing practice scale, formal and written. Meetings should be effective, with frequency proportional to practice scale (ie, larger practices need FAR more meetings than small practices.) Financial and volumetric benchmarking data have to be timely and equally well understood by both lay managers and physician owners. A means of tracking forward progress with projects is essential. (As a provider you keep dated chart notes on each patient … your manager should have an analogous, transparent system in place so that you know where each project stands.)

Appearances still count. Readers above a certain age may remember Deputy Barney Fife (played on TV by Don Knotts) as the overly excitable sidekick to the town sheriff (played by Andy Griffith). At the first sniff of petty crime, Barney (the hare) would be dashing all over the little town of Mayberry, begging to put his one allotted bullet to work. Andy (the tortoise) always sorted things out calmly by the end of the episode. The collected, effective administrator listens calmly as a provider downloads the "emergency" of the hour, settling an overwrought surgeon's nerves, and assuring with a tone of confidence that all will be well. Less effective managers will send their excitable, thoroughbred doctor into outer orbit, validating the provider's anxiety while dropping everything else to investigate.

• • •

So don't be hustled by an administrator or manager who only appears to be a flutter of activity. Sometimes slow and steady wins the race. Like Mike the carpenter, some of the most productive workers in eye care move slowly but accomplish much.

CHAPTER 14

Feedback

The Fine Art of Boosting Staff Performance

John B. Pinto

Most workers in eye care will report that they love ongoing, honest feedback on the job they're doing. And most surgeons and managers know that giving their workers feedback is one of the most important parts of *their* job as a boss.

But because great performance appraisal and feedback requires great measures of honesty, appropriate confrontation, and tact on one side ... along with openness, a willingness to listen, and nondefensiveness on the other ... neither side, in truth, is very good in this critical area of practice management.

Appraising and communicating staff performance effectively, in a way that results in durable improvement, bumps up into old inhibitions covered elsewhere in this book: the insecurity, resistance to change, and defensiveness that is inherently present in most ophthalmic settings.

Pinto JB. *Ophthalmic Leadership: A Practical Guide for Physicians, Administrators, and Teams, Second Edition* (pp 89-92).
© 2022 SLACK Incorporated.

This is not rocket science. We all know the right things to do in this area. We all know what works. What's simply needed from time to time is a reminder to get back on track. Here it is.

Do Not Give Feedback Unless You Know How to Take It

If you're going to effectively appraise another's performance, you need to be able to take a dose of your own medicine. Think of it this way, if you're a surgeon reading this. How did you feel the last time a patient told you, "Doctor, I'm not sure the surgery you did worked … I'm not seeing any better." Chances are you closed down and ran up a defensive flag in response, saying back something like, "Well, we told you many times there were no guarantees with any surgery." This response, while humanly understandable, is less effective than, "You know, you may be right … let's take a look and see what we can do." Until you can see the difference between these two completely different ways of responding personally to feedback, you won't be very effective when it's time to provide an employee with your opinion on their work.

Observe First Hand

To be highly effective as an advice giver, you have to know the nuances of the job skill you're critiquing. This, as with everything in this chapter, is commonsensical … but commonly overlooked. Here's an example from my field work. A surgeon-client will complain about their technician, saying, "Amy is doing a terrible job working up patients for me." I'll then ask the doctor if she's ever directly observed Amy in action, in the room, during a patient work-up. Invariably, the client's answer is, "No." Whether you're a department head, an administrator, or a practice owner, you can't provide believable feedback on a given task until you've observed it directly.

Be Kind

Remember that being "brutally honest" is more often an excuse for brutality than a profession of truth and transparency. People remember acutely exactly how you make them feel. Do this quick three-step exercise:

1. Pick any random person you supervise (could be your clerk, could be your 15-year-old).
2. Consider how, in all of your past interactions, you have made that person feel. Accomplished? Belittled? Frightened of you? Proud?
3. Ask yourself, "How does the way that person feels when we're together affect my ability to influence their performance?"

Start With the Ending in Mind

The desired ending with any staff member is, of course, *better performance and longer tenure, at lower cost.* So start with that goal in mind. Do not be like the otherwise highly intelligent surgeon who will walk up to a quivering, first-year tech who has just made a benign error and berate them in front of their peers. The outcome of that? The tech will avoid the doctor, decline opportunities to advance or learn new skills (for the doctor to then berate), and if they stay at all will demand a higher salary in exchange for a hostile environment.

Know Your Audience

You can be more forceful and direct in your feedback with some staff. Less so with others. The crusty 70-year-old patient van driver who fought a war, buried three wives, and swears like a sailor can be told abruptly that one more speeding ticket means the end of his career. The 20-something receptionist who was daddy's princess at home, praised-on-high for a C+ average, needs gentler treatment.

Emphasize the Positive

Ken Blanchard, famous for his classic book *The One-Minute Manager,* wrote that managers should first give a one-minute praise before commencing with any reprimand or negative feedback. In a later book, *Whale Done,* named after his observation of killer whale training at Sea World, Blanchard recanted this praise-plus-reprimand advice. His updated urging is that all performance feedback should be overwhelmingly affirming: positive reinforcement and relatively mild redirection. An example of the latter would be this. Instead of saying, "Jill, you did a terrible job with those last two refractions," you would frame the feedback (the "redirection" in Blanchard's terms) in the context of past, excellent performance and say, "Jill, those last couple of refractions didn't measure up to the near-perfection I've seen from you for the past few months. Thanks for anything you can do to spring back to the great ability I know you have."

Widen the Reviewer Base

Even if you're a worker's direct supervisor, you should encourage your employee to develop an "accountability" group at work—people they can turn to for feedback on job performance and interpersonal skills. This works whether the employee in question is a lay staffer or a senior provider. Think of this in your own context. If you're an administrator, you might select a handful of trusted colleagues and invite them to give you feedback on your performance. This might be your practice's MP, a veteran billing supervisor you are especially close to, and the practice accountant. And don't just fish for compliments or a soft critique. Invite honesty from the start and foster this with a consistently nondefensive response. (Again, the phrase, "You know, you may be right," is an effective way to let the advice-giver know that you're ready to hear more.)

Err on the Side of Overly Frequent Feedback

Giving and getting negative feedback—even positive feedback—can be anxiety provoking for most people. So treat it as you would any other phobia (like flying). Desensitize yourself by giving, seeking, and receiving feedback more often. Instead of the high drama of the dreaded annual review, provide feedback throughout the year in shorter, less formal settings and augment this with frequent, sincere expressions of appreciation.

CHAPTER 15

Getting Things Done

Keys to Prioritization and Implementation

John B. Pinto

As an ophthalmologist, by the time your formal training is completed, and after accounting for vacation time, you only have about 8000 work days left to accomplish your professional mission. In these 8000 days you have to build a staff team, construct a business enterprise, refine your mastery over a complex body of clinical knowledge, and use this mastery to serve perhaps 30,000 different patients—all to improve the functional vision of about 60,000 eyes. That's it ... just 8000 days. This works out to about one hour per eye over the panoramic span of your career, which is rather a nice way to think of things.

This time passes swiftly. If you're the average doctor in their mid-40s, you only have about 4500 workdays left. In another decade, you'll only have perhaps

Pinto JB. *Ophthalmic Leadership: A Practical Guide for Physicians, Administrators, and Teams, Second Edition* (pp 93-97).
© 2022 SLACK Incorporated.

3000 workdays remaining. And by the time you finish this chapter, you'll have used up another 4% or so of *one* of those precious days.

So ... what can you do to extract the most value from each of these fleeting days? The first answer is to prioritize. And this prioritization flows downhill, from profound life goals to unremarkable practice minutia:

Life goals (eg, buy a mountain vacation home to retire in one day)

↘ **Practice goals** (eg, increase income by $35,000 per year)

↘ **Practice projects** (eg, get more optometrist referrals)

↘ **Practice tasks** (eg, call Dr. Edwards for lunch)

If you keep your eyes open to opportunity, hundreds of alluring new ideas arise every year—you only have time in your life to seriously pursue a fraction of these ideas. How do you know which opportunities are important? You have to know your long-term goals, which provide a critical context for focusing the limited hours of your day, and the limited days of your working life.

Consider the following scenario. Imagine you're a 48-year-old general ophthalmologist who dreams of owning a five-partner subspecialty practice. You want to be the MP of this group and work hard in this role for 20 years if your health can hold out. You want to continue performing cataract surgery, and pass along to your colleagues just about everything else. These goals are consistent with the following actions:

- Going to the Academy meeting and sitting in on courses related to being the MP of a group practice.
- Directing your administrator to strengthen their financial training to be ready for managing a larger organization.
- Getting good at delegating to middle management staff in the practice.
- Calling a recruiting firm to cast a net for your first partner-track associate.
- Hiring a personal trainer to increase your energy levels.

These goals, to own a larger group practice, would *not* be consistent with the following actions:

- Going to the Academy meeting and taking courses related to medical retinal care. (You'll be delegating such cases in the future, remember?)

- Directing your administrator to learn now to scrub into surgery as a backup for your lead scrub tech. (Such work would be a distraction if they're going to be running a business for you.)
- Holding on to lots of detailed projects instead of delegating. (You're going to be too time-poor to do everything well by yourself.)
- Failing to follow a diet and exercise regimen that will keep you vigorous well into your 70s.

Here's a practical pop test: Ask if your actions in this past week, day-by-day, have been consistent with the outcomes you desire. If not, you'll want to align these to the greatest possible extent. Before reading further, fill out this simple grid:

Actions I Have Taken in the Past Week	The Larger Goal I Hope to Accomplish Through This Action …
I visited an old friend from my residency (who performs cataract surgery faster than I do) to learn how I can shift from two cases per hour to three or four cases, to make it financially viable to develop a modest ASC.	I would like to have my own surgery center one day and can't afford this unless I'm a more efficient surgeon.

Were the activities you wrote down in the left column in accord with the goals you wrote down in the right column? If not, what does this tell you about the way you're prioritizing your time? Do you need to adjust your goals (perhaps defining them formally for the first time in years), or better direct your actions to match your goals?

Sometimes the focus of your time and attention is not driven by your desires alone, but is bounded by practical realities. Let's say you would indeed love to develop an ambulatory surgery center (ASC). You've bought every book on the subject and go to every possible ASC course. You have hired a few consultants to review the prospects and get the same answer back each time: "You can't develop an ASC because (1) your case volumes are too low to support such a center, (2) your market is so small that you'll never build to sufficient case volumes, and (3) the regulations in this state prohibit the development of private ASCs." In light of these facts, it would be foolish for you to keep attending ASC courses, reading ASC how-to guides, and hiring advisors. Adjust your dreams; find another kind of practical ancillary service (an optical perhaps, or an augmented diagnostic testing pod) and put your energies into these more achievable goals.

Managing Your To-Do List

You don't gulp down an entire steak dinner in one bite; instead, the meal is divided into discrete courses, and each mouthful is cut one at a time. Practice projects should be carved up the same way. Once you have prioritized the outcomes you desire, and have developed a list of projects, it helps to break each project down into its component parts.

A number of computer programs have emerged to automate your to-do list. Microsoft Project is a robust program designed for projects with hundreds of subroutines ... as would be the case if you're a general contractor building a new office tower. Microsoft Outlook is a much simpler program, packaged with Microsoft Office, that allows you to arrange projects by initiation date, departmental area, or responsible party. Perhaps the simplest and most familiar approach is to use Word for Windows to create the grid shown here.

Sample Action Grid

Action (Dated)	Who (One Person)	Deadline	Progress Notes (Dated)
October 2—Replace the worn carpet in the Akron main office	Susan	November 20	October 15—Carpet samples reviewed and order placed October 30—Installation scheduled for November 13 November 10—Date pushed back due to flood damage repair work

Here are a few simple rules to accompany the use of such a grid:

- Date all action items, which should be a complete thought, even someone from outside of the practice should understand what you have written down in simple, subject-predicate format.
- Each item should have a single owner, not a committee.
- The deadline should be a specific date in the calendar, not "spring."
- If an item is approved but tabled until later, enter the "tabled to ____" date in the deadline column.
- Make sure that all progress notes are entered and dated *by each responsible party* on a networked or central/open-access PC at least 48 hours in advance of regular management meetings … then you can use the grid as both the agenda and minutes for such meetings.
- Highly confidential items should be moved to a separate grid.
- Completed items should be removed to a separate archive file and reviewed periodically by the practice's managers to assure that completed projects continue to be closed.

Whatever system you use—from a worn out legal pad to a dedicated computer program—it's critical to foster an *accountable* environment, where each action item's "owner" feels truly responsible for their line items, and where there is a formal consequence for not carrying out an agreed task. By starting with a clear understanding of the desired long-term outcomes for your life and practice, you'll find yourself and your staff spending more time on purposeful activity, and less time on busy-work that robs each day of the precious hours you need to accomplish your dreams.

Practice the traits and conduct you want to become habits. On more than one occasion I've had coworkers ask how I consistently sound welcoming when answering the telephone. The simple answer is—it's habit. You don't think about applying the brake when you put your car in gear in a parking lot because it's habit. Likewise, don't think about applying the charm when you put your mouth in gear. If the person on the other end of the telephone line is spoiling for a fight and you answer with a pleasant tone, you've just taken a step in disarming them. It may not be enough, but you can be confident knowing you've started the process to do all you reasonably can to resolve any issues. No one wants to talk to a sourpuss, and unfortunately most people don't have good experiences with "customer service." Put yourself in their shoes. Chances are you've made a phone call when you were mad as a hornet. Talking to someone whose tone was pleasant and who attempted to work with you brought the ire down at least a notch or two. There have been a number of times that the tone and words of my habitual greeting have taken the patient somewhat by surprise. It's rare for one of those conversations to end without an improvement in the patient's deportment. And if *you're* the one spoiling for a fight, maintain a positive demeanor and make sure you have facts. Discuss whatever it is with the individual(s) with discretion and an open mind. I personally would prefer to give someone the benefit of the doubt and be wrong than fly off the handle and be right. A discussion that explains, educates, and informs accomplishes more than a browbeating. Usually.

Manners should be thought of in the same phrasing as the American Express card advertisement—"don't leave home without it." There's no place good manners *don't* belong. *Please* and *thank you* deserve lots of use. I still remember an occasion when an employee thanked me for their paycheck, then said "I don't know why I'm thanking you, I worked for this." The statement was correct, but the thanks were also. Just because someone is performing the job duties for which they receive a paycheck doesn't mean "thank you" shouldn't be voiced. If you appreciate the attention to detail that went into a project or the tact that a difficult patient was addressed, say so. Make an effort to say hello or ***at*** least smile and nod a greeting. Make it a habit and it will become second nature. It might even catch on! Don't be so focused that the people around you feel ignored or invisible. The same goes for the doctors in your practice. Being at the top of the food chain doesn't make them immune to the desire to be noticed and appreciated. A sincere "thank you" is good for the soul. And if it's not accepted in the same nature that it was extended, well that's not something you can control. You can't "control" people or their actions—you control your actions/reactions, but you set a standard for others to follow.

I've had my share of conversations I've come to classify as inertial conversations—the irresistible force meets the immovable object. The patient/employee/doctor/spouse/parent/child is determined to be right and nothing you can say or do will change it. At some point in the conversation you will realize you might as well play a solo game of table tennis. That's when you wrap it up, agree you're not going to agree, and move on. Moving on isn't always easy, but don't think of it as quitting. Think of it as regrouping while waiting for a better opportunity. If the merit of the topic remains, opportunities to reintroduce it will present themselves. Do not waste your energy on a battle to prove "right-ness." A victory is doubtful, and if there is a victory it will be very hollow and more lost than gained. Whether it's a compliance issue with a ranking member of the staff or a policy matter with a subordinate, when your information has been provided and the requirements have been explained and you realize it's an unending discussion that's going steadily downhill, let it go.

Being right and being a good leader are not always mutually inclusive. If you make a mistake, acknowledge it, take steps to correct it, and take steps to prevent it from happening again. That's what you expect from your subordinates, and that's what they should see from you. They know you're not perfect and they know they're not perfect. No one is, but let's all give it our best effort. This is all part of leading by example. If you "don't make mistakes" (HAHA) or if you humiliate staff members when they do, then don't be surprised if what started out as a minor error ends up on your desk as a giant, ugly fiasco because someone was afraid to inform you or tried to cover it up.

Leading by example is not walking unprotected into battle and expecting subordinates to blindly follow. Your example should mean something. Don't ask someone to do something you wouldn't do. And you should have at least a basic understanding of ***how*** they're going to do what you're asking them to do. One of the benefits of starting out as the "manager of me" when the young doctor and younger office manager started out years ago, was that I did just about everything. I checked patients in, while answering the phone, while checking eyewear prescriptions, while taking histories, while checking patients out, etc. Oh, and don't forget posting charges, payments, and adjustments to a paper ledger and balancing at the end of the day. So even if I don't do all those things today, I have an understanding of what it takes to fulfill those duties. Do not do things you wouldn't accept from your staff—another part of leading by example. It also fits in with manners and developing habits of positive traits. Be cordial, speak kindly, work together. Being friendly does not mean you *are* friends, but it does give you a better vantage point. Good leaders can be relied upon by those who are following. Life happens, and your people need to know they can come to you when issues arise without fearing your response. Good employees will appreciate your flexibility when you can accommodate their requests ***and*** when you can't. If you aren't willing to offer flexibility there may not be much offered in return.

You don't always get what you give in a positive fashion, but it certainly tips the scale in your favor. You can save yourself, the practice, and the staff stress by being aware of the pulse of the staff instead of only finding out when there's a need for admin 911. This keeps you in the loop, making you less vulnerable and better prepared. Keeping up with the highs and lows of your staff reminds them of their importance to you on both a personal and personnel basis. The balancing act is knowing enough of what's happening to be in touch, without being overwhelmed. The lines of communication need to remain open and flow in both directions, maintaining an atmosphere of compassion that will inevitably be shared with the patients in your practice. "It's a small world" is not just a song for theme parks, and you want it to work to your advantage. Sharing what's happening with the staff with those higher on the food chain, on an edited scale, reminds them of the humanity of employees and might avoid discomfort at times. Not long ago I had an opportunity to view grandbaby pictures brought in by a long-time employee. I had a vague recollection of a tragedy with a previous grandchild and didn't recall any details regarding a pregnancy. Fortunately they provided all details regarding an adoption opportunity with notice of just a day or two as we admired the new blessing. It was obviously a very important and emotional occasion for them, and something they looked forward to sharing with their coworkers. I would have been mortified if someone in the community asked about the baby and all I had for a response was a dumb look. Love covers a multitude of sins and a sense of humor covers a multitude of flaws. If they hadn't shared the unexpected nature of the new grandchild or if I had been otherwise caught off guard I probably would have employed self-deprecating humor. Life throws punches at all of us every day and we need to be able to "roll with the punches." Not taking ourselves too seriously is a good way to roll, because most situations don't land in the "life or death" segment on the scale of importance. Showing your humanity and fallibility *and* your ability to continue functioning when fully exposed is the embodiment of leading by example.

Starting at the beginning of a fledgling practice afforded me many opportunities and challenges. About 5 years into this adventure, a change took place that had significant impact on my career. The doctor informed me one day that they had hired an administrator. They provided a basic description of the background and credentials of the individual they had hired, and told me the individual had requested the two of us meet before they came on board. A thousand different thoughts were flying through my head as this was happening and the voice of pride just kept repeating "NO!" I think I maintained my composure and decided I would meet the inevitable head-on and hopefully with some grace. I learned several things from my administrator at that first meeting and I'm still learning from him today. Jim introduced himself, gave me some professional and personal background on himself, and paved the way for a team approach. He told me our combined skills would be very beneficial to the practice and each other. He wanted my input on the strengths and weaknesses of the practice, and changes I would like to see made. I was a little surprised but cautiously optimistic. My pride was still stinging, but time has a way of healing. In his first week on the job Jim was able to get the doctor's approval for at least a dozen items I had been presenting for years. I knew I could either feel miffed that he accomplished things so quickly or I could be thrilled that progress was being made. I chose to be thrilled … and that was the start of a long, successful collaboration. It's another version of "make the best of a bad situation," but it was never really a bad situation. It could have been if I had chosen to resist, but the addition of Jim as our administrator is one of the high points of my career. It has enhanced my opportunities and challenges, provided even more instruction and education, and made the structure of the practice even stronger. One of his well-worn phrases is: "Perception is reality." Look at things from all angles and you might be surprised at all the positives you can glean from what initially appears to be a big mess.

Be prepared for times when the following quote seems to apply to your practice: "We, the unwilling, led by the unknowing, are doing the impossible for the ungrateful. We have done so much, for so long, with so little, that we are now qualified to do anything with nothing." It might not all happen at once, but it will happen. Investigate the "why" of the unwilling and address it. Is it lack of information or training, fear of failure or reprimand, mentally/physically/emotionally unprepared for the task or is it "I don't wanna?" Each of those reasons can be addressed to the benefit of the employee and the practice. Does the unknowing know they are unknowing? Again, address the reasons.

Maybe it's a forest-for-the-trees situation and a renewed perspective is needed. Why is it impossible? If it's accomplished it wasn't impossible after all, and everyone involved in the accomplishment should receive credit. Ungrateful?? Yikes, that is ***not*** good. Do your best to avoid the perception of "ungrateful." Again, a job done well should be appreciated *and* compensated. And if the perception is incorrect, find out what's behind it and address it. It's much easier to get rid of a thistle in your practice when it's little than when it's a great big thorny clump of prickliness. So much for so long with so little—appreciate your talented, dedicated, hard-working staff. If they're truly doing this, grease the wheel before it starts squeaking. Evaluate their needs. Are they being stretched too far or does the variety of tasks keep things interesting? It would be unfortunate if one of your dependable, valuable wheels fell off before you noticed it needed greased. Doing anything with nothing is another sign of skillful and effective employees. Give them reasons to stick it out with you beyond the paycheck. Everyone will benefit.

Attitudes can be contagious, have one worth catching. We're all human. Our feelings get hurt, and we feel overworked, underappreciated, and sometimes downright ignored. Yep, and life goes on. It's all about how you handle it. Grumbling staff is a downer for everyone, so don't be one of them! A negative attitude will create a feeding frenzy and take precious time to turn it back around. In fact, the time invested to return back to neutral will be exponentially more than the time it took to get to negative. And even then you'll have flare-ups for some time to come. Take the issue in stride, move on, and continue leading by example. It's much easier to expect someone to follow your example and instructions willingly if you're already demonstrating the desired behavior. And it will be much easier to spot and weed out the negative attitudes when you aren't dealing with your own. You know your "buttons," and you know who has the propensity to push them, knowingly or otherwise. Before you start to go into launch sequence, take a (mental) step back and breathe. Put things in perspective and move forward—positively!

CHAPTER 17

Coaching and Motivating Office Staff

John B. Pinto

Pity the average ophthalmic practice administrator. Running an efficient and profitable practice is like cooking an elaborate 12-course dinner for the most discriminating patron imaginable. And then doing it all over again, only better, the next day. And the next, and the next, year after year, for the rest of your career.

Perfection, while expected, is impossible, of course. Disaster is always imminent. And the most frustrating part of your job as a leader is that you have to cook up this perfect practice using decidedly *imperfect* people—techs and receptionists and opticians and doctors and billers—whose ingredients never include a consistent or sufficient measure of:

- Ethics and honesty
- Intelligence

Pinto JB. *Ophthalmic Leadership: A Practical Guide for Physicians, Administrators, and Teams, Second Edition* (pp 105-108).
© 2022 SLACK Incorporated.

- Loyalty and trust
- Spirit and exuberance
- Teamwork
- Adaptability to change
- Productivity
- Grace under pressure
- Punctuality and timeliness
- Accuracy
- Attention to detail
- Ability to learn
- Stamina and endurance
- Professional appearance
- Intuition
- Involvement
- Follow through
- Volunteerism
- Sensitivity to others
- Ambition to improve

In truth, just how your practice turns out each day depends largely on how many of these desirable traits you can hire and retain. It's easy to coach a tech to take a more accurate intraocular pressure. But can you as readily coach them to be more interested in their career, to be more thoughtful in handling expensive instruments, or to be more ethical?

While a few of these worker attributes can be taught, most are either innate in an employee or have been embedded long before you showed up to be their new boss. And most of these traits are difficult to judge during the typical employment interview. But let's assume you've already picked a pretty great team. What can you do to get the most from them?

While your original training may be in accounting or marketing or medicine, the most important daily skills you must bring to the job must be much broader, and often very intuitive. You have to be able to motivate talent, improving the weakest half of your organization, while vigorously rewarding the strongest half. Building on the previous cooking analogy, you have to be much more than a chef, who after all is working with static ingredients. You have to be a coach—molding the ever-shifting, fragile human ingredients to better serve your patients.

After more than 40 years of watching some of the most talented managers and practice owners at work, here are some of the top skills they apply.

First and foremost, great practice managers are constantly improving themselves. To do this, you have to do more than simply reading the business literature or attending national meetings. You have to start by being nondefensive. Sharp managers readily accept constructive, even negative, feedback from team members. Doing so is self-reinforcing … when you say, "You know, you may be right!" to a critic, you'll start getting feedback that's faster, more useful, and more honest.

In order to get this feedback, you can't be talking all the time. You have to listen. This is sometimes easier to do one-on-one than during group sessions, such as department meetings, where your staff are looking to you for all of the answers. Be sure to build into every group meeting a formal time for brainstorming or going around the table for input.

Most workers are pretty good about picking up on your opinion of their talents and will perform accordingly. If you're sending signals that say, "I think you're going to blow this assignment," chances are a worker will live down to your expectations. So, no matter how many times a staff member has disappointed you, assume that they have hidden talents that you have just not been able to bring out yet.

This can yield surprising results. The next time you hand out an assignment to someone you're on the fence about, try this. Accompany your request with the statement, "Mary, in the past I think I've unfairly misjudged your abilities. I know you can do this project. In fact, I'm sure of it. Let's start with a clean slate for you here at Smith Eye Center."

Try to not be the kind of boss who supplies all of the answers. Yeah, you're probably the smartest and hardest working member of your team—that's why you're a leader. But your practice will go farther, and you'll have more time for major issues, if you teach people to solve most of their own problems.

Always emphasize the positive. Catch your staff doing things right and encourage more of this, rather than dwelling on what's been done wrong. This is often difficult for managers and doctors who hold themselves to high expectations—and give themselves a healthy daily dose of negative criticism. The same negativity you apply to yourself just naturally spills out with others. While you may think that this will evoke the desired improvement in performance, the opposite is actually the case. Most employees will simply shut down under negative reinforcement, shrinking from trying to learn new skills, and missing opportunities to improve by taking on duties that are at the edge of their competency.

Fearless, fair, and well-timed confrontation is a critical administrative coaching skill. Even while remaining positive, it is important to call attention to performance gaps and not sweep important behavioral gaffs or technical errors under the carpet. Every great manager must find their own balance in this area.

The tipping point between tough and fair is decidedly *not* static. Every worker changes over the course of their career, and your threshold and timing for bringing things up has to be flexible. On top of this, your own skills and perceptions change over time. Knowing when to apply the correct, nuanced pressure in the right areas separates exceptional managers from those who lose nearly as many points as they gain with their staff and boards over time.

One key to finding this balance is to make sure that you first understand a staff member's or doctor's motivations and goals before you come down hard on their behaviors. When you listen to a staff member, also watch for nonverbal clues. Try to pick up on how they're responding to you.

When giving feedback and handing out assignments, especially to a newer member of your staff, try being a little more "suggestive" and a little less "directive." By being just a little too directive, especially with people you have not yet learned to read, you can bring out a defensive response that will take weeks or even years to overcome.

In most practices, managers spend nearly as much administrative time directing doctors as they do leading lay staff. Although it can be difficult, especially as a younger manager, work on being as comfortable confronting these superiors as you are in confronting subordinate staff. Most doctors, especially those who are insecure and bullying, have far more respect for their managers who are fearless and stand their ground on difficult issues.

Context is critical whether you are addressing problems or opportunities. Before describing a performance deficit or a desired new goal with a member of your staff, make sure that you both agree on the strengths and weaknesses of their past performance. Then, make sure they understand what's in it for them if they are able to reach a new standard or goal. At the end of a "coaching moment," make sure you have your colleague's commitment. When appropriate, put things in writing and even have staff sign off their commitment formally on major initiatives.

Keeping all of this in mind, your side of a conversation with a senior technician might include:

- "Great! I think we're both on the same page with this. Just a little more attention to the detailed steps of each technician skill and you should be able to wrap up the final draft of the protocol manual."
- "Think a little more about the timeline for getting this done, and by the end of the week please drop me an email with a sample of some of the edits we've discussed and your best guess for a final deadline."
- "Once you're done, this is going to make training new staff so much easier and faster."
- "You've really turned a corner in your career here at Smith Eye Center ... based on your progress, I think you could be ready to manage one of our satellite offices within the next 2 years."

Finally, realize that your coaching style may not fit the needs of every worker. With experience, you'll pick workers who can not only perform their core job functions well, but who will be responsive to your particular approach to supervision.

CHAPTER 18

Assembling a Practice and Personal Advisory Team

John B. Pinto

Ad • vice: Noun ... recommendation regarding a decision or course of conduct ... from Middle French avis "opinion," probably from the phrase ce m'est a vis "that appears to me."
—Merriam-Webster Dictionary

As a surgeon, you render advice hundreds of times a week. Hundreds of thousands of times in a career span. You advise patients in your exam room, staff in the lounge, fellow doctors at medical conferences, and your golf buddy Bob on the 15th hole.

Of course, it's a two-way street. You're also on the receiving end of advice, or should be. As a physician you have many more advisors than the typical person ... colleagues down the hall, your administrator, scores of vendors who teach you how to use their products, the mechanics and technicians who keep all the fiddly bits working. Plus, various professionals who help you make more money; save it; count it; and keep as much of it as legally possible from the IRS, unworthy heirs, and plaintiffs' attorneys.

Pinto JB. *Ophthalmic Leadership: A Practical Guide for Physicians, Administrators, and Teams, Second Edition* (pp 109-112).
© 2022 SLACK Incorporated.

The anthropologists got it wrong. Man is not a maker of tools, but a maker of opinions, traded widely in this modern world.

That's the set-up for a brief discussion, courtesy of my retired pal Dr. Herve Byron, who suggested the topic and urges you to ask: "Do you have enough of the right advisors, are they integrated as a team supporting you, and do you use them the right way?"

• • •

Here is a look into many of the advisors you may have.

- *General business attorneys.* This person (and you should have one, lead, go-to person … even if you employ a firm) should have grey hair, a super-organized assistant, be slow to anger, and skilled in their ability to extract justice from those in your world who will from time to time prey upon you, your business, and your family. Like your GP, they will know when to handle your matter personally, and when to call in the…
- *Specialist attorneys.* The most fortunate doctors have few of these on retainer. They come in every variety to unravel all the modern tangles we manage to get into: tax issues, bankruptcy, divorce, partnerships, contracts, regulatory compliance, employment law, and so on.
- *Accountants.* If your financial matters are blessedly simple, you are joined at the hip with one, widely skilled, affable-if-a-bit-dull, numbers professional who can handle everything. But in today's increasingly complex world, accountants are specializing to a similar degree as attorneys and doctors. There are forensic accountants to testify before a court, analysts to drill down into arcane business math problems, as well as the familiar kinds who help you close your books at the end of year. Career-long relationships are not unusual. If you are a young doctor, pick a young accountant (who is backed up by a senior partner for the tough stuff.)
- *Personal financial planners.* These come in lots of flavors and skill levels, from the highly trained and skilled professionals who will provide unbiased counsel and help you stay on a conservative retirement track, to wannabe's with a $25 certificate, a nice suit, and marching orders to churn your account. Use recommendations from your most financially successful friends to find a fee-only planner who feels "just right" from the first meeting onward. If the stakes are high (or you're nearing retirement) don't be shy about getting a second or third opinion on the strategy you're taking.
- *Practice management consultants.* I have an inherent conflict to say much about this, since I am one, but here goes. I admire most of my colleagues. Just like the surgeons we work for, we learn something new from every assignment, we learn from each other in this "microguild," and we get better at our jobs over time. I wince reading reports I wrote 25 years ago for clients, probably the way you wince at old postoperative patients dating to the 2nd week you were learning phaco. Practice management consultants are typically generalists. We've seen lots of case histories go by, and get good at recognizing patterns. Just like you, we do our best work for doctors with real problems (or opportunities), doctors who are either nice people (or at least only temporary pains-in-the-rear because of a tough patch they've hit), and doctors who remember to say "thanks" when the treatments we apply work especially well. Every practice should have one of these, but that's just my advice.

- *Billing, coding, and compliance advisors.* Every surgeon should also have one of these vitally important experts in orbit around their practice. For the typical, well-run, Medicare-biased practice, a peek in the charts every two to four years is simply good hygiene and housekeeping. For practices with chronic difficulty in this area, more frequent review is indicated.
- *Personal physicians.* Most ophthalmologists I know haven't had an eye exam in years. And unless they're in the midst of a health crisis or being treated for a chronic condition, they similarly skip the traditional annual exam. Self-treatment has its limits. Even if you're in the pink, your "personal board of directors" should include an internist or GP who you think is even smarter than you. Keep searching till you find one.
- *Mental health professionals.* I live in California, where they've just passed a new law that says everyone has to have a personal shrink. Or so it seems. Seriously, ophthalmology is a very emotionally challenging business conducted by generally very high-strung people. Most benefit from counseling of one kind or another (as we all do, probably.) Rather than an infrequent touch-and-go landing in a crisis, which is all the average person can afford, consider using your psychologist, psychiatrist, pastor, or counselor as someone you see every few months, even when life is completely wonderful. Think of it as flossing for your brain. And when the next personal crisis arises, you'll already have a strong, trusting relationship with someone who can immediately grasp your new issues rather than take a few warm-up sessions to develop rapport.
- *Personal trainers and coaches.* I think this is another California invention. In Vermont, your average guy goes out, chops some wood, shovels some snow, and the daily workout is done. In California, "cords" of wood are really little and made of fiberglass for our artificial fireplaces, and snow is something we import from Canada to SeaWorld around Christmastime so the kids can fall down and make angels for a day. Out here we need someone to tell us how to work up a sweat, and maybe you do, too. Like most professionals, half the value of an athletic trainer is to provide a source of external discipline. At 5:00 AM in the morning. Ugh!
- *Nutritionists.* If you have a weight control problem that hasn't succumbed to exercise and self-care alone, or even your new personal trainer, consider a nutritionist. Although you're a physician with lots of education and common sense, you'll be introduced to new topics and tactics, one of which may just be the silver bullet you've been needing to add weight, lose weight, or just be more energetic.
- *Massage therapists.* The practice of ophthalmology—and particularly ophthalmic surgery—is fraught with opportunities for repetitive motion injury, back and neck strain, and a host of musculoskeletal aches. In addition, being economically productive in modern practice obliges a far more hectic and stressful workday than a generation ago. A wonderful prescription for these low-grade, chronic assaults on your physique and your psyche is regular massage. Some surgeons I know reward themselves with this immediately after every surgical session to work out the kinks and decompress.
- *Occupational/physical therapists.* Sometimes massage alone is not enough, or is not addressing the underlying cause of your physical strain at work. If you are

developing neck or back pain (and especially if you have progressed to the too-common stage of tingling fingers and other signs of the frank harm your posture is doing to your career longevity), consider a consultation with an occupational or physical therapist. Have one or the other come to your office and surgical facility to observe. Together you will be able to collaborate on creative solutions, such as ocular extension tubes on your operating microscope, or sandbags to prop your wrists on at the slitlamp, taking the pressure off your lower back and neck. If you're a woman, they'll tell you to stop seeing patients while sitting "side-saddle" out of modesty ... and to simply get in there and straddle the patients like the guys do.

- *Instructors in general.* As a busy professional, you don't have the time to learn the guitar on your own, dabble awkwardly with oil painting, grind through a $299 language learning website, or figure out how to drive your new sports car with vigor. Being self-taught is a virtue for those who are time-rich and dollars-poor. If you are reading this, chances are high you are neither of these. A professional teacher of any kind who can come to your home or office, assess your skills, and efficiently push you to the next level will save you precious time and frustration. If it's important enough to you to want to learn, do it right, do it fast ... do it with a professional.
- *Architects.* The most talented architects I've met are among the most interesting and intellectually balanced people I know. Consider the skill set: math, engineering, complex building codes, changing materials science, aesthetics, economics ... along with a rather large dose of psychology to deal with clients. It's too bad you only need them a few times in your life.
- *Handymen (and women).* As I write this, Bruce is downstairs hammering away at the pipes. Bruce is pretty much a regular around our house, which after 80 years of hot summers, salt air, and earthquakes needs Bruce even more than Bruce needs the job. Even if you live in a new house and work in a new office building, you still need a guy like Bruce to keep up appearances, get after the stray stucco cracks, or at least pound on the pipes, smile a lot, and look busy when you walk past him.

• • •

The list is much longer still, of course ... recruiting firms and insurance brokers ... the 12-year-old who launched your website ... and the 73-year-old perfectionist who can get your surround-sound system finally set up just right. But you get the point. The quality of your life and the success of your business can be measurably improved with the right professional team, and ruined with just one wrong choice.

Most of these experts should not operate independently, but rather, be arrayed by you into teams for best effect. For example, you and your accountant, attorney, and practice management advisor should confer jointly on big issues. It's vital that your accountant, administrator, and personal financial planner be in the same room with you at least once a year to orchestrate a plan on your behalf. Depending on your health status, your various fitness and health advisors should each know what the other is recommending.

Advisers. You gotta have 'em in today's complex world. Pick the smartest and most attentive ones you can find. Fire the dullards and those who seem ungrateful for your patronage. Give the best ones your loyalty and regular rewards ... the best of which is to take their advice as seriously as you'd like your patients to take *your* recommendations.

CHAPTER 19

Keeping Yourself in 24/7 Turnaround Mode

John B. Pinto

I once talked to a doctor who had *doubled* his clinical and surgical output in the space of just a few months. Why? Because he was told in clear terms by his colleagues that he wasn't pulling his weight and was at risk of losing his partnership status. *Fear makes things happen.*

I once visited with an administrator who, because they were on the verge of losing their job, doubled down on their career commitment and singlehandedly found missing profits for their board (after several years of inattentive dabbling). They've trimmed staff hours, closed down a satellite, and worked with each surgeon in their group to boost marginal revenue. *Fear makes things happen.*

After seeing scores of examples like this go by, I made up the acronym "FMTH." many years ago. *Fear makes things happen.*

Pinto JB. *Ophthalmic Leadership: A Practical Guide for Physicians, Administrators, and Teams, Second Edition* (pp 113-115).
© 2022 SLACK Incorporated.

With the proper motivation, we're all capable of digging deeper. I'm seeing more FMTH at work today than ever before, as managers and doctors alike are peddling faster in the midst of the great recession and looming health care payment reform.

It's only human nature that we wait for the last possible minute before getting our game on. But why wait for a frightful environment to become more assertive in your attentiveness, your energy, and in your raw output?

Many years ago, in response to a prior economic downturn, I wrote a book, *Turnaround.* As the title suggested, it's a book about turning around faltering eye practices. One of the core tenants of the text is to *not wait* for economic difficulty before getting serious about your career and business. By adopting a permanent "turnaround mindset," you are actually likely to snuff out business disasters before they even arrive.

Here are five practical examples of how to do this in your own practice setting:

1. Get out a sheet of paper (or a blank computer screen). Imagine you were going to lose your highest producing doctor in the next 90 days. Spend a few minutes writing down everything you would do to mitigate this loss and preserve profitability. Don't stop until you have written down at least 25 smart ideas. Now go over your list from the top … are there any tactics you should be applying *today* to boost company success that you don't have to wait to implement?
2. Ask yourself as a practice leader: "Do I strike the right balance between telling our people that the future is going to be bright … and telling them the future is going to be much tougher than the past?" If you're too much of a Pollyanna, you'll lull the team into so-so performance. If you freak folks out with too many dire predictions, they'll freeze. Find the right tipping point, with enough "sunshine" to promote confidence and sufficient "dark cloud" warnings to spur performance.
3. Imagine there was a new law in your town, saying that every ophthalmology practice had to terminate ***one*** staff member this month. Who would you pick? How would you cope with their absence? Would the result of this mental experiment be a net rise or fall in profitability for your practice? If you answered, "Our profit would rise," ask yourself just one more question: "Why haven't we terminated this staff member before now?"
4. Pick your least satisfactory vendor. Spend a couple of minutes writing down what makes them so bad … and why you stick with them anyway. Write and implement a plan to improve or replace this outlier. (As it turns out, a lot of management in already-pretty-strong businesses is nothing more than the role of predators in nature, constantly culling the weakest link.)
5. Having a permanent turnaround mindset isn't just enterprise-based, of course. You can turn the same habit of thinking on *yourself.* Scan the wide spectrum of your abundant management talents. Pick out one thing you are weakest at. (PS: If this exercise stumps you, ask your grumpiest, most hypercritical doctor to help you out.) Then ask yourself, "Why am I still weakest in this area? What is it costing our practice? What is it costing my career progress? What new resources would I need to get better in this one, weakest area?" Use the resulting answers to make near-term improvements. And then ask yourself the same questions all over again next month.

• • •

Thirty years ago, I worked for a brilliant nuclear physicist. With a PhD at 18, "Freddie" was part of the original team that developed the first atomic bomb. As CEO of our nonprofit research institute, Freddie played his board and managers like a fiddle, perpetuating a myth that at any moment the institute was going to go bankrupt and collapse. Fear of this kept all of us in a lather, in a state of perpetual exertion looking for ways to make new scientific discoveries, boost donations, and save costs.

Fear makes things happen. Harness FMTH, even if you and your practice have nothing in particular to be afraid of. Yet.

CHAPTER 20

Helping Your Managers Manage

The Hallmarks of Superior Supervision

John B. Pinto

Here's a true story exemplifying even the best practice management environments.

A Huey Cobra helicopter was just finishing up a nighttime practice run. The pilot was working on their low hover maneuvers at the air base when they tipped the tail rotor sharply backward, snapping off the tail boom. Without the tail that keeps a helicopter from spinning around in circles, the helicopter took off like a pinwheel, sliding down the runway doing 360s in a brilliant shower of sparks. As the Cobra passed the tower, the following exchange was heard:

Tower: (urgently) "Sir, do you need any assistance?!?"

Cobra: (calmly) "I don't know, tower. We ain't done crashin' yet."

Pinto JB. *Ophthalmic Leadership: A Practical Guide for Physicians, Administrators, and Teams, Second Edition* (pp 117-120).
© 2022 SLACK Incorporated.

Sound familiar? Few business management environments are as vexing as ophthalmology. The simple, common sense routine of running any business enterprise—being nice to the customers and getting paid for what you do—must rub shoulders with the immense complexities of third-party reimbursement and the even-greater complexities of ophthalmic care, itself. Every day can feel like a slow-motion crash landing. Like the helicopter pilot, the best practice supervisors need to be calm and serene, even in the midst of disaster. Let's talk about the other attributes of great supervisors.

Departmental supervisors are those middle managers who take direction from an office manager or administrator to translate the doctors' policy decisions into daily activity. Most practices with only a few lay staff members can get by without mid-level supervisors. They only need one lay leader, the "office manager." But with any more than about eight or 10 staff, the span of control becomes too wide for a single office manager and it pays to nominate supervisors over the natural departments: clinical services (the techs), patient accounts (billing), reception, marketing, optical, and surgery center.

Unlike your practice administrator or office manager, department supervisors are on the front lines of running your practice. The right supervisors can make any administrator look great. Poor supervisors will undermine the effectiveness of even the most outstanding administrator and can take down a practice much more abruptly than the helicopter in the story.

During a recent client conference with a group of experienced managers at the table, we brainstormed about the attributes of great supervisors. Here's what emerged.

- *Direct job knowledge.* It's not absolutely necessary that a practice administrator know how to post a charge in the computer system. But it's essential that the billing department manager be the most savvy person in the practice when it comes to patient account matters. Supervisors in most environments should be *working* managers. The chief technician should be on the clinic floor working up patients with their crew at least 2 or 3 days a week. The optical manager should be serving the customers.
- *Delegation.* Almost all supervisors are brought up from the ranks. They know the job. And as working managers they still spend most of their time *doing* the job. But they need to balance this with the ability to delegate. One of the most common complaints leveled at otherwise excellent supervisors is that they have difficulty delegating. Your supervisors should continuously strive for a balance between doing and delegating.
- *"Action today" oriented.* While every manager needs to keep the keep their eye on the future, your practice's supervisors should not be spending a lot of time pondering the long-term destiny of the practice. They should not be compiling endless, overly-elaborate to-do lists, which commonly lead more to procrastination than organization. Instead, they should be executors, working with their teams to plow through the week's tasks.
- *Grace under pressure.* Middle-management supervisors are squeezed in a four-way vice, pressured by patients, doctors, their administrator-boss, and their own staff to get things right. Like the helicopter pilot, great supervisors are understated, upbeat, and calm.

- *Accountability.* Too often, the pressure of pleasing so many parties at the same time can lead to overpromising. Great supervisors are able to gauge the needs of the job at hand against their resources and be realistic about what they need in terms of time and staff to get the job done.
- *Communication.* It should go without saying that superior supervisors are great communicators, starting with being very good listeners. Although most supervision puts a premium on verbal communication, your practice's department heads should also be able to write clearly. Any practice with more than a handful of staff needs to transition from being a purely verbal culture to writing down agreed protocols and procedures and using frequent memos to keep everyone in the loop.
- *Discipline.* Supervisors bear and uphold the operational standards of the practice. If these standards are wobbly because of an undisciplined supervisor, the practice itself starts to melt down.
- *Tough love.* Holding staff members to the operational standards of the practice takes more than discipline. It requires the ability to be tough with the people you manage. If a staff member arrives inappropriately dressed, they still get sent home, even if it means they'll have to drive 40 miles round-trip and the clinic will run behind that morning.
- *Fairness.* Staff, when they're being well managed, will always tell me something like, "Susan, my manager, is great. She's the toughest boss I've ever had to work for, but she's also the fairest." People do their very best work when they are supervised by someone who's inordinately tough, but combines that with inordinate fairness.
- *Openness.* People love working for managers who are open to their ideas. People hate working for a boss who will only take their own counsel ... or worse, will twist things around and take all the credit for the ideas of their staff.
- *Forgiveness.* All staff make mistakes. They're human. So they need to be redeemed after every mistake. Nobody likes to work under someone who holds a grudge for an error made last week. Unless an error has been made that deserves frank termination, every staff should be able to erase their personal error scoreboard by at least the end of the week and start out the following Monday with a clean slate.
- *Adaptability.* Superior managers may as well wear a button that says, "I Love Change!" Rather than being rigid and bristling at the thought of policy changes or alterations in the routine, they welcome every change for the better and get their more resistant staff to support unpopular changes.
- *Organization.* The very best supervisors I've ever met, in more than 2 decades of field work observing practices first-hand, are working parents who have raised two or more kids. I'm the father of just one son, so I certainly don't qualify, but I'm convinced that if you can properly manage a few kids as a primary caregiver, you can just as well organize the world. Be sure to ask candidates for any supervisory position about their parenting style—you'll learn a lot about how they'll manage your staff and how organized and coordinated they'll be. I like to call supervisory applicants at home, at about 7:00 PM when things get especially hectic, to see how organized they really are.

- *Guardianship.* Even the most robust practices are still relatively fragile as business organizations go. The best supervisors see themselves as protectors of the organization, the patients, the staff, and the doctors. If they see something that's wrong, they act directly to correct it. If they think the practice is heading down the wrong path (eg, wrong doctor, bad office location) they speak up.
- *Mentoring.* Supervisors are coaches, cheerleaders, and mentors. Staff protegees are well served if their supervisors have the patience and knack for passing along their knowledge, and at the same time create a hunger for career development. Your practice's supervisors are the chief career advisors for each person they oversee. Every annual or semi-annual written staff evaluation should include a section on career development goals signed off by both the employee and their supervisor.
- *Team playing.* Not only are supervisors the leaders of their own small departmental team, they are also members of the larger team called the "practice." Beyond technical skill and leadership, your supervisors should have the ability to defer to the needs of the group. For a front desk supervisor, this means not allowing warfare to break out between receptionists and techs. For the head of the marketing department, it's making sure that everyone is truly prepared for the new ad campaign that's coming out on Sunday, and not slaughtered with calls and patients in the weeks that follow.
- *Sacrificing.* Sure, there's the glory. And the bump in compensation. But these rarely pay back completely for the stress and demands of being an effective supervisor. Managers have to be open to early and late hours, open to criticism, and open to the adverse consequences of making the occasional crummy decision.
- *Maturity and respect.* Every supervisor has the right to express their opinion. But sometimes, the organization and its board need to bypass opinion and make an unpopular decision. The mature supervisor publicly respects the decisions of the doctors and administrator, even when they privately disagree.
- *Humility.* In a world where you're generating dozens of decisions and requests a day, you're going to make mistakes. Managers (and doctors and administrators!) should readily own up to their mistakes, which will only cause staff respect to grow.
- *Personal reserves.* Ask your supervisors how much they're giving of themselves to the practice. Most will probably answer, "Why, 100% of course!" This is the wrong answer. If any of your supervisors are having to give 100% of their personal best to get the job done, they're working too hard. The adroit manager only gives about 90% so they consistently have some gas left in the tank during crisis periods … that, given that this is ophthalmology, is rarely very far around the corner.

• • •

Consider sharing this list of ideal standards with your own supervisors. As a group exercise, customize it to fit your special setting and requirements. Use the results to check periodically that everyone in an overseer capacity is living up to your practice's expectations.

CHAPTER 21

Are You an Entrepreneur?

Take This Simple Test

John B. Pinto

Lots of people are called "entrepreneurs," from the kid at the end of your street selling lemonade, to Henry Ford. And if you're an ophthalmologist running your own practice, you probably think you qualify as an entrepreneur. But are you really?

What defines a doctor-entrepreneur? Is it starting a solo practice on your own, in the face of adversity? Taking over a small practice and making it larger? Adding a new elective procedure and handling all the details from service development, to promotion, and pricing? These are all vanguard activities that would make you stand out from the crowd of eye surgeons who take a safer path. And these are certainly examples of "little-e" entrepreneurism. But to my way of thinking, to be a "BIG-E" ***Entrepreneur,*** you need to take your business enterprise to the next step: From a business that lives and dies based on your personal, daily inputs to an enterprise that no longer needs your daily production or presence.

Pinto JB. *Ophthalmic Leadership: A Practical Guide for Physicians, Administrators, and Teams, Second Edition* (pp 121-128).
© 2022 SLACK Incorporated.

Self-Exam

Here's a simple self-exam to determine if you're a "BIG-E" or "little-e" entrepreneur, or if you might be more suited to join an existing enterprise rather than failing to thrive in one that you own. There is no value judgement in this exam; it is equally honorable to score high or low.

Vision and Opportunism

Doctors at every place in the entrepreneurial spectrum have the ability to creatively take in the facts and data of their business environment, dream about the future, and invent in greater or lesser detail the endpoint they then aim for. Which of these best fits you?

____ 1. People who know me well often kid me about how I have my head in the clouds. I really enjoy imaging my practice in the distant future, and am very comfortable thinking in terms of a 5-, 10-, even 20-year plan. I really don't mind if it turns out that my long-term vision was incorrect—I just really need a big goal to strive for. When I see a clinical or business trend, I'm often among the first to jump on it. ***(5 points)***

____ 2. I can readily think of my practice in terms of 3 to 5 years out, but beyond that the picture gets a little fuzzy. I don't think we can reliably predict the environment any farther out than that, and I'd rather not get my hopes up for nothing. I'm neither the first nor the last person to adopt new ideas and trends. ***(3 points)***

____ 3. I prefer to wake up and simply take each day as it comes. I've never really been one to plan my life or career out more than the next year. When I see a new trend, I like to wait to see how it pans out, and not be the first one to jump in … it might just be a fad. ***(1 point)***

Positive Versus Negative Orientation

Super-entrepreneurs tend to be extremely positive people. They see the glass as half full and believe that even the most difficult circumstances will somehow lead to an otherwise undiscovered opportunity. Which one of the following three descriptions best fits you?

____ 1. I have found that life pretty much hands you what you can handle and overcome—even the toughest breaks. I may get down from time to time when disappointments arise, but this feeling is fleeting, and I bounce back stronger than ever. I mostly wear a smile, even at times when most people would be down. My staff are attracted to my positive outlook on life, and I really enjoy getting folks to see the bright side whenever problems come up. ***(5 points)***

____ 2. I am a realist. So when problems come up in the practice, I groan like the next guy. However, for the sake of the team, I put on a smile when

I have to, even if down deep I'm really worried and pessimistic. I really appreciate being around "up" people who can keep me from thinking the cup is half empty. ***(3 points)***

____ 3. I believe that life is basically difficult and unfair, unless you happen to get lucky. It can really bug me to be around highly optimistic, positive people ... I mean, who's kidding whom? Life's tough. Keep a low profile, be careful, and you won't get hurt. ***(1 point)***

Ability to Drive to the Finish

All the business brilliance in the world has to be combined with years and years of hard work to see your plans come to life. Each of these years contains an opportunity to throw your hands up and quit pressing so hard. Giving up prematurely on a satellite, an associate doctor, or a marketing plan is a lot easier than gutting it out and making things work. Strong entrepreneurs keep marching forward when others would quit.

____ 1. When a project is looking dim, that's when I really shine. I just can't bear the thought of quitting something our practice has made a commitment to accomplishing. My clinical and business career is full of examples where pushing just a little harder and longer, no matter the cost, gets the job done. ***(5 points)***

____ 2. When I'm faced with adversity I'll push for a while, but not like some people I know. I'm all for giving projects our best shot; but when it seems we might be going in the wrong direction, I change course pretty quickly. ***(3 points)***

____ 3. When projects get too tough, that's a clear signal to me that it's time to quit. There's only so much we can do, and if we take on too much we're going to fail. It doesn't take much for me to say, "Let's try something else, this isn't working." ***(1 point)***

Risk Taking

Some of us love risk ... others are risk-adverse. Most are between these two extremes. The classic entrepreneur will mortgage their home to the hilt to start a long-shot business. Risk must obviously be weighed by an intelligent judgement of the odds involved, the consequences of failure, and the scale of off-setting benefits.

____ 1. I *love* taking calculated risks. So long as the odds are even remotely in our favor and the potential payoff is big, I'll roll the dice and go for it. If it's legal and ethical and the practice payoff is huge, I'd risk almost anything if it could help us accomplish our long-term dreams. ***(5 points)***

____ 2. I don't feel comfortable putting it all on the line, but I'm OK proceeding with policies and projects for the practice that we can reasonably survive in the event of failure. ***(3 points)***

____ 3. I break out in a cold sweat and my heart races just *thinking* about taking a business or clinical risk. ***(1 point)***

Delegation

This is one of the most important attributes of any entrepreneur, but especially in medicine, where it's common to say, "It's faster to do this myself" or "Sally couldn't do this quite as well as I do without lots of experience." Unlike a car wash or furniture store, it's much harder to build an ophthalmology practice and turn it over to non-owner employees to run for you and generate a passive profit. But that's exactly what the entrepreneurial doctors of the future will be doing.

_____ 1. Anything that others can do for me, I delegate avidly. That goes for clinical, surgical, and business chores. I know that if I would simply stop and take 30 minutes to teach someone a task, I can potentially save myself hundreds of hours over the course of the next few years. ***(5 points)***

_____ 2. I am pretty good at delegation, but still find myself from time to time doing routine, mundane tasks that others in the practice could be handling for me. ***(3 points)***

_____ 3. Nobody can do things as well as I can, so I rarely delegate. ***(1 point)***

Business Versus Practice Orientation

Some practices run their operations like a 1950s nonprofit foundation, with little regard for the bottom line and every decision based solely on the quality of care. Other (thankfully few) practices are on the opposite side of the spectrum, ignoring quality in the interest of profits. Over the last 2 decades, it has been increasingly necessary to shift somewhat from a "foundational" model to a "bottom line" model. Just where you place yourself on this continuum is obviously a sensitive and difficult decision for every eye surgeon today.

_____ 1. I absolutely respect and honor my role as a clinician, providing the very best care I can to my patients. But having said that, I know in today's world you have to run an ophthalmology practice like a fine-tuned business, and that's exactly what we do. ***(5 points)***

_____ 2. I would say that an increasing number of our decisions are driven by the bottom line, but that still leaves us running things kind of casually around here. ***(3 points)***

_____ 3. Even at the risk of business failure, I run my practice the old-fashioned way and I'm not about to change. ***(1 point)***

Reproducible "Systems" Thinking

Medicine is both an art and a science, and a great deal of spirited discussion is now playing out about what the balance should be between the two of these. Scaling up, training extenders, and delegating requires that entrepreneurs take a systematic approach to care … doing things the same, predictable way each time to the extent possible.

_____ 1. I think of our practice as a finely tuned assembly line, in the good sense of that concept. We try to break down every step of the patient visit, and have it go as predictably, smoothly, briskly, and pleasantly for the patient as we can. Everyone here knows the agreed "one best way" to do just about everything. ***(5 points)***

_____ 2. I have made this practice a little more systematic and organized than most, but I allow our doctors and staff a wide degree of latitude in how they treat each patient. ***(3 points)***

_____ 3. We are clinical artists. I treat each patient encounter as a highly customized event, based on the patient's personality and their unique needs from us. We really don't think in terms of "pathways," "branching logic trees," or "algorithms" ... we just take care of each patient based on what seems to be right for them at the time. ***(1 point)***

Process Documentation and Control

Let's compare professional surgeons to professional airline pilots. Somewhere long ago you read a cataract textbook or two enumerating the step-by-step process of safe and effective surgery. But odds are long, after of thousands of cases, that you have anything like a how-to checklist for surgery today, because it's all become a rote routine for you. And the pilot? There are manuals and checklists galore, even after thousands of hours of practice. Medicare is a lot looser than the FAA, obviously. And this same laxity resonates to your practice's business operations, unless—as an entrepreneur—you've recognized the value of process documentation and controls.

_____ 1. I have insisted that we prepare and regularly update an operations manual for the practice. This is used for training, procedure auditing, and regular staff recredentialing. ***(5 points)***

_____ 2. Many of our important procedures are written down, but at least half of what each staff member does is in their heads and passed on verbally to new staff members. ***(3 points)***

_____ 3. We only have a few handwritten crib notes, the rest of what we do is not documented in any way. ***(1 point)***

Staff Selection, Training, and Development

Being entrepreneurial and growing at faster rates requires that you replicate your ace technician's or billing clerk's skills in successive staff ranks, and that you do this efficiently and consistently—so that everyone is taking pressure checks and posting charges in the same, optimal way. To do otherwise results in error, frustration, and costly rework.

_____ 1. We put lots of time and care into the selection of staff here, allowing in only those workers who have a willingness and ability to learn our way of doing things. We quickly weed out new staff who can't step up to our pace, fit into our team mode, or who insist on importing the bad habits they learned at their last job. In fact, we're so good at spotting raw talent and "trainability," that we no longer rely on finding experienced job seekers, which saves us a lot in labor costs. It's not unusual for us to put 5% of a typical work week into training ... 2 hours or more. ***(5 points)***

_____ 2. Of course, we think that staff selection and training are important, but frankly we're so overwhelmed with day-to-day patient care that we don't put much time into the hiring or training process. We follow our instincts, hire the best people we can find at the time, give them a week to settle in, then it's sink or swim. Lots of our new staff drown and leave well before their probation period is over. ***(3 points)***

_____ 3. We almost always hire staff who have experience from somewhere else and let them run with the way they've done things in their last job. It means we have to pay top dollar, and there's not that much consistency, but it makes life easier for our managers to not have to waste their time training workers from scratch. ***(1 point)***

Process Improvement

Even in the most successful, mature companies, constant and ongoing improvement is essential for continued prosperity. Every owner and manager—ideally every single member of the team—should be questioning every process and subroutine for opportunities to reduce costs or improve quality.

_____ 1. In our practice, there are no sacred cows and everything we do is subject to scrutiny. We not only do this formally by ourselves, but we invite patients, visiting doctors and managers from other practices, consultants, and regulatory officials to tell us how to do a better job. We're not defensive when hearing criticism. And we don't just listen, we rapidly implement every reasonable suggestion. We see the job of "improving" like housework—something that never gets permanently done. ***(5 points)***

_____ 2. From time to time we ask ourselves, "Could we do this or that better?" We read articles and go to meetings, and frequently we'll find a pearl here or there. But you know, there's probably not that much more we could do to improve without driving everyone crazy. ***(3 points)***

_____ 3. I guess we're pretty complacent around here. It takes a major clinical blunder or patient complaint for us to stand back as a team and reinvent the way we do things. We certainly don't go out of our way looking for outside advice. And even when we improve something, things often shift back to the way they were. Old habits are hard to break. ***(1 point)***

Fiscal Management and Resource Apportionment

In bygone days of 50+% profit margins, financial planning and cash flow management was relatively easy. There were plenty of reserves to fund any reasonable practice initiative. Today, ophthalmology is typically a ±35% profit margin business. And we are on an all but inevitable glide path to the lower percentile levels seen in "normal" businesses. Business growth takes time, expertise, and capital. Lots and lots of capital.

____ 1. The doctors here realize that to grow we have to invest profits back in the practice. To accomplish this, we have a lot of personal discipline. We have each learned how to sacrifice and live on a lot less than we make. We know that if we invest wisely, the practice will thrive. We may take a personal pay cut this month and even this year, but we're confident that over the next 10 years, we'll be dollars ahead, provide better care, and be more secure in our market. ***(5 points)***

____ 2. Doctors in our practice take a middle path. We are certainly willing to fund obvious money- making opportunities, but the payback period had better be within the next year or we would just as soon take the money home personally. ***(3 points)***

____ 3. The doctors take every available penny out of the practice. Even though we've been in business for years and years, we're still caught short during lean months and have a hard time making payroll. Our facility is getting a little shabby. We're short of some equipment. It feels like we're starving the golden goose. ***(1 point)***

Succession Modeling, Planning, and Execution

Every individual ophthalmic career has a beginning, a middle, and a finite end. Not so practices, which with planning can live on, constantly improving and growing, for many generations. Some eye surgeons see their practices as a personal money machine, something they would just as soon discard at the end of their career rather than taking on the hassle and uncertainties of bringing in one or more successors. Other ophthalmologists think in bigger terms. They see their practices as institutions that should outlive them, serving future doctors, staff, and patients. Like proud and responsible parents, such doctors are more than willing to make personal sacrifices to see that their practices live on and succeed.

____ 1. It would be a very great disappointment to me to not have my practice thrive and grow after I'm retired. To this end, I've already worked out the timeline for phasing in the next doctors. My plan even includes a way for me to earn a little passive income during the last years of my practice, and to have a private office to come to and work on my novel after I've retired from medicine. ***(5 points)***

_____ 2. It would be nice to see some young doctors carry on with my practice after I'm out of the picture, but if that means the cost and risk of taking on a long string of trial associates like my old medical school roommate, forget it. Maybe in the last 3 years of active practice I'll try to find a successor, but not at the cost of topping up my retirement savings. If it doesn't work out the first time, or maybe the second, I'll just work until I'm ready to walk away, and hand the keys over to one of my local colleagues for salvage value. ***(3 points)***

_____ 3. I see the business nuts and bolts of my practice as a personal tool to use so long as I'm professionally active, and then discard. I worked hard to build this practice with little help from anyone else. Let the next guy figure it out for himself. ***(1 point)***

• • •

Now add up your total score, and see where you seem to fit in the ranges below. The maximum score is 60, the minimum 12:

50 to 60 points: Consider yourself a "BIG-E" Entrepreneur. You may have the drive, perspectives, and attitudes necessary to build a larger, multigenerational, multilocation, multisubspecialty practice that at some point in the future no longer needs your personal input. Such a business could provide you with a passive source of income or allow your personal take home pay to rise, even as fees and margins fall, by hiring employee providers to increase your practice's total output well beyond your individual capacity.

25 to 49 points: Perhaps you're a "little-e" entrepreneur, which is the vast majority of eye surgeons. You still want to build a great business, deliver outstanding care, and may even be successful in passing it on to successors who pay you a small buy-out for what you have created. But nearly all of your income from the practice will be active—generated by your own personal efforts—not passive. As fees fall along with normative profit margins, and you reach the limits of your personal time and output, your income will inevitably fall.

Under 25 points: You may be more comfortable, happy, and successful in a modest practice, operating at relative stasis, where there's a lot of room for customization and complexities can be kept under your personal control. Alternately, as medical economics change and put a premium on efficiency and scale, it may be appropriate for you to consider joining a more entrepreneurial practice, rather than building a larger company on your own.

Please keep in mind that wherever you score on this informal self-evaluation is perfectly ok so long as you're true to your personality, your aspirations, and the practical realities of your local marketplace. And please realize that there's an important age-related factor in all of this. It's not at all unusual for doctors younger than 40 and older than 55 to be quite averse to being entrepreneurial, and doctors 40 to 55 to be more risk taking and vanguard. It may be interesting for you to bring this evaluation tool out every few years to see if your perspectives change ... and in what direction.

CHAPTER 22

How to Recruit and Integrate a New Doctor

Lauren Simon and Amelia Rogoff

Adding a new associate is both an exciting and serious venture for you to embark upon as a leader. It is a sign of both accomplishment and successful strategic planning for your practice. Your growth is at the point where expansion becomes inevitable. With this addition you can absorb the extra patient volume and act on any opportunities for expansion, while increasing profitability. Most importantly, the new associates are the required ingredients to the succession planning of your practice. You are selecting not only a near-term follower but a potential future leader in your practice.

Pinto JB. *Ophthalmic Leadership: A Practical Guide for Physicians, Administrators, and Teams, Second Edition* (pp 129-135).
© 2022 SLACK Incorporated.

Recruiting a physician has become a more challenging and complicated process in recent years. This is true not only for the practice adding an associate, but also for the physician candidate who is likely uninformed of the process and has different considerations than you did when you were in their place.

Today's candidate is looking for professional security, which is perceived to be found more in a larger, "safer" group setting than in a solo physician practice that has the worry of personality conflict. These larger groups offer subspecialists the security of automatic in-house referrals without having to go out and hustle for referral sources. Additionally, with continuing declining reimbursements and the uncertainties of tomorrow's medicine, the newly graduated physician is concerned with how this will impact on their practice.

Choosing a larger, financially stable group with professional management, that has implemented strategic planning allowing for these changes, is highly attractive for someone still green on the business side of medicine. It is also safe to say that today's physicians are less concerned with their careers being the center of their lives, they want to spend more time with their family and friends than their predecessors. With this in mind, you can still develop your new associate to become highly-motivated and an exceptionally effective future leader.

During the selection process it is important for the practice to follow these guidelines:

- *Decide exactly what you are looking for.* Does it make sense for you to add a medical retina specialist who is willing to do comprehensive ophthalmology therefore bringing an additional revenue source for the practice? Would a Mandarin-speaking physician help bring in a completely new patient source? Are you looking for a partner or an employee? Ask yourself these poignant questions before starting the process. Remember, you are probably in touch with the kind of leader you are, and the kind of people who respond to your style of leadership ... be sure to factor this into your recruitment activity.
- *Reviewing CVs.* Do not consider only where the candidate did their residency and/or fellowship. Look for hobbies and interests and community service. Is it important to your practice if the candidate has written many papers? If not, then don't be impressed by a long publications list.
- *Telephone interview.* Consider utilizing a video conference call instead of a traditional phone interview. This will not only give you a personal connection in future conversations, but will allow you to assess a candidate's demeanor and body language. Be prepared with both your questions and answers for the candidate. It is during this process that you can start assessing if the candidate has the right "chemistry" for your group. The bottom line in making your final decision will always come down to chemistry. It is during this first interview that you should take notes on the candidate's career goals and what factors are influencing their decision when choosing a practice.
- *On-site interview.* This is your chance as a practice to shine. You will typically pay for all interview costs for both the physician and their spouse. The candidate should be met at the airport by a member of the group who is already familiar with the candidate. This person should point out shopping, restaurants, and other areas

of interest on their way to the hotel; first impressions are lasting. Have a personalized basket ready in their room. Make sure the candidate has adequate time with the administrator of the practice, so they have the chance to ask questions regarding flow, finances, staff, patient allocation, and growth of both the group and their projected practice. It is often the feedback from the administrator and staff that offers the best assessment of the candidate's interpersonal skills and their career and personal aspirations.

The candidates should always bring their spouse, the decision process will never come to fruition if the spouse doesn't have first-hand knowledge to discuss every aspect of the group and the community. It is their geographic preference (and often solely the spouse's) that will likely make their final decision. They should always have enough time to explore the community both with a trusted realtor (who can also give helpful feedback) and on their own. A cocktail party/dinner party, preferably at one of the physician's homes is always an opportunity to get to know the candidate on a social level. A wrap-up/review session should be planned. This will give you the opportunity to assess the candidate's level of interest and address any new questions.

- *Have a contract prepared.* It is nice to have a contract ready when the "right" candidate is about to join your practice. If there is a high level of interest on both sides you need to keep the momentum going. A formula for partnership should be addressed in the initial contract.
- *Post interview process.* Did the candidate write a thank-you email to all the partners and the administrator? During the few days after the interview, gather the feedback from everyone who had communication with the candidate, especially any technicians or ancillary staff. Complete reference checks on the candidate. Write an email to the candidate expressing your interest on pursing the relationship.

  The candidate will also want to obtain references for your group. It is important for you to be prepared when the candidate asks to speak with past associates. Know in advance those who you do and those who you do not want the candidate to communicate with.
- *Keeping a competitive advantage.* Do not compare candidate's salaries locally, as you are competing nationally. There are too many ophthalmology jobs available and too few candidates. You need to offer an attractive income and benefits package that is complete, detailed, and competitive to attract physicians at different phases of their career.
- *Maximize your pool of candidates.* Often practices focus on one candidate, and in the process they may lose other qualified candidates. Always choose your top few candidates. You will likely succeed in hiring the one that both fits your criteria and accepts your position. You must keep in mind that most candidates are looking at and evaluating additional opportunities as well. Your first choice of candidates may not always be your only choice.
- *Choosing the right candidate.* Educational background and surgical skills are very important traits to look for, but a personality fit is the most essential piece of the puzzle.

- *Contract negotiations.* Give and take is essential during this process! You will learn much about how the candidate manages stressful, challenging situations. The candidate will be expected to compromise, and so will the practice. Know where you have flexibility and where you do not. Take great care throughout the negotiation process and always keep in perspective that your legal council is employed by you. Don't let your advisors lead you down a path that can turn friendly dialogue into a battle of ego. While the contract is made to protect the employer, it also has to be fair to the employee. This is a delicate process and both sides need to be clear on the prize. It needs to be a contract that you, yourself would be willing to sign.

  Recruiting a physician is not easy and there is always risk on both sides. Ultimately it is a leap of faith for all. A candidate may seem to be the perfect fit in every way, and for some unforeseen circumstance the physician always has a chance of leaving. You can decrease these odds by being thorough in the initial assessment of your candidate.

Recruiting Highlights

To determine how closely your job opportunity matches the candidates' top priorities, have each candidate prioritize the items listed here. This will give you a better idea of what influences the candidates' decisions and what the most important elements of a new job are to the candidate and their family.

Cultural/Social Influences

- Schools systems
- Safety
- Recreational needs
- Hobbies
- Civic opportunities
- Religion
- Family and friends

Economic Influences

- School loans
- Cost of living
- Tax implications
- Present income vs future income
- Future ownership vs employee

Geographic Influences

- Climate
- Urban
- Suburban
- Rural

Professional Influences

- Academia or research opportunities
- Administrative/leadership opportunities (eg, future medical directorship)
- HMO-capitated clinic
- Private practice (owner)
- Private practice (employee)
- Small group
- Large group
- Private equity

Successfully recruiting a physician who is truly a good fit for a specific opportunity is expensive, frustrating, and very time consuming. Using a professional recruiter who has extensive knowledge exclusively in the ophthalmic field helps reduce, if not eliminate, many of the time-consuming and stressful components of hiring a physician.

Successfully Integrating a New Doctor Into Your Practice

Yes, recruiting a doctor was probably a bit more challenging than you had anticipated. You approached the hiring process systematically, deliberating on all the important skills and experience needed for the position, as well as the type of personality that would work best with you and your practice. You combed through many CVs, and strategically selected the appropriate candidates to interview. You made the offer, negotiated the contract that made both parties feel like they had won, and have finally hired the perfect addition to your practice. You may finally believe that you can actually sit back and enjoy the benefits of your new hire. Wait for it … the important work has just begun!

Adding a new doctor to your practice can afford you incredible growth opportunities. Although seemingly complex and extremely time consuming, the time and effort that you put into the integration and adjustment period will pay major dividends in the long run. It will be well worth your while, as well as jump start the initial comfort level and success of your new doctor.

First Things First (Putting the Cart Behind the Horse)

Your administrator/office manager must perform the following duties without delay to help facilitate a seamless and rewarding transitional experience for the practice and your new doctor.

1. Coordinate all of the new doctor's state licensure. Credential the associate with the various payers (eg, Medicare/Medicaid) and other participating insurers. Your Medicare/Medicaid representative must be contacted to add the new doctor to your current profiles. Also, prepare a list of the additional third-party payers of your new doctor to be notified, and include all companies (HMO/PPO) that you have agreements with. Your new associate needs to be enrolled in all of your outstanding payers. If this is not done in a timely fashion, a lapse in billing and collection will be created for the new doctor and subsequently affect the bottom line of the practice and the morale of your new doctor.
2. Make all necessary insurance arrangements, including malpractice. You might need to reevaluate your coverage and find out what is needed to protect you and your practice from potential malpractice claims.
3. Any other insurance arrangements including worker's compensation, primary health, major medical, group disability, and/or group term life also need to be updated and or notified.
4. Sign your new associate up for practice facilities including, but not limited to, any hospitals and surgery centers used by the practice.
5. Get them acquainted with the equipment used and supplies that might be needed, including furniture for the new doctor and additional clinical supplies and surgical instruments.
6. Make introductions for the doctor to potential referral networks and community leaders, either in person or through a letter format. The doctor might also want to put together a list of their own future prospective networks that they would like to have contacted.
7. Select your most experienced and qualified technicians for the new physician. This will enable them to acclimate to their new environment at a faster pace.
8. Be as clear as possible with your (attainable) goals for patients seen, productivity, and attraction of new referral sources and new patients. Put everything in writing, as things are always open to misinterpretation if left verbally only.

Put Your Best Foot Forward (Little Things Mean a Lot)

- Place "Welcome to Our New Doctor" signs on the reception counter. Include a photo and a brief bio on the sign.
- Profile the doctor on your website. The doctor's bio should include his degrees, area of specialty, hobbies, and any other personal touches that might enable patients to bond with them.

- Don't hesitate to send out a news release and a photo to local media. Many newspapers publish a "People/Profile" section and/or a "Lifestyle" section. Use the exciting news of your new associate to promote your practice and spotlight your business in the local community.
- Prepare and mail out announcements of your new associate's arrival to include, but not be limited to: active as well as inactive patients, and all local physicians including optometrists, opticians, and primary care physicians. Community business leaders, Chamber of Commerce, and an internet directory should also be updated.
- Supply a list of names and numbers of local advisors for your new doctor's consideration including, but not limited to: realtors, attorneys, accountants, doctors, and personal insurance agents.
- Notify answering service and all other pertinent office personnel of doctor's name, employment date, and cell phone number.

Plan for It

Plan for the arrival of your new associate from the first day of work. The new doctor needs to know who and how often they will meet with other associates to discuss performance objectives. Take the time to allow the associate to ask questions, as well as listen to their feedback. It is imperative to take the time and write down your expectations and review them with your new associate.

Honesty and timely action are the best policies in all relationships. Make sure all promises and contract agreements are met without the associate having to ask about them. Keep an open door policy. Share all pertinent practice information with your new physician. Let the associate see how you run your company.

Work closely with the new associate as they start seeing patients and in surgery before sending them out on their own. Conscientious supervision, along with precise expectations, will lead your new associate and your practice to a more effortless adjustment, and to eventually thrive in the process.

CHAPTER 23

Leadership Leaps for Women in Ophthalmology

Marsha Link, PhD

While it has been over a decade that the content of this chapter, "Leadership Leaps for Women in Ophthalmology," was initially written, much of the material still has relevance. In the interim, there have been important "leaps" by competent, motivated women who have exercised their leadership talents in a variety of ways.

Progress Has Been Made

There has been progress, albeit somewhat slow, toward gender parity in corporate America. At the beginning of 2020, the representation of women in companies across America was trending in the right direction. For example, an article

Pinto JB. *Ophthalmic Leadership: A Practical Guide for Physicians, Administrators, and Teams, Second Edition* (pp 137-148).
© 2022 SLACK Incorporated.

published by McKinsey and Co entitled "Women in the Workplace 2020" reported the most pronounced positive trend was in senior management. Between January 2015 and January 2020, representation of women in senior and vice-president positions grew from 23% to 28%, and representation in the C-suite grew from 17% to 21%.[1]

The ophthalmology space has also seen growth in the number of women who are now in top leadership roles in companies, at the CEO or vice-president level, as well as in top leadership roles in professional organizations and societies. In the clinical arena, the number of female ophthalmologists who have completed residencies or fellowships, presented at professional meetings, or participated in research studies has increased. Despite these advances, women are still in the minority in top leadership roles. Additionally, access to leadership development for entry and mid-level managers is still not widely available. There remains the need to build awareness and intentionality in helping women develop professionally and rise to top levels of leadership within ophthalmology, as well as in other sectors.

The Impact of the Pandemic

Not only have women been challenged by the underrepresentation situation, but the impact of the 2020 pandemic has posed additional challenges for women who aspire to hold and grow into leadership roles. Consider these statistics. Since the onset of the pandemic in February 2020, more than 2.3 million women have left the labor force, compared to nearly 1.8 million men who left in the same time frame.[1] During this crisis, women were unusually impacted by the additional stress and demands placed on them because of increased responsibilities. A study by McKinsey and LeanIn[2] found that during the pandemic, women worked, on average, 3 more hours each day than men. These hours were devoted primarily to child care, family, and personal responsibilities. These extra hours, in addition to the hours spent in the work day, add up to 20+ more hours per week ... the equivalent of another half-time job!

For those already in leadership roles during the pandemic, women were faced with difficult choices. Because of the demands of leadership positions and the uncertainty of the future, women who had progressed in their leadership capacity and experiences found themselves in a position where their ambition and progress might slide backward. Of the more than 40,000 women surveyed in the McKinsey and LeanIn study cited above, one in three mothers considered leaving the workforce or downshifting their careers. This staggering statistic has implications for developing and having access to women leaders of tomorrow. Only time will tell if these decisions by women will negate the progress thus far achieved in advancing women leaders.

The Impact of Diversity, Inclusion, and Belonging

In recent years, the focus on diversity, inclusion, and belonging has ignited interest in helping people in underrepresented groups become more engaged in leadership roles. Women remain in the category of those who are underrepresented, even though we are gaining ground. This increased interest is due, in part, because it is not only women who have awareness of the underrepresentation, but it is also men in top leadership roles, as well as Boards of Directors, who are understanding the value of having a more diverse group of individuals in their organizations. Diverse individuals in both business and in the clinical arena bring knowledge, competencies, and unique perspectives that can differentiate an organization and better address the diverse customer and patient populations that are served.

One way in which this new movement has expanded in the ophthalmology space is through the efforts of OWL, Ophthalmic World Leaders. During my tenure as President of OWL, the Board of Directors of OWL made the bold and decisive move to change the name from "Ophthalmic Women Leaders" to "Ophthalmic World Leaders." This change was initiated to address the idea that women are not the only group that is underrepresented in the ophthalmic environment. The awareness that there are others who have valuable contributions to make, precisely because of their unique combination of skills, experiences, and ideas, is being addressed in many sectors, including ophthalmology. The idea that diversity is an asset, when more women and others with different perspectives are engaged and welcomed, has gained momentum. When implemented even more robustly, this idea will benefit customers, patients, and those who work in ophthalmology.

Hope Is on the Horizon

The future of ophthalmology is bright! The capable and progressive minds that work in this space are a catalyst to provide opportunities for women and others who have previously been underrepresented. In the closing content I discuss "Future Leaps," suggesting concrete and practical ways for women to take charge of our own leadership development. While it is still important that each individual develop their own plan for making "leadership leaps," it also behooves top leaders (whether male or female) in every organization to open their minds and hearts to the idea that women and others who are underrepresented will add great value.

Management and employees need to work in concert to ensure that leadership development efforts are not only encouraged but designed and implemented. This will require behaviors that foster trust, collaboration, and thoughtful decision making to ensure that the leaders of tomorrow are the best people, be it male or female, to move the research, products, and services to address the eye care needs of the patients we serve.

To conclude this chapter update, let me use a quote from Socrates that describes my hope and vision for all of us who work in the ophthalmology space:

> *The secret of change is to focus all of your energy, not on fighting the old, but on building the new.*

Let's work together to build a new environment in ophthalmology where the ambitions, talents, and strengths of everyone are acknowledged, developed, and used for the benefit of those we serve.

• • •

This book is about leadership. This chapter is about ***women in ophthalmology*** who are currently leaders in their respective spaces: administrators in ophthalmology practices, ophthalmologists who work in private and academic settings, and industry professionals who work in leadership functions in both large and small companies.

Perhaps you are wondering why a topic about women's leadership is included in this book. Consider the following:

- In 2009, women made up 59.2% of the US labor force, after peaking at 60% in 1999. The percentage of women in the labor force has been relatively stable over the past several years, but it is estimated that from 2008 to 2018, the percentage is projected to increase by 9%.[3,4]
- Among women aged 25 to 64, who are in the labor force, the proportion with a college degree roughly tripled from 1970 to 2009.[5]
- In 2008, the Center for Women's Business Research estimated that there were 10.1 million privately held, women-owned firms in the United States … accounting for 40% of all businesses in the country.[6]
- In 2009, women accounted for more than 50% of all workers in several industry sectors, including health services.[5]
- It has been over a decade that ophthalmology residencies have had at least 50% women students.[7]

It is clear from these data that women contribute much in the world of work, and in health services. Why then, is it difficult for women to achieve the "leadership leaps" necessary to attain top positions where their skills, knowledge, and expertise can be leveraged to the benefit of themselves and the environments in which they work? The answer is complex, with many factors impacting the ability of women to rise to positions of power and influence.

This chapter provides food for thought about women's leadership, or lack thereof, in the field of ophthalmology. I've based this on input from conversations with 15 professional women who work in ophthalmology in one-on-one, structured interviews. Five women are currently administrators in ophthalmology practices, five are clinicians who work in private practice and/or academic settings, and five are professionals who work in a variety of leadership functions in industry. (A list of the participants is at the end of this chapter.) These women represent a diverse demographic group in terms of age, geographic location, job function, marital status, and motherhood.

Leadership: What Is It All About?

Trying to define leadership is a difficult task. If you Google "current number of books on leadership," 12,200,000 options appear. If this is not confusing enough, consider that there are at least eight major leadership theories, including great man, trait, contingency, situational, behavioral, participative, management, and relationship theories,[8] and perhaps more that have yet to be formally named.

In the interviews with these 15 women, their definitions of leadership and characteristics they attributed to outstanding leaders were very similar. What rich and insightful comments these women provided! All three groups viewed leadership as the ability to create unity among many toward a vision that will enable both individuals and organizations to achieve their goals, translating good intentions into great actions.

In the process of creating that unity, great leaders communicate the vision clearly and passionately to others so that those they lead will be motivated and inspired to engage in the vision. If leaders believe deeply in the vision, then the belief is "catching."

Great leaders have the ability to ascertain what others need, can build bridges, and raise people up, recognizing that not everyone contributes in the same way; leaders who are empathetic, yet firm and decisive when the situation demands, earn the trust and respect of those they lead. Leaders are courageous during times of change, have a risk tolerance that is healthy, and are self-aware, including owning what one does *not* know, as well as being able to give and receive feedback in a constructive manner.

In listening to these descriptions of leadership, some characteristics surfaced that one does not routinely see in the literature describing leadership: humility and humor. Several women spoke about great leaders having the capacity to set egos aside, avoiding using position and power as the primary means of influencing others.

Some indicated that humility is sometimes considered a "weakness," but that in great leaders being humble many times draws people closer to each other and to the leader. One participant shared a concept learned from one of her mentors. It clearly shows behaviors congruent with humility, and also provides a great example of a leader who understands how to share the glory. She said, "When applause is coming, a leader pushes others to the front of the room; when darts are thrown, the leader is at the front." While leaders love success, those who are capable of sharing success with others and are willing to take the heat when necessary, are clearly valued by these women leaders.

Humor, the other quality mentioned, was linked to the idea that leaders do not always take themselves seriously. Furthermore, when mistakes are made, great leaders can admit them and trust in themselves and others that a corrective course can be found. Often, using humor is a valuable tool in managing mistakes.

It was not surprising to note that some of the qualities that were mentioned appear to be those that are typically ascribed to women: communication, building bridges, being empathetic, sharing success, and valuing humility. Also mentioned were strong interpersonal skills, ability to build consensus and collaborate, good organization and multitasking skills, willingness to say "I don't know," strong observational skills, ability to be the "glue that holds the organization together as well as the grease that keeps the wheels turning," and humility.

The interviewees also noted that women may have some areas where "stretching" is required to maximize their leadership talent. For example, in attempts to promote collaboration and consensus, women may have difficulty challenging the status quo or may avoid conflict because some women tend to seek and enjoy harmony. Women may not appear as forceful as men, being prone to overapologize and fail to keep the competitive spirit and perseverance when roadblocks appear or gender bias operates.

It occurred to me that one of women's unique contributions may well be the ability to bring a different set of leadership concepts and behaviors that can be integrated into the models that both men and women have historically embraced.

I am reminded of Anna Quindlen's essay *Redefining Leadership*,[9] in which she contends that by its very nature, women's leadership is about redefinition (ie, bringing new ideas about ways to lead that can help both men and women develop new and perhaps more effective ways of leading). She also notes that since women have historically not held top leadership positions, women are less wedded to the shape of the table if they haven't been permitted to sit at it. Thus, women have the opportunity to redefine what leadership is all about, for the benefit of women *and* men.

Taking the Leap, or Not: The Rewards and the Challenges

The path to leadership is not simple, nor is it necessarily a linear journey. Many of these women were fortunate to have one or both parents as role models, either because the parents were leaders or they provided inspiration and opportunities to help these women develop the confidence and skills to become leaders. Other women identified particular persons with whom they had worked as helping create their leadership talent. For many women, making a conscious decision to strive for leadership positions is not easy, particularly if they don't believe they are capable of achieving top leadership roles. Thus, women can sometimes be their own worst enemies by marginalizing their potential. However, it was clear that the interviewees rarely thought of themselves as lacking the motivation, drive, confidence, or skills to become the leaders they are.

These women were extremely similar in their descriptions about the rewards of being a leader. The common themes that merged were: watching individuals and/or organizations grow and thrive, knowing that I am a part of the process; loving what I do and mentoring others; effecting positive change and seeing the vision become reality; building an incredible community of people I didn't know previously, creating lasting friendships and colleagues; having autonomy, visibility and influence about strategic decisions; raising two independent children, exercising leadership skills both at home and at work. Two comments full of impact that describe the rewards of leadership came from an ophthalmologist who commented, "I get more than I give in my leadership role." And from an industry professional who said, "It is great to be able to steer the ship!"

The rewards of leadership are many, but these women also recognize the challenges, some of them unique to women. While there were divergent opinions about the existence of gender bias, there was consensus that raising the question about promoting women leaders in ophthalmology was good. Opening up the discussion about this issue is needed because sometimes it appears that no one wishes to address it. This symptom of recognizing that few women are in leadership roles in ophthalmology, but not addressing it, is similar to knowing that an elephant is in the room, but no one wants to openly admit it is there!

Women face interesting challenges when it comes to developing leadership. Among the challenges mentioned were: women's failure to believe they are capable of being a leader, failing to dream big because we are too practical, inability to adequately network and break into the "fraternal order" that men create, a tendency to overcompromise, learning how to communicate when challenging the status quo to avoid being perceived as too confrontational, striving for perfection, and difficulty saying "no" because women feel they have to prove themselves more than men and, therefore, try to do it all.

Even in today's cultural environment, one particular challenge women face is the dilemma of how to combine a professional career and motherhood. While not all women interviewed had children, the majority did. There was considerable discussion about the difficulties women have integrating these two dimensions in their lives. Even women who have supportive partners or households with two professionals face this challenge, deciding when to take time off for child-bearing and how to balance rearing children and family life with one's professional life. This situation will remain for a long time, given the data from the Bureau of Labor Statistics that show that from March 1975 to March 2000, the US labor force participation rate of mothers with children under 18 years of age rose from 47.4% to 72.9%.[3] Many women realize the time they take off puts them at a disadvantage. Those who return to work and strive to "catch up," work tremendously hard to achieve greater leadership roles, but often become weary and discouraged in their attempts to regain their professional momentum.

Catherine DeAngelis, MD, MPH and editor-in-chief of the *Journal of American Medical Association* writes in her article, *Moving Toward Equity,* that women who bow out of the work environment to bear children are doing so at an age when most men are revving up their careers. She notes that if we can collectively begin to acknowledge that women do things differently and allow, or even help them achieve their full potential, we could stop wasting so much intellect and creativity.[10] Women are sometimes passed over for leadership because they have, or plan to have, children. One example of this was provided by an interviewee who described a situation in which she was a top candidate for a new job that represented a promotion, but was passed over because she just became a new mom. Another person, a man, was hired to fill the position though he was less qualified. She felt disappointed and marginalized. This bias, whether overt or covert, is present.

Other women have elected to choose a work environment that best fits the work-life balance they want to achieve. However, finding those environments can be challenging. One of the younger women in the group mentioned that she recognizes that people in her generation don't perceive long-term job stability being as important as people have in the past, partly due to the fact that the world of work is ever-changing. She feels that perhaps women in this generation are putting more emphasis on family and not feeling the need to be married to work. As these examples point out, there is not one answer to the topic of balancing personal and professional goals. Even for the woman who is single, the work-life balance can present challenges.

Leadership Leaps for You: Practical Ideas From Women Leaders in Ophthalmology

Even with the challenges identified previously, these 15 women have successfully traveled the road that has taken them to leadership roles. The rich and varied experiences of these women provided not only insights into what leadership is all about, but their respective routes provide inspiration and practical ideas that can help those who have leadership aspirations.

I have extracted a few valuable tips that were offered during the interviews. These may be helpful tools to help you achieve your leadership goals. As you read the list, check off items that are particularly applicable to you. Rereading those you checked can become a reminder for you as you embrace your own leadership development.

_____ 1. Practice "gracious self-promotion" and do not let frustrations and skepticism get you down.

_____ 2. Do not be afraid to speak up and take on projects and do a good job with them while you remain strong, confident, and competent.

_____ 3. If you want a leadership role, decide what you need to do, where you need to be, and just do it! Figure out if this is worth it for you.

_____ 4. Find a partner who values who you are and helps you achieve what you can become. Few of us can do it alone.

_____ 5. Women don't always support each other, and we should. Women bury the hatchet, but too often leave the handle sticking out.

_____ 6. Trust the instinct inside you when you have maxed out on a job and take a risk to move to another job that may offer opportunities, even if it is a lateral move.

_____ 7. Never compromise your ideals or values to get to a higher place.

_____ 8. Believe you can be a leader and proactively manage your career vs letting others drive it.

_____ 9. Work hard to build your network, create your own path and "blaze a trail" if necessary.

_____ 10. Do not be afraid to lead in ways that are natural for you, and do not be afraid to experiment.

_____ 11. Learn how to navigate the organization and become visible; some women see themselves as the passengers and not the navigators.

_____ 12. Dare to be different, invest in further training, accept a challenge, and be a problem-solver.

_____ 13. Be persistent and never give up, but always learn from mistakes.

_____ 14. Do what you love, and the money will come. When you get it, give back.

_____ 15. Be professional and unbiased, lead by example, be ambitious—but know your stuff.

____ 16. Step back; assess your behavior, strengths, and weaknesses; then participate in continuous learning; use ASOA, classes, a coach, or a mentor to improve and grow.

____ 17. Enjoy the ride! Take time to figure out the balance in life you want and commit to implementing that balance.

Future Leaps: So What Is Next?

Many women have managed to reach top levels of leadership with poise and confidence. There is room for optimism, especially if we look at constructive ways of moving into the future so that more women achieve the leadership roles they want and deserve.

Leaps to the future include:

- *Taking charge of your own leadership development.* Too many women are not intentional about making decisions about their personal and professional lives. In the inaugural *Woman to Woman* column in the *OWL* (Ophthalmic Women Leaders) *eNews* in May 2010,[11] I challenged women to take responsibility for their own development. In subsequent columns in the *eNews,* I suggested that women articulate their personal and professional goals congruent with their values, and create a plan to achieve them. It is important to "work the plan" conscientiously, keeping in mind the need to balance all the dimensions of life that are important. Women need not rely on others to create development opportunities for them, they will do best by embracing this responsibility with an attitude of hope for continually improving themselves. Not all women will choose the same plan. Integrating one's personal and professional values and goals depends on individual preferences and it behooves us all to avoid passing judgments on those who choose a particular path. One size does not fit all!
- *Developing a plan for increasing your networking and/or visibility.* Women sometimes wait for others to create opportunities for networking or becoming engaged in activities that will increase leadership potential. Men tend to do a much better job of seeking and finding these outlets. Additionally, historically, women have not been promoted in these ways. For example, in the article, "Why Men Still Get more Promotions Than Women," in the *Harvard Business Review,* the authors note that in a study of 4000 persons identified as high potentials, women received mentoring more than men; however, the type of mentoring received was different. Men were "sponsored," ie, advocating for the mentees in ways that provided visibility and engagement that would take them to the next level. Women, on the other hand, were provided feedback and advice by the mentors, but were not sponsored in the same ways as the men.[12]

- *Advocating for more research on women's leadership.* While there is a growing body of literature on women and their leadership styles, preferences, and behaviors; more is needed. If we are able to make strides in understanding what makes women unique, as well as understanding those factors that create strong, competent women leaders, it will be more likely that we will advance the cause of women leaders in ophthalmology and elsewhere. Implementing research on women leaders is similar to what has occurred in research on older adult development. Until recently, there had not been a significant pool of research candidates because people historically did not live long enough to be studied when they reached their 80s, 90s, and beyond. Likewise, until recent decades, the number of women leaders has been minimal. However, the number of women leaders is increasing, though too slowly. Through research, we may learn to strengthen the leadership talent in both women and men in ways that will add value and bring innovation to individuals, as well as to the organizations in which they work.
- *Proactively create venues and programs where both women and men can dialogue about the rewards and challenges of leadership.* No one has all the answers about leadership and how to achieve it. However, if we have open, candid conversations with men ***and*** women about our beliefs, perspectives, and struggles, we can make progress. Perhaps the leaders of the ophthalmology professional societies and organizations might consider initiatives where this kind of dialogue can occur. When we seek to understand, support each other in the journey, and work toward positive outcomes for both genders, then we will truly become more interdependent and find avenues to capitalize on the strengths and contributions of everyone—while breaking down barriers and misunderstandings.

• • •

I offer my sincere thanks to the 15 women administrators, clinicians, and business professionals who participated in the interviews. Sharing of their personal and professional experiences with candor and sincerity have made this chapter possible. I wish each of them, and those reading this chapter, much success and happiness as each of you continue to make leadership contributions in your respective environments. These are extraordinary women and ophthalmology is better because of each one.

Interview Participants

Ophthalmology Practice Administrators

- Jolynn Dobson Cook, RN, COE, Administrator, Laurel Eye Clinic in Brookville, Pennsylvania
- Beverly M. King, COE, Practice Administrator, Fishkind Bakewell Maltzman Eye Care and Surgery Center in Tuscon, Arizona
- Tina Pinke, COT, COE, Administrator, Pinke Eye Center in Shelton, Connecticut

- Candace Simerson, COE, CMPE, President and Chief Operating Officer, Minnesota Eye Consultants in Bloomington, Minnesota
- Lesley Spektor, BS, BCS, Administrator at Center for Excellence in Eye Care in Miami, Florida

Ophthalmologists

- Lynn Gordon, MD, PhD, Associate Dean Diversity Affairs, David Geffen School of Medicine, UCLA; Professor of Ophthalmology, Jules Stein Eye Center in Los Angeles, California; President, Women in Ophthalmology
- Kristiana Neff, MD, Assistant Professor of Ophthalmology, University of South Carolina School of Medicine in Columbia, South Carolina
- Audrey R. Talley Rostov, MD, Northwest Eye Surgeons in Seattle, Washington
- Jennifer Simpson, MD, Associate Clinical Professor of Ophthalmology, Gavin Herbert Eye Institute, University of California in Irvine, California
- Erin Stahl, MD, Assistant Professor of Ophthalmology, University of Missouri School of Medicine; Children's Mercy Hospital in Kansas City, Missouri

Industry Professionals

- Jane Rady, BS, MS, MBA, Divisional Vice President Business Development, Abbott Medical Optics in Santa Ana, Missouri
- Heather Ready, BS, MBA, Vice President of Marketing, AcuFocus in Irvine, Missouri
- Elisabeth Sandoval, BS, MBA, Vice President, Global Marketing & Strategy Surgical, Bausch + Lomb in Aliso Viejo, Missouri
- Julie Speed, BS, MBA, US Director of Marketing, IOLs & Refractive Education, Alcon, Inc. in Fort Worth, Texas
- Ellen Troyer, MT MA, CEO of Biosyntrx in Colorado Springs, Colorado

References

1. Women in the Workplace study; lorman.com/blog/post/women-in-the-workplace-2021.
2. Women in the Workplace 2020; leanin.org/women-in-the-workplace-2020.
3. Bureau of Labor Statistics. *TED: The Editor's Desk: Women in the Labor Force, 1970- 2009*. Retrieved August 1, 2011 from http://www.bls.gov/opub/ted/2011/ted_20110105.htm
4. Bureau of Labor Statistics. *Women at Work: BLS Spotlight on Statistics*. Retrieved July 30, 2011 from http://www.bls.gov/spotlight/2011/women/
5. Bureau of Labor Statistics. Labor force statistics from the current population survey. *Women in the Labor Force: A Databook* (2010 ed). Retrieved July 30, 2011 from http://www.bls.gov/cps/wlf-intro-2010.htm
6. Center for Women's Business Research. *Key Facts about Women-Owned Businesses*. Retrieved July 7, 2011 from http://www.womensbusinessresearchcenter.org/research/keyfacts/
7. Chang DF. Gender bias: The Heidi Roizen study. *EyeWorld*. July 2011, 13-15.
8. Cherry K. *Leadership Theories—8 Major Leadership Theories*. Retrieved July 7, 2011 from http://psychology.about.com/od/leadership/p/leadtheories.htm

9. Quindlen A. *Redefining Leadership.* Retrieved June 26, 2011 from http://www.drexel.edu/vision 2020/equality/insights/Quindlen/
10. DeAngelis C. *Moving Toward Equity.* Retrieved June 26, 2011 from http://www.drexel/edu/vision2020/equality/insights/Wuindlen/
11. Link M. Discovering key dimensions of personal and professional growth, March 2010; Dimensions for systematically getting your plan initiated, May 2010; Tips for re-balancing the dimensions of life, October 2010. *Ophthalmic Women Leaders eNews, Woman to Woman Column,* http://www.owlsite.org.
12. Ibarra H, Carter NM, Silva C. Why men still get more promotions than women. *Harvard Business Review.* 2010;1-6.

CHAPTER 24

Top Issues That Administrators Have With Their Doctors

*John B. Pinto; Craig N. Piso, PhD;
and Candace (Candy) S. Simerson, COE, CAHCM*

There was this ophthalmologist ...
and when he was good he was very, very good.
But when he was bad, he was horrid.
(With apologies to Henry Wadsworth Longfellow)

The Set-Up

The three of us—a consultant, a psychologist, and a practice administrator—had the privilege of co-presenting for the first time as a team at the 2011 Hawaiian Eye meeting on the subject of "practice development." This topic was generic enough to give us license to cover just about anything we wanted up to the last minute ... and to go with the mood and requests of the audience.

And so we did.

In the midst of the day's upbeat presentation to about 150 administrator attendees, we asked workshop participants to write down and turn in a short answer to a difficult, highly charged practice development question: "What are some

Pinto JB. *Ophthalmic Leadership: A Practical Guide for Physicians, Administrators, and Teams, Second Edition* (pp 149-153).
© 2022 SLACK Incorporated.

things that the doctors in your practice do that hold back the growth and development of your organization?"

Their responses, which you'll read here, will come as no surprise to those who are practice veterans, but may shock readers who live a more cloistered life. In Part One we share a roughly rank-order abstract of the brave comments generously shared by 58 of our Hawaiian Eye participants during "Development Day," which Candy and Craig co-chaired. Part Two is a generalized discussion of what you might consider doing if *your* practice is held back by some of the same issues discussed in Part One. Part Three is Candy's closing remarks on how important it is to face up to the challenge of vanquishing these doctor-driven challenges.

Part One: Doctor Behaviors That Hold Practices Back From Greatness

1. *A lack of teamwork.* This was the most common catch-all criticism, and ranged from not responding to emails or following agreed rules to the point of being baldly dishonest. Examples shared included doctors saying "Yes" in the board room or to the administrator, and then undermining on the clinic floor what was agreed. Some doctors were described to be changing policies without telling others. A central theme expressed was concern about an all-too-common double standard: Doctors (especially owners) not personally demonstrating the kind of work habits and team building behaviors that are expected of lay staff (eg, arriving late to clinic, hoarding charts, and/or giving certain staff the cold shoulder while lavishing undue praise on favorites). One respondent wrote: "Our doctor discounts obviously valuable staff members, while inflating the value of others who don't deserve his praise."
2. *Poorly developed communication skills.* Providers were cited for jumping to conclusions without listening to all sides, finishing other peoples' sentences for them, butting heads with management rather than communicating more productively … and especially a hesitancy to confront or engage in difficult conversations.
3. *Being rude, condescending, and belittling with staff.* Some providers were described as seeming to derive pleasure in finding fault with others and meting out criticism that is out of all proportion with the scope of a given problem. One participant wrote, "We are so afraid of what he's going to say next that we go out of our way to not talk to this doctor at all. Another wrote, "Our doctor is very kind and appropriate with patients, but is rude and inconsiderate with staff members. Sometimes such behavior can be consistent, but it's more often unpredictable and presents as frequent mood swings. Blaming and fault finding. Arrogance."
4. *Unreasonable expectations.* An example cited was a variety of perfectionistic behaviors, a disconnect between demanding high performance from the team while not being willing to release the resources needed to staff up to needed levels.
5. *Overt "anger management" issues.* This is always a serious problem, but particularly adverse when it takes place in front of patients.

6. *Being inconsistent and indecisive from day to day.* "My doctor has an inability to plan ahead and think about the future." Eye care is typically provided in 5-minute units from room to room, so it's not unusual for doctors to be lost in the now rather than thinking a year down the track and anticipating future needs.
7. *Old-fashioned selfishness.* Not considering the needs of others, a "me first" approach to all practice decisions.
8. *Excess controlling behavior.* "One of our doctors is a control freak." Being a know-it-all. Negative reactions to new ideas unless they came from the offending provider.
9. *Passive-aggressive behaviors.* Pot-stirring. "If a crisis isn't brewing, our doctor will create one."
10. *Being suspicious, to the point of paranoia.* Trust is a vital component of working groups if they are to function effectively, and trust has to be built from the top of the organization.
11. *Disengagement with, and disinterest in staff and their lives.* This issue is one of degrees. Too much or too little engagement with support staff can be problematic. A "Goldilocks" approach is indicated, which requires judgment, sensitivity, and limit-setting.
12. *Defensiveness (an inability to accept constructive coaching) and lazy work habits on the part of young doctors.* Some time ago the term "precocious sweatophobia" was coined by one of us to describe the habits of providers who were curiously less workaholic than the previous generation. When a young provider with commendable work–life balance replaces a retiring high-volume senior doctor, this can create headaches for administration and frank financial collapse for the practice.
13. *An "ADHD-like" distractibility.* Respondents described this in a lot of ways: "An inability to stay on task … a poor sense of time … procrastination … poor time management … thinking in distracted, round-about terms, out loud rather than forming his thoughts privately and then directing staff or patients clearly … asks for management to research something and then ignores the findings as though he's forgotten he ever asked for the help … tells multiple staffers to do the same task … gives conflicting orders to two different staff members."
14. *Overt discourtesy to patients.* As evidenced by answering personal cell phone calls in the exam room, arriving late for clinic, and blowing off reasonable patient questions.
15. *Being over-committed.* Taking on too many projects at once.
16. *Paperwork gaps.* Attendants wrote: "Coding 'any old way' instead of what's correct … holding onto charts … not finishing chart entries at the time of an individual exam, but instead pushing all of the notes and dictation to the end of the day … multiweek delays with dictation."
17. *An unrecognized need to retire.* "Our surgeon's skill is getting shaky and he's getting forgetful … hard to tell him this, though."

Part Two: Personal Responsibility and Problematic Physician Behavior

Ophthalmologists need to be picky, perfectionistic, and detail-oriented. They are trained to be alarmed by small, even microscopic problems. In daily practice, however, this advanced skill set is overgeneralized and misapplied to staff, marking others as "the problem" and stirring staff resentment by demanding perfection. Tensions are created when a physician is close-minded, rude or disrespectful, overly controlling, and especially if he is imposing a double standard. Such problems sometimes stem from a provider's blind spot within the domain of personal responsibility (ie, the provider is looking in the wrong direction, applying the wrong lens, and choosing the wrong focus—external rather than internal).

Ophthalmologists wield powerful influence within their practices, and with this power comes a potentially burdensome responsibility. Physicians are imbued by society, patients, and staff with super-human powers, leaving providers feeling inherently burdened with the lion's share of responsibility. (Since power and responsibility go hand in hand.)

This can set the stage for dysfunctional interactions between physicians and between doctors, patients, and staff, resulting in many of the issues outlined previously. Tension-producing interactions follow when any physician seeks to take charge without accepting commensurate responsibility. (And is it any wonder that in the current financial and legal environment, any provider is loath to take on more responsibility?)

Jim Collins, who wrote the classic text *Good to Great,* asserts that a key component of great leadership is demonstrated through the "window and the mirror": Looking unselfishly through the "window" to give full credit to staff when things are going well, and looking courageously in the "mirror" to take responsibility when things go poorly. In a more recent text, *How the Mighty Fall,* he described the first three stages of business failure, which are applicable, perhaps, to problematic physician behavior:

- Hubris born of success
- The undisciplined pursuit of "more"
- Denial of risk and peril

Accordingly, here are three self-diagnostic questions each physician should ask and answer. These same questions can be used by practice administrators to coach their physician-leaders:

- Am I a servant leader, humbly striving to serve a mission greater than myself, or do I impress others as being primarily concerned about my own welfare and prosperity (eg, using my position authority in ways that demean, frustrate, or hurt others)?
- Do I demonstrate a democratic leadership style in which others feel empowered, valued/appreciated, and encouraged to find/express their voice, or do I show more of a dictatorial approach (eg, unilateral decision-making, "double standard" behavior, controlling others without holding myself equally or more accountable)?

- When I become frustrated, anxious, irritable, and tired, do I take responsibility for my reactions to others, graciously trying to become part of the solution, or do I blame others (eg, expecting others to change/adjust to improve my moods and feeling states)?

Frequent self-assessment with these questions will provide an ongoing barometer of the degree to which your power and responsibility are in synch. Remember: Real power in leadership comes from your ability to generate loyal followership. Accordingly, the physician who does the best job of controlling himself in an authentically responsible fashion is most effective at influencing change in both people and circumstances.

Part Three: Practice Leaders Start With Themselves to Address Problem Behaviors

Dealing with conflicts arising from behavioral issues is an ongoing challenge for administrators. When these situations occur, each party (doctors and managers alike) is certain that the conflict is entirely someone else's fault. Generally speaking, even in the toughest issues described here, all involved parties have contributed to creating the issue. As a result, it is impossible to reach a successful resolution unless *everyone* is willing to step back and take a role in contributing to the needed solutions.

In order to get past the point of self-deception, someone (generally the administrator or MP) must proactively accept the reality of the problem, take ownership, and then take positive steps with all involved parties. This obliges setting aside time, building a foundation of trust, engaging in honest conversations, and active listening.

It is much easier for an administrator to ignore behavioral issues than deal with them. The provider exhibiting any of the adverse behaviors described here is likely your boss. Unfortunately these behavioral problems rarely resolve without intervention … they get worse and become more disruptive over time. It takes courage to lead, to be proactive, and especially to expose yourself to potential censure or termination by a physician you are trying to redirect.

As a leader, you *may* be able to positively influence the behavior of others, but you can absolutely control your own feelings and behaviors. When inappropriate behavioral issues first surface, don't wait for the provider who has acted out to spontaneously change. The provider involved may not be aware that their behavior is unacceptable. If your practice is saddled with a provider who was not sufficiently screened or oriented when they were hired, take the time to review expectations and goals, set boundaries and roles, and outline rules and consequences. Then, with progressive discipline, hold your providers accountable.

CHAPTER 25

Curing the Blahs

Has Your Practice Lost Its "Organizational Vigor"?

John B. Pinto

There's a time for backing off and slowing down the intensity with which you run your practice. The muggy "dog days" of summer are excuse enough for getting a little lazy and de-energized and hammock-bound. But taken to extremes in your practice, a lack of energy and vigor can put your enterprise at grave risk. Just a 10% drop in productivity—flowing from more vacation, lightening up your clinic loads, or taking a half-day off each week to sharpen your golf game—will result in a 20% or greater drop in profitability.

This wasn't always the case in ophthalmology, where 50+% profit margins, high allowable fees, and low operating costs allowed us all to "dog it" and still do just fine.

Pinto JB. *Ophthalmic Leadership: A Practical Guide for Physicians, Administrators, and Teams, Second Edition* (pp 155-159).
© 2022 SLACK Incorporated.

Loss of organizational vigor stems from many causes, sometimes business-based, often personal. Just one disengaged or mildly depressed manager or doctor can put the entire practice in a funk. Falling behind a competitor, which should stimulate you to dig deep, can lead some practice owners to quit trying. Certainly, the talk each year of pending fee cuts is enervating.

These personal and business sources of reduced vigor can leverage each other. I sometimes arrive on the scene after a practice has already entered a figurative "death spiral," from which it's hard to pull out.

Let's explore some practical ways you can re-invigorate yourself and your practice before you ever get to this point. As you'll read, the most effective cures for a stale practice either involve doing something more, something less, or something new … ultimately changing people, services, habits, or systems to shake things up.

• • •

Change Leadership

We hold national elections every 4 years. In much the same way, the average practice administrator is also employed for only about 4 or 5 years (a bit more if they win "re-election"). Such managers are rarely forced to move on because they are no longer competent—indeed, most go on to new heights of performance in their next practice. In most cases they move on because their strengths no longer coincide with the changing needs of the organization, or because the honeymoon is over and they have accumulated enough "black marks," fairly or unfairly, to no longer enjoy the board's confidence. It's the same for a practice's managing partners. If you have a case of the practice blahs, the first thing you should do is ask, "Is it time for fresh leadership here?" Sometimes it's not a matter of replacement, but reinvigoration. Sending your leaders to workshops and seminars can extend their tenure and their value to the organization.

Add a New Doctor, a New Service, or a New Office Location

Adding a young doctor to an older, solo surgeon's practice can be like adding a puppy to your household. At first, your old dog is gruff and growling, but with time he becomes more youthful and energetic. If you're in the doldrums, find something new to shake things up. This doesn't have to be a new doctor. Upgrading technology, adding a new testing modality, or learning a new surgical maneuver can breathe new life into bored providers and staff, while augmenting revenue. A new office location—even a half-day satellite a few miles away in an underserved geographic pocket—can get out the cobwebs.

Subtract a Service or Satellite

Perhaps your lack of energy is simple exhaustion. Sometimes practice perfection is more a matter of subtraction than addition. It's likely that 60% or more of your profits come from 40% or less of your practice's services. Closing a satellite office or winding down a low-volume, money-losing LASIK service may free up time, energy, and capital to focus on what you do best (and enjoy most).

Take a Sabbatical

Are you feeling stale? Almost ready for retirement but not yet willing to hang it up? Taking an extended break away from the practice may be an intelligent prescription, nothing less than 6 weeks and ideally 2 months or more. Yes, it's costly. But much less so than personal burnout or a continued low-grade failure to thrive with vigor in your profession. Most of the surgeons I know who take sabbaticals, even if they originally thought they were near retirement, come back with new ideas for their practice, vastly more energy than when they left, and a retirement calendar that has been pushed back by years.

Hold a Retreat

Sometimes your entire group needs to recharge. It's obviously not practical to take your collective workforce on sabbatical with you, but you can't afford ***not*** to periodically gather the troops for a long weekend to review strategies and operations and gird yourselves for the path ahead.

Provide Free Services Locally or Internationally

While it may sound counterintuitive that giving away free services will help you and your staff get recharged, almost nothing feels as great as helping others, and to do so with absolutely no compensation. You don't have to travel to Africa to get energized by mission work. Chances are great that within a 5-mile radius of your practice there are hundreds, if not thousands, of people who need your help desperately.

Track Your Numbers and Get Excited by Positive or Negative Trends

Whether the news is great or grim, you should track the metrics of your practice monthly. Routinely reviewing positive economic or volumetric performance can be a confidence-building springboard for even greater output. Negative news can be even more motivating. National leaders, from presidents to dictators, have long understood that fear is galvanizing. With all the dire reimbursement rumors floating about today, harness the resulting fear and use it to stimulate new levels of group and individual productivity. In addition, read up on trends in the industry and use adverse forecasts to motivate needed change.

Release Negative Staff or Doctors From Your Practice

While the judicious use of fear can be an effective leadership tool, too much scary talk will kill morale and stop practice performance in its tracks. Frank negativity or defeatism (ie, "times are not only tough, but hopelessly so") will only accelerate the adverse consequences of any rough patches your practice goes through. Reform or remove naysayers.

Make Staff Suggestions Mandatory

As an owner or manager, you may be running out of fresh ideas for practice improvement. Do not think you're the only ones responsible for original thinking. Create a culture which obliges one new idea per month from *every* staff member. Make the suggestions, as well as your feedback, public. And be sure to reward staff with a fair percentage of any resulting revenue enhancement or cost containment you achieve with implementation of the best ideas.

Identify Your Closest Competitor and Work to Best Them This year

In competitive sailing, sometimes it's hard to race the whole fleet. It's far better to just concentrate on gaining on the boat in front of you. It's probably impossible for you to know your competitor's revenue, their case volumes, or profits precisely, but you almost certainly know that they're ahead of *you* in the race. Catching up and pulling ahead will give you the confidence to then look ahead on the racecourse and find the next competitor to challenge.

Set a New Personal Goal That Will Force You to Change the Way You Practice

Prudent surgeons live on far less than their personal incomes. Because of this, there can be very little of the inner drive required to spur you on to new heights. The quickest way to solve this problem is to set a new personal goal. Clients who take up flying their own airplane, who dream of a spectacular vacation home, or who take up a time-consuming hobby instantly reset their internal measure of success and kick up their performance. As bourgeois as such dreams may be, supersizing your home to a mansion or upgrading from a prop plane to a jet forces you to adopt an entirely new and invigorating pace. If your personal passions require more time than money, working fewer hours will force the entire practice team to creatively increase productivity.

Start Building a Practice War Chest

Even if you're not exactly sure about the next business initiative you'll be undertaking, adopt the discipline to harbor capital reserves equivalent to 5% to 10% of annual profits. These funds can be kept within your corporate or partnership shell (talk to your tax advisor) or sequestered personally in an ear-marked fund. With tens or hundreds of thousands of dollars set aside, you'll look at business opportunities much less conservatively and will be more likely to leap at new projects with greater abandon (and less anxiety) than if you were funding out of today's cash flow or debt financing.

Take the Time to Dream

When you were younger, and your destiny was still quite unclear to you, you probably spent a lot of time staring out the window (when you should have been listening to your freshman chemistry professor) dreaming about what you would be when you grew up. Most adults are too busy to do this any longer. It takes a little discipline to return to the creativity of your youth. Perform this simple exercise. For the next month, block out one solid, 30-minute period every workday for unstructured thinking. Do this by arriving at the office 30 minutes early each day. Have a computer or yellow pad at hand and record any ideas that come up. Don't worry if the screen or page is blank for the first few sessions. Keep at it for 20 days, completely alone, even if it bores you. Chances are, this will be the most interesting and productive 10 hours you will spend all year.

CHAPTER 26

Is It Time to Replace or Tune Up Your Office Manager or Administrator?

John B. Pinto

Few practices stand still. In the past several years, some practices have grown rapidly with the fast-rising demand for geriatric services—even as LASIK volumes have cratered. Most practices have at least slowly increased in revenue and enterprise complexity. A few spiral downward, either by design (as when a doctor decides to slow down) or by neglect. Whatever the direction of change in your practice, it's unlikely the practice administrator who was a *perfect* fit when they were hired is still well-matched today.

Pinto JB. *Ophthalmic Leadership: A Practical Guide for Physicians, Administrators, and Teams, Second Edition* (pp 161-164).
© 2022 SLACK Incorporated.

Ensuring a Match

The skill sets of your practice manager or administrator should be in line with the needs of your practice today, as well as anticipated future needs. Let's say your practice's profit margins have been thinning for the past few years. The dip from 50% to 40% profits might have been barely noticed. But now the margins are approaching just 30%, the staff are overdue for another pay raise, and your aging office is ready for a facelift. You clearly have a *financial* problem. And you may need a new administrator or manager, with skill sets that line up with your most pressing kinds of problems. But in this example, you should discriminate. You may need a manager who has sharp accounting skills, who can contain costs. Or, you may really need a manager whose core competency is in marketing, to boost the top line of the practice, making the new costs more affordable.

Seven Warning Signs

Here are seven warning signs, by no means a complete list, that your ophthalmic practice manager may be in trouble.

1. *Your manager lacks a sufficiently broad skill set.* No manager is a complete package. The clichés are true: Strength in finance and accounting is classically antithetical to good human resource development skills. A manager with outstanding sales and marketing skills can be befuddled when looking at the bottom line. And outstanding strategic thinkers often overlook day-to-day operations. But to the extent possible, your manager should have balanced skills, and perhaps more importantly, the ability (and humility) to know when to call on outside expertise.
2. *Your manager is not sufficiently committed to their career.* It's ordinary for a practice manager to spend 50+ hours per week on the job, even in smaller practices. They should be among the first to arrive and among the last to leave. It's rarely helpful for a manager to work part-time, and be routinely missing on 1 or more days per week, unless the rest of the management team (the head tech, optical manager, patient accounts manager, etc) are extremely high-functioning and can work autonomously.
3. *Your manager has burned their bridges with staff or doctors.* Let's face it. Even the smallest practice is an emotionally and politically charged environment. Even a superior manager who starts out with 100 points may slowly have their leadership capacity diminished by the corrosive barbs of competing staff member or doctors. Enough judgment errors, and a harsh physician board may lose sufficient confidence in an administrator to let them work independently and do their job.
4. *Your manager has simply lost interest.* Talented managers need stimulation. If you have a mundane, no-growth practice, your manager may not have enough to do. Finding a special project or leasing your manager out to referring optometrists as a consultant may perk your manager up. Make sure your practice has objective performance benchmarks, which a manager can strive to reach to relieve their boredom.

5. *Your manager is in over their head.* The signals from a drowning manager are often overlooked. Competence can and should be measured. Are deadlines made, written down, and kept? Is your manager in command of the myriad details? Inasmuch as written and verbal skills are at the heart of management, does your manager have the communication skills (including *listening)* to be able to run the practice? Bluntly, are they smart enough for the job?
6. *Your manager fails to delegate.* Doctors are too quick to applaud super-hero managers who take on every detail of every project. One practice I serve is still recovering a year later from its loss of a manager who failed to delegate. Authority and responsibility should be sufficiently distributed throughout the practice so that no one person is "mission critical."
7. *Your manager fails to groom their eventual replacement.* As vital as an administrator is to your organization, it's critical that this manager work to continuously groom their understudy. Mentoring a junior manager in training is understandably skipped by insecure managers, and relished by strong, secure managers.

Terminate or Remediate?

It's quite common for physician-owners to wring their hands and delay making a decision about their faltering manager. Whatever you may say about the perfectionistic tendencies of ophthalmologists, at the core they usually have a soft heart and an aversion to conflict, which can drag out the "What are we going to do with Francis?" decision. When doing administrative remediation and recruitment work for clients, one of the first questions we explore is "How long has your current manager's performance been unsatisfactory?" The answer commonly exceeds a year.

The strongest practices don't make any fewer senior management hiring blunders, but they do make their mistakes *faster,* and are willing to fix or cut an underperforming manager. It may be perceived kindness to give "Francis" yet another try, but at the same time you may have 10, 20, or more staff members and their families (not to mention your own!) dependent on optimal performance at the top. It's lax leadership to put 10 or 20 careers in jeopardy just to avoid one confrontation. And such confrontation need not lead to termination.

It may be that your now underperforming manager was elevated to their position just a little too soon. Find an honorable way for them to step back into a more junior role for a few quarters or years. If your practice has grown rapidly, outpacing the career development pace of your relatively junior office manager, the easiest solution may be to bring in a more seasoned administrator and let that individual determine the best slot for your out-paced manager.

Perhaps your manager is not performing satisfactorily simply because they do not have performance guidelines. The basics should include a position description, a written set of operational enhancement goals for the next year, and specific financial targets for the practice. If your administrator does not have a roadmap and directions from the doctors, they are likely to drive your practice to an unintended destination.

The Rising Performance Bar for Managers

Practices are more complex, and have more moving parts, today than ever before. Happily, most managers, with the help of groups like the American Society of Ophthalmic Administrators, have all the resources they need to stay ahead.

The most common skill deficit I see for working managers (most of whom have come up through the ranks of the practice, and not through formal business training) is in the areas of finance, accounting, and budgeting. As fees continue to stagnate and slip and profit margins thin, it's imperative that both managers and managing partners develop real skills in this area.

The Rising Costs for Practices

When it's time for a new manager, the typical small (ie, two to five doctor) group practice is exchanging a $70,000 per year office manager for a $100,000+ per year administrator. This fact should feel as threatening to the underperforming manager as it feels encouraging to strong managers. For practices, there is an increasing mandate to secure competent management staff, because practices within a competitive market are no longer just competing doctor-to-doctor, but manager-to-manager for dominance. Managers must be given the time and dollar resources to attend meetings, take field trips to other successful practices, and purchase study materials. This, combined with higher base salaries, an increasing trend toward bonus compensation, and even equity participation for superior managers, is driving up costs for practices. I believe this will continue to contribute to a trend of the aggregation of some smaller practices into larger practices—organizations that can collectively afford exceptional management talent.

Increasingly, the practice with an underperforming manager will simply lack the one strategic asset that is increasingly the most needed to stay ahead, even if this same practice has superior clinicians, superior equipment, a great team of support staff, and a long history of past successes.

CHAPTER 27

"Can't I Just Manage My Own Practice?"

Alternatives to Employing a Practice Manager or Administrator

John B. Pinto

I've long written and lectured about the vital role that lay managers play in ophthalmic offices large and small. Indeed, as the medical management world continues to become vastly more complex and competitive, there is more need today than in the past to employ a competent administrator. Heck, some of my very good friends manage practices ... and I hope they're still friends after they read this.

That's because there's a reasonable counter-argument, that may read like heresy in a book dedicated in part to serving practice managers: *not every practice needs a manager.* In fact, there are a number of practices (some quite large) that seem to get along fine for years without an administrator on board.

Let's see if this counter-argument might apply to your practice.

Pinto JB. *Ophthalmic Leadership: A Practical Guide for Physicians, Administrators, and Teams, Second Edition* (pp 165-168).
© 2022 SLACK Incorporated.

One of the chief reasons for not having a lay manager is cost. The lay office manager or administrator does indeed cost a significant percent of practice revenue and profits.

As you can see from this table, there can be a strong incentive in smaller-scale practices to forego an office manager because their cost is an outsized percentage of collections (and profits). For the smallest practices, like the $500,000 practice shown, even though the cost is high, it's nearly always impractical to *not* have an office manager, because in such settings this person is not just a supervisor but is rolling their sleeves up and providing direct patient care or handling all of the billing work.

Practice Annual Collections	Typical Skill Level of Manager or Administrator	Typical Fully-Burdened Wage/Tax/Benefit Costs	Management Costs as a Percent of Practice Collections
$500,000	Low to moderate skills, often no formal business training	$50,000	10%
$1,000,000	Deeper skill-set, often coming from longer experience in the field	$65,000	6.5%
$2 million	More experience and special talents in areas of importance to the practice (eg, personnel, marketing, billing)	$90,000	4.5%
$5 million	Can often be the same person as found in a $2 million practice, but with longer work hours	$115,000	2.3%
$10+ million	Often highly sophisticated with masters-level education and many years of experience, strong financial background and the ability to work quite independently	$170,000+	Can be well under 2%

And it's similarly unrealistic at the other end of the spectrum to run a $10+ million, multidoctor practice without a savvy administrator, for several reasons. At this larger scale you need a sophisticated business head in-house. There are simply too many moving parts to be supervised by even the most engaged MP. And, with multiple doctors, you sometimes simply need a respected referee. Besides, as a percentage of collections and profits, the cost of a professional manager is relatively low.

For practices in-between these two extremes, and particularly for practices in the $2 million to roughly $5 million range, it has proven not only possible, but practical, to get by without an administrator. Several factors have to be aligned for this to be done successfully.

First, you need an extremely engaged doctor-owner who is willing to put in 8 hours or more per week as the MP of the practice. Next you need lots of communication, and much of this should move to the formality of putting more in writing: agenda and minutes for meetings, position descriptions, written project and to-do lists, and procedure manuals.

When operating without an administrator, it helps if you work in a less challenging environment, with lower growth rates, little external competition, and a minimum of doctor-to-doctor controversy within the practice.

In practices of this intermediate scale that forego having an administrator, you need a second tier of high-functioning middle managers; this will typically include department heads for the technical team, optical, reception and patient accounts, and marketing. Formal meetings are essential, with the MP and department heads gathering at least once a month—semi-monthly is better. Such meetings are so important that I now call running a practice administrator-free the "executive committee" model of practice administration.

There are several pathways leading a practice to going without an administrator. The most common in my experience is a series of failures in recruiting or keeping a manager. Such practices start out administrator-free by default, not by active choice. Other practices make an active choice to do without an administrator, or they wean themselves from having a manager as their administrator semi-retires and withdraws slowly.

The advantages of running a mid-sized practice without a designated administrator can be compelling:

- A "flatter" organization—one layer of management is removed
- Happier middle managers—who enjoy a direct reporting line to a doctor-owner rather than an intermediate supervisor
- Higher-functioning middle managers—because they have to learn to work more independently
- Lower costs and higher profits—you can bring a six-figure salary straight to the bottom line

Of course, there are downsides. Many practices without a strong administrator at the helm rely more heavily on outsourcing subject expertise in marketing, billing, or personnel management or other areas to management consultants. Used to excess, these external resources end up costing more than one competent, multidisciplinary administrator.

In my experience, most practices that operate without an administrator do so for a finite number of years, and then go back to the orthodoxy of a full-time administrator. They do this either because the MP's enthusiasm and time availability have waned, or because the practice has outgrown this administrative model. In many cases, practices that never really found the right person for this critical role, eventually come across a great candidate, and return to having a manager.

Chances are great that you really *do* need a professional manager on staff. However, as you should with every expensive practice resource, challenge that assumption regularly. Do you need a higher-level individual or is an MBA overkill for your solo practice? Do you need someone working full-time? Could you share your manager part-time with another compatible practice in the community and split the salary costs? Could your manager really cover your practice half-time, and sell hours on a consulting basis to other local practices, recouping a large percentage of her salary? I believe we'll increasingly see these and other creative approaches in the years ahead, as we strive to stay one step ahead of fee reductions and inflationary pressures that will be coming around the corner very soon.

CHAPTER 28

Questions to Ask Before Accepting Your *Next* Job as Practice Administrator

John B. Pinto

Good judgment comes from experience.
Experience comes from bad judgment.
—G. Warren Nutter, 1923 to 1979,
industrial and political economist

Until recently, the typical ophthalmic practice administrator changed jobs every 5 or 10 years, and some stayed on in the same position for decades. That may be changing. As the overall health care environment becomes more volatile, so too will your career fortunes.

Even as things stand today, over the course of the next 12 months, you probably have a 10% or greater chance that you will be looking for greener pastures. But as they say, the grass on the other side of the fence is not always greener. Sometimes it's Astroturf ... and sometimes its rocks and dirt clods.

Although I hope you're ecstatic about your present posting, and you'll never really need what follows, let's discuss how you can avoid one of the largest mistakes of your professional career and joining the wrong practice ... *just in case.*

Pinto JB. *Ophthalmic Leadership: A Practical Guide for Physicians, Administrators, and Teams, Second Edition* (pp 169-172).
© 2022 SLACK Incorporated.

Here are 10 signs to be aware of as you interview, and are interviewed by, your next practice.

1. Where is the practice going in the future? In the ideal practice you might consider joining as administrator, the partners meet annually to refine a 5- or 10-year plan. The practice collects robust data on not only internal trends, but also competing practice and regional institutions. Things are nearly as favorable if your prospective new board wants you to write a strategic or business plan early in your tenure. Only a minority of practices of any size ever have the discipline to write down their goals formally, so it's not a black mark against a practice if it doesn't yet have a plan. But beware the interviewer who tells you, "Oh, we don't go in for planning that much around here. We just run from week to week. The doctors are impossible to pin down, and even if they agreed for 1 day on a plan, they would get into a big argument about it the next day."
2. Are you an intense, career-focused leader who would love to help a practice grow 10% or more a year? Then be sure to ask your interviewer about the practice's historic and desired growth pace. Mismatched growth ambitions are a common source of frustration for doctors and managers, alike. And if your prospective employer says, "Yes, of course we want to grow ... as fast as possible," be sure to ask these follow-up questions:
    a. "Are the owners willing to forego income to make investments back into the practice, or is this the kind of practice where every available dollar of profit is withdrawn as doctor compensation?"
    b. "Are the owners comfortable with the kind of overt promotion that growth may oblige?"
    c. "Are the owners willing to put in extracurricular time for outreach, community lectures, staff training, and everything else needed to grow?"
3. If you're a finalist for any administrative position, you should ask for and receive a copy of the practice financials. If any practice is unwilling to share these (even an eyes-only copy), walk away ... you can't trust an employer who is so uncertain about their judgment of people that they can't trust you. Look over the balance sheet. The total assets (inclusive of the recoverable accounts receivable, which is sometimes left off such documents) should materially exceed the total liabilities. The "quick ratio" (simplistically, current assets divided by current liabilities ... if this term is unfamiliar to you, click on http://en.wikipedia.org/wiki/Quick_ratio) should materially exceed 1.0. What if you examine the books and find that the practice has $200,000 in current assets and $400,000 in current liabilities, or a quick ratio of 0.5? Unless you are professionally prepared to take on a frank turnaround situation, run.
4. Practice profit margins (defined as profit available for MD/DO compensation divided by total practice collections) should be at or above 30% for an urban or similar high-cost/low-pay general ophthalmology practice, and most subspecialists. This figure should be 35% or higher in suburban and rural settings. Retinal practices should have a 40% or higher profit margin. If your prospective practice has lower profit margins, it's like an airplane flying close to the ground ... any pilot error can quickly result in a crash landing.

5. Staff mood and morale, and the overall tone of the practice is harder to gauge than numbers, but what do you feel when you walk in the office? Are staff warm and welcoming, shy, or worse—aloof? Trust your gut. If the vibes are wrong, look elsewhere. You can train staff to do any task for the practice … but you can't train them to be happy. Ultimately there are only two kinds of people, "givers" and "takers." Choose a practice and a board of doctors that is generous and giving. Past is almost always prelude. What's been the fate of your predecessors? Odds are, their fate will likely be yours in a few years.
6. Beyond the ambitions and skills of the owner-physicians, the most important predictor of practice success is the local population to provider to ratio. We now have about 20,000 people in America for each actively working ophthalmologist. If you are considering offers from two otherwise-equivalent employers in two different markets, select the practice with the more favorable ratio. Here's an example. Denver has about 8000 people per ophthalmologist and is terribly competitive—not only are there fewer customers to go around, but local managed care organizations can readily pit one practice against the other for lower costs. This is compounded by a more youthful market (with fewer older adults and less eye disease to treat).
7. Owner age distribution and succession factors can be a major go/no-go factor when evaluating a new practice. This is obviously not a problem if you would be working with a young soloist or with a larger group where ages are widely ranged. But for all other practices you would like to see that succession is not going to pose an undue difficulty in the years ahead. This is particularly critical in practices located in less-attractive markets, where ophthalmologist recruitment is becoming much more difficult of late. If you have 20 years left in your own career and are taking a job as the administrator of a practice of four docs in their late 60s … in northern Michigan … you had better have a back-up plan.
8. Your potential employer's attitude toward capital equipment, office facilities, and similar high-ticket investments should be critically reviewed before you accept a job. This is a classic, too-hot, too-cold "Goldilocks" issue. Excess outlays for all the latest gadgets is poor policy, especially at the current crossroads of the profession. But it's equally poor business judgment to underinvest in the practice. If you think the current office facilities are cramped and shopworn, just consider how shabby and frayed your own career will become in a few years working there.
9. Are you underqualified for the job? Too much responsibility, too soon in your career, will lead to frustration for your employer and failure for you. At the other end of the spectrum, you may be inclined to accept too little responsibility, either because of burnout from a prior position or simply because of the present environment where jobs are more scarce. Try to match your experience and career commitment with the needs of the practice, erring slightly on the side of a bit more than you can handle today to stimulate your own growth and development as an executive.

10. Owner harmony is an obvious basis for judging a potential practice to join. Does the practice have an MP, which can make your job as administrator vastly more effective than reporting to eight separate doctors? What's the practice's communication and conflict resolution style? Some practices will serially hire a string of new managers hoping to find someone who can keep the doctors in line or somehow "make" everyone behave like adults. Even if you arrive with a degree in psychology and a whip, your effectiveness will be far less than if you can start out with a group of mature adults who communicate in an accountable fashion, and who have a history of working out tough problems as a team.

• • •

In going over this list you may not only find a few pearls to help you make your *next* career decision but, even better, ferret out those aspects of your current position that are least satisfactory, so you can make improvements and stay put.

Be sure to see the big picture. If any one or two of these factors are adverse, but everything else is swell, the prospective job may still represent a great career move. Indeed, if you are an uber-manager and ready for a challenge, the most adverse factors outlined here may actually signal a great fit.

CHAPTER 29

From Bench to Boardroom

The Path From Scientist to CEO

Adrienne Graves, PhD

This chapter ends with five pearls for leadership, but I'd like to provide you with a context for how I arrived at these.

It was during my undergraduate days at Brown University that I developed an interest in visual science. Intrigued by a course on sensory processes, I went on to do my first vision research project during my senior year. I remember being thrilled to hang out with graduate students in a dark basement laboratory. I was running an experiment on the "McCollough Effect," a curiously persistent color aftereffect. I became passionate about the research and the challenges of understanding the complexities of the visual system. I felt certain that I was embarking on an exciting path of vision research in the academic world.

Pinto JB. *Ophthalmic Leadership: A Practical Guide for Physicians, Administrators, and Teams, Second Edition* (pp 173-177).
© 2022 SLACK Incorporated.

As it turns out, I was indeed going down an exciting path, albeit one with some significant hairpin turns. I did pursue my passion for vision research, but as a young scientist I had no idea that I would eventually do this from within the business world. And I certainly had no idea that I would end up one day as a corporate CEO.

So, how did this happen? Here's a brisk look at my journey from scientist to CEO, with experiences along the way that prepared me for a spot in the boardroom.

Following My Research Passions

After graduating from Brown, I spent a year in Boston working for Dr. Anne Fulton, a pediatric ophthalmologist at Harvard Medical School and Children's Hospital. I helped set up Dr. Fulton's electrophysiology lab and learned to assist her in clinical electroretinography. It was an exciting year in many ways—it reinforced my passion for vision research and sparked an enduring interest in clinical visual disorders.

In the quest to follow my research passions, I applied to PhD programs in visual science. I chose the University of Michigan for its excellence in ophthalmology and visual science, particularly its interdisciplinary vision research programs. I was fortunate to have Dr. Daniel Green as my advisor and mentor. Dr. Green was working on electrophysiological studies of the retina, and had appointments in ophthalmology, electrical engineering, and psychology.

After working for a year on Dr. Green's studies of retinal adaptation, he encouraged me to find my own particular research passion. At the time, stepping beyond my mentor's research guidance was daunting ... but it ended up further enhancing my love of science. I became fascinated with Hubel and Wiesel's studies of visual deprivation and development (for which they later earned a Nobel Prize). For my PhD thesis I developed and studied an animal model for anisometropic amblyopia—a topic completely different from my advisor's field.

While I was writing up the results and putting my dissertation together, I was invited to give a presentation at a vision research conference in Belgium. It was there that I met scientists from the University of Paris, who—remarkably to me at the time—invited me to join their lab for my postdoctoral studies. The thought of living in Paris provided an instant motivation to rapidly finish my thesis: *Behavioral Studies of Spatial Vision in Normal and Amblyopic Cats.*

The Paris Experience

Moving to Paris opened up new worlds for me in many ways. It certainly reinforced my passion for visual science. I began my postdoc at the Visual Neuroscience Laboratory at the University of Paris, combining psychophysical and electrophysiological methods to study the development of depth perception in cats.

Life in Paris was exhilarating—it is a stunningly beautiful city and I loved exploring its many treasures. I was exposed to high fashion, foie gras, wine that actually tasted good, and fascinating people from culturally diverse backgrounds. Learning

French, however, proved to be more challenging than I had imagined. It was agonizing to maneuver relatively ordinary tasks (eg, finding an apartment, opening a bank account) with rudimentary French. I gradually made progress (painfully slowly, or so it seemed) and eventually was able to speak French proficiently. But even so, I knew I wasn't able to express myself as eloquently or as precisely as I could in English. It's hard to be as quick or as witty when speaking a foreign language. That realization has stayed with me, and I believe it has given me an empathy for those who must do business, discuss complex issues, or negotiate while speaking a foreign tongue. Many years later I would stress to employees that an understanding and compassion for the language challenges of nonnative speakers is critical to working effectively in a global business environment.

The Business World Calls

As I was starting my third year in Paris, I received an unexpected call from a recruiter in the United States. When she said she was representing a pharmaceutical company in Ft. Worth, Texas, I was taken aback. I didn't know anything about the pharmaceutical business or about Texas! But when she told me that her client, Alcon, wanted to hire a scientist to start a visual function laboratory, I was intrigued. So off I flew to Texas for an interview ... and so began a ***serious*** turn in the road for me in a number of ways. I had never even considered working in industry. At the time I didn't know any other visual scientists who had chosen the industry path, but I saw the Alcon job as an opportunity to pursue vision research in a new setting.

When I started at Alcon, some aspects of my work didn't change. I was still doing basic research, interacting with visual scientists and ophthalmologists, and attending some of the same scientific conferences. But the new and exciting part was that I was expanding my research interests. I quickly learned that glaucoma was the largest market within ophthalmic pharmaceuticals, so I began to learn as much as I could about the pathophysiology of glaucoma and the animal models for studying it.

Since I had some experience with animal psychophysics, I thought it might be possible to teach Alcon's glaucomatous monkeys to perform an automated perimetry task; that would allow us to correlate their IOPs with their visual fields, look at therapeutic responses, and eventually correlate these data with anatomical findings. I contacted Drs. Ron Harwerth and Earl Smith at the University of Houston, who were friends and colleagues from my early graduate school days. Experts in animal psychophysics, they were immediately excited by the "monkey perimetry" challenge. They modified a Humphrey field analyzer and successfully trained monkeys to fixate on central and peripheral visual stimuli. This led to a wealth of investigations on visual functions (eg, perimetry, color vision, ERGs, contrast sensitivity) and corresponding ganglion cell losses in monkeys with experimental glaucoma.

I was thoroughly enjoying life in the pharmaceutical business. I was still immersed in vision research, but was able to broaden my scientific interests and knowledge base. More importantly, I became fascinated with clinical trial design and the drug development process. I was fortunate to be given roles in clinical development, project management, and in liaison positions with sales and marketing teams internationally. The opportunity to learn key components of the pharmaceutical industry was stimulating and rewarding—like getting a PhD all over again.

A "Start-Up" Opportunity

After 9 years at Alcon, I joined Santen Inc—a US subsidiary (newly formed at the time) of Japan's Santen Pharmaceuticals. Although the company had a 100+ year history in Japan, US operations were just beginning. This was a huge move for me in many ways. At Alcon I was part of an established infrastructure, but at Santen I joined a small team of 10 employees before the headquarters had even been built. Why did I take this chance?

I saw the move as a unique opportunity to help start a company, develop its first products, and build a team from scratch—without some of the financial risks typically associated with start-ups. And it was a chance to more directly see the impact of my contributions.

I started putting together a research and development (R&D) team and rapidly initiated clinical development in the United States. Despite being an extremely small group, we received our first FDA approval less than 5 years later. From that point we achieved three FDA approvals in less than 4 years. Along the way I was given the responsibility for Global Clinical Development at Santen, and I began managing the groups in Japan, Europe, and the United States.

Seven years after joining Santen, I was asked to take on the role of President and CEO of Santen Inc. This was *truly unexpected,* and my first reaction was to decline. I had never thought about running a company and I wondered whether I could be an effective CEO. None of the CEOs I knew were scientists.

Scientist as CEO?

As I considered my decision, I thought about the role of CEO and discussed it with leaders in our field. A well-known executive pointed out that a CEO has to be comfortable with uncertainty and problem-solving ... skills a scientist has honed. Scientists relish questions and challenges, and typically have strong analytical skills. However, scientists usually like to delve into a single topic and understand it as thoroughly as possible; scientists tend to be uncomfortable making pronouncements without "sufficient data," while a CEO rarely has complete information when making decisions. Fortunately, I had left bench science many years earlier, and had already developed and embraced a broader, outward-looking perspective.

The CEO Role: Opportunities and Challenges

Taking on the CEO role was initially intimidating, but it led to a steady stream of experiences and learning opportunities—and certainly many challenges. I had run R&D

organizations and had interacted for many years with sales, marketing, business development, and manufacturing functions, but the CEO role required a change of focus.

A major challenge was immersing myself and learning key aspects of the non-R&D functions. However, I found that a passion for learning, along with a genuine interest in understanding the components of our business, made for an exhilarating time. A willingness to ask questions—even when they seemed basic—was probably quite helpful. I think this came naturally to me, since scientific training is essentially about asking questions, identifying missing information, and figuring out how to get answers.

There were also challenges in managing multiple functions and being comfortable with the role of overall leader. While I had managed groups previously, they had all been related to my own expertise. As CEO, the ability to assemble the right talents and then rely on their expertise is key. A priority for me was building an executive team with not only the proper experience, but also a passion for working together to grow the company. It took me some time to realize and embrace the fact that I was not just a member of the team—I was now leading it. While many of my decisions continued to be consensus-based, being CEO required me to actively set the tone in terms of strategic decisions and corporate culture. It seems obvious to me now, but it was an interesting part of transitioning to the CEO role.

Despite the numerous challenges, I came to realize that scientific training was in many ways an advantage in running a pharmaceutical company. What skills can a scientist bring to the CEO role?

1. *The ability to embrace and enjoy problem solving.* A CEO faces a series of "problems" on a daily basis. Scientists have learned to be comfortable with unknowns and new challenges.
2. *Comfort with research.* As a scientist I was interested in learning about new research findings, examining new technologies, and assessing the challenges faced by the R&D team. Science is still the foremost element in a pharmaceutical company. It is a significant advantage for a pharma/biotech CEO to have a keen interest in and understanding of science.
3. *Paying particular attention to the pipeline.* The lifeblood of a pharmaceutical company is its pipeline. Having a passion for exploring new opportunities is key, as is an informed expectation for the likelihood of success of any given project.
4. *Flexibility and openness to change.* Good science starts with a hypothesis, but great science happens when one can recognize an unexpected result and act on it. Many breakthrough discoveries were unintended consequences that only a keen and unbiased observer could see. I believe that comfort with the "unexpected" translates well in the business world. Planning is essential—but news about a competitor, economic changes, or new regulatory hurdles can rapidly alter a plan's course. The ability to recognize and incorporate new information is key to successful operations.
5. *Passion for learning and discovery.* As a scientist, vision research still excites me, as does understanding disease processes better in order to develop new therapies. It has been thrilling to experience numerous advances in ophthalmology, but there are still unmet needs in major areas, including glaucoma, retina, and dry eye. Following the research advances in ophthalmology—and having the opportunity to influence the development of sight-saving therapies—is still a thrill.

Section III

Leadership's Nuts, Bolts, and Basic Training

CHAPTER 30

The Mission

How the Physician-Leader Can Help Keep Staff Focused

Paul N. Arnold, MD

The sole meaning of life is to serve humanity.
—Leo Tolstoy

Vision leads the leader. Vision comes from within the leader. True vision must meet others' needs.
—John C. Maxwell in *Qualities of a Leader*

I don't know what your destiny will be, but one thing I know: The only ones among you who will be really happy are those who will have sought and found how to serve.
—Dr. Albert Schweitzer

Begin with the end in mind. What is the goal of your medical practice? What is the mission of your unique practice of ophthalmology?

There is a profound link between pursuing your purpose in life, your mission, and experiencing happiness on this earth. With a sports team, there must be an understanding of the goal and selfless teamwork. In your practice, there must be an understanding of the goal of the practice and how each staff member works together to accomplish that goal. And just as each team has a coach or team-leader, the practice must have an acknowledged leader. Who better to provide "the big picture" goal than the physician-owner of the practice? Who has a greater stake in getting everyone to row together in the same direction than the physician-owner?

Pinto JB. *Ophthalmic Leadership: A Practical Guide for Physicians, Administrators, and Teams, Second Edition* (pp 181-186).
© 2022 SLACK Incorporated.

As one who works alongside the staff caring for patients, answering for scheduling and billing problems, the doctor is also the best member of the team to relate to staff how all "the little things" fit into the big picture. Communication is key. The doctor cannot put the practice on autopilot, assuming that someone else (eg, the administrator, section supervisor) will guide the practice according to the vision they have for the practice. The physician-leader must take responsibility for communicating this vision to everyone.

Our mission in a medical practice is to serve patients. The staff can serve patients directly and indirectly—that is, personally *and* by helping the physician to serve patients better (indirectly). One way of defining every staff position is "to help the doctor help patients." With this in mind, the receptionist can see how she must not only compassionately care for each patient presenting to the front desk, but must also schedule the follow-up appointment in such a way that the patient won't have to wait inordinately to see the doctor because the schedule was over booked, frustrating the doctor as well as the patient. The technician can see how getting accurate information in the work up serves not only the patient, but helps the doctor decide on appropriate therapy in a timely fashion.

We not only serve patients personally and by helping the doctor, but we serve them as a corporation. Our business can serve them in the community—by supporting worthy eye-related proceedings, by donating to worthy causes as a practice, and by sponsoring cultural events that sustain the whole community.

However, all of this service to patients must begin with an understanding of your unique practice mission. Once again, that requires communicating your vision to your staff.

This type of communication is obviously easier in a smaller practice. For the sake of this discussion, let's assume a single physician practice or one with a clear physician-owner. All of the points I will be making can be extrapolated to a larger practice by adjusting the frequency and scale of the meetings. Ah, that dreaded word, "meetings"! Communication in a medical office cannot take place without meetings. So let's discuss them.

What is the best interval for staff meetings? Every day! Or, as frequently as is practical for the office. There are different types of meetings made of different groups of staff. Allow me to outline the meetings that should be held regularly:

1. *Daily "stand-up" meetings.* These are called "stand-up" meetings because they are meant to last no longer than 15 minutes, and may be as short as 5 minutes. On days the physician-leader is in the clinic, they may lead them; on days the physician is in surgery, another doctor or the administrator or office manager may guide the discussion.

   The focus of the stand-up meeting is simple—analyze what the schedule looks like today and how the flow of patients worked yesterday. Focus on problems and solutions. Highlight jobs well done, suggest improvements for errors or inadvertent predicaments, discuss the best way to handle problem patients. Relate these to your vision and values (more on that later).

The stand-up meeting is a good way to teach staff how to prepare for certain patients and how to anticipate your needs in performing particular procedures. This preparation will help streamline patient flow through your day, and the education will help improve future days.

In a smaller practice, the stand-up should involve all staff. In larger practices, they may just be a gathering of the "front (administrative) office" or "back (clinical) office" with their respective departmental supervisors.

2. *Weekly "management meetings."* The physician-leader should gather all the team leaders together to make sure they are all working together interdepartmentally. This is where issues involving coordination between different sections of the practice can be ironed out. Personnel issues can be brought to light and discussed. The needs of various departments may be opened for insight from other leaders of the practice.

   If the various departments are not meeting on a daily "stand-up" basis, they should meet with their team leader on a weekly basis. This is where topics from the management meeting may be brought to the other staff of those specific departments. Furthermore, the staff from each section can bring to their team leader issues that might need to get back to the other leaders at the next management meeting.

   In larger practices, the management meeting may be held with all physicians or partners of the practice. If this proves too unwieldy, the physician director or president may be sufficient to provide the physicians' representation. Really large groups may have an executive committee of three to five partners who help direct the managers at such meetings.

3. *Monthly "sit-down" staff meetings.* These are so-called because the whole staff gathers and sits together. These meetings last longer and get into more detail about issues affecting the practice. They may last from 30 to 60 minutes. It is necessary to temporarily close the office and turn the phones over to an answering service, so that no one is absent from the meeting nor is anyone distracted by immediate patient care.

   This type of meeting allows the practice leaders to delve further into the details of particular issues, like coding, the new EMR system, clinical educational issues, the financial health of the practice, technical training, the new doctor, etc. These are educational opportunities for the entire staff. By devoting time and attention to developing the skills and knowledge of your staff, they will better assist you, the physician, and more effectively serve your patients. Practices with more than 50 employees may find it difficult to meet with everyone on a monthly basis. Quarterly gatherings can serve the same purpose. Find a large hall or auditorium that you can use for these big group meetings. Providing lunch or breakfast can serve as an incentive for attendance at the sit-down meetings no matter how large the group.

4. *Monthly "doctor meetings."* In a practice with three or more doctors, it is wise to hold a doctors meeting at least monthly. In busy offices, there may not be enough quality time to exchange more than the standard pleasantries with your physician coworkers. We need to talk seriously to our partners about the business. These discussions

may focus on larger strategic issues, as well as clinical and personnel topics. Even if no big issues require discussion, keeping the lines of communication open between physicians is helpful. Some groups find it useful to meet for a regular breakfast or lunch on a particular day each month, for example, a "first Friday lunch." In larger groups, the physician partners may divide the practice business responsibilities: the "numbers guru" could serve as the primary financial analyst, the most relationship oriented partner could take on the personnel management, the most "handyman" of the group might take the lead on plant and equipment issues, etc. These doctor meetings are a good time to report to each other on these topics to keep everyone up to speed.

5. *One-on-one meetings.* These may be planned, regular meetings that the physician-leader has with particular staff (eg, the administrator, the ASC director, the optical director) or may be ad hoc with any staff member who may have a concern that requires the physician-leader's attention. Providing big picture direction is an essential asset for the physician-leader. While it is very important to delegate the proper responsibility to each of these departmental leaders, being a sounding board or provider of second opinions for your directors is another advantage of these one on ones. If possible, a daily meeting with the administrator is beneficial. This can be a good way to wrap up the day for both parties, especially if there has been a stand-up meeting to start the day. The exchange of information might include things like staff performance, the flow of the schedule that day, the day's collections, or the status of any ongoing project. At the very least, this meeting should take place weekly.

   The practice may incorporate other business entities. If so, the physician-leader should meet one-on-one with the ASC director and optical director once a week, when possible. These meetings allow you to focus on particular issues without burdening the rest of the management team with some of the arcane details of these unique departments.

I should emphasize the distinction between "micromanaging" and providing direction. Delegation within the practice is necessary, but delegation does not mean the doctor can abdicate responsibility for leadership. The physician-leader must provide the framework within which the manager manages.

The physician-leader should see another purpose in these meetings—to master the art of listening. These are the best opportunities for staff to express their insights and observations to you. These are prime opportunities for you to learn about each staff member, their unique characteristics. Without knowing your audience, it is very difficult to communicate effectively. Seek first to understand, then to be understood.

The physician-leader's job is to help keep everyone focused on the goal, to keep everyone marching in the same direction, to keep everyone singing from the same sheet of music. Without a unified vision, each staff member heads off in a different direction, creating disunity in the practice. With an authoritative road map, questions and conflicts can be resolved more easily, and staff and patients know what to expect from everyone in your practice.

Where does that roadmap or that sheet of music come from? It is essential to develop the *practice vision,* or *mission statement,* with the help of key staff members. This should be a one-sentence embodiment of the big picture goal of your practice. Example: "The team at Arnold Vision seeks to provide the highest quality of vision restoration in a caring, supportive setting."

In addition to the *vision,* it's important to elaborate a set of *values*—characteristics that should guide and exemplify all members of your team (ie, quality, state of the art, caring, personal, professional, comforting, patients first…). Certain aphorisms can illustrate these values (ie, High Tech—High Touch; People don't care how much you know until they know how much you care; Cure sometimes, but Care always; The little things don't mean much—they mean everything!).

Development of the practice vision and values is a process.

Begin by putting together a small team of key employees, especially those who have worked in the practice for some time and understand the general culture of the physician-leader and the practice. It is fine for the doctor to start the process with this committee, letting them know what the goal of this exercise is, and how you will go about accomplishing it. They may guide the group along by asking Socratic questions about the mission and values the committee members see as the heart and soul of the practice. The administrator is usually the best person to chair this group, to see the process through to completion.

Once the committee has hammered out the mission statement and list of key values, the paper goes to the full staff for review and critique. After obtaining staff feedback, the document is finalized and presented to the entire staff as the practice's statement of guiding principles.

• • •

After production of the practice *vision and values,* they must be put into action. Never just post this statement in the break room and forget about it! Do post it in a prominent place so that all staff will regularly see it. Review it at meetings—ask individual staff members to recite the mission statement, or describe what one of the practice values is and what that means to them. Refer back to it when discussing ongoing issues or projects, show the staff how this or that action relates to the vision and values of the practice.

Most importantly, let the staff know that these are the objective standards that they will be evaluated by in their job reviews. The formal job description is the basic measure of performance, but all employees should also be held to the standard of the vision and values of the practice. Every team leader reviewing a staff member should employ this standard. Without knowledge of the mission, no one will know if it has been accomplished.

The physician-leader must be the embodiment of these values. We've all heard the truisms: lead by example, practice what you preach. Nothing will render your guiding principles moot faster than a leader who does not try to live them. Expediency is a corrosive—do the hard right thing rather than the easy dishonest thing.

Another potential pitfall for the physician-leader is vacillation. If one is regularly changing the meaning of what defines "true north" for the practice, the staff will be lost. Consistency is a virtue in leaders. You must be an accurate compass for your staff and patients.

Do not worry about achieving perfection in leading your staff. Frank Lloyd Wright seemed to think doctors had it easier than architects when he said, "The physician can bury his mistakes, but the architect can only advise his client to plant vines." Perhaps our staff, in following the practice's vision and values, can be like the vines that conceal our imperfections.

In summary, the job of the physician as a leader is to help define the practice mission and help keep the staff focused on the achievement of that goal. This is best obtained by regular, effective communication with your staff and by your own excellent example.

CHAPTER 31

Effective Practice Leadership

Balancing Authority, Power, and Responsibility

Craig N. Piso, PhD and John B. Pinto

The price of greatness is responsibility.
—Winston Churchill

You can delegate authority but not responsibility.
—Stephen Comiskey

With great power there must come great responsibility.
—The Official Spider-Man Credo

Most of the chapters in this book have been prompted by workplace challenges that every client surgeon faces to one degree or another. This chapter is no exception.

Let's explore a West Coast ophthalmic setting, where we have highly experienced and committed surgeons who have been trying—without result—to help their manager find the right balance between tough and fair ... between the authority and power and bluster needed to get the job done, and the responsibility and sensitivity it takes to use that power wisely.

At the roots of every practice challenge, a unified board needs to establish every policy and goal for the company. Each of these policies and goals should advance the interests of the company, and not the unilateral interests of individual

Pinto JB. *Ophthalmic Leadership: A Practical Guide for Physicians, Administrators, and Teams, Second Edition* (pp 187-191).
© 2022 SLACK Incorporated.

doctors. Once the board's desired outcomes are clear—and clearly well-intended—the administrator carries the ball going forward. But managers in today's enlightened world are not just mute executors. They have a duty to challenge their boards to better decision making.

If a practice manager disagrees with his board, he has three progressive, step-wise choices. First, he can raise concerns backed up by facts and attempt to secure a revision of policy. This is a vital, valuable duty of any administrator and should be welcomed by every board.

If a revision is not secured, the competent administrator will next typically accept the policy and support it publicly and vigorously. If a policy is deemed by the administrator to be illegal or materially against company interests, and it cannot be changed, the administrator has a duty to leave the organization.

A board's goals are always going to fall into two crisp domains: *objective* goals (eg, collections, patient volumes, profit margins, market influence, staffing levels, service mix), and *subjective* goals (eg, working environment, morale, style of operation, tone of the office, and the like).

The administrator's ability to understand and achieve the desired practice outcomes is always tougher for the subjective goals. Everyone can agree on what a 40% profit margin looks like and can measure it. It's harder to communicate what's meant by staff harmony or high morale or empowerment. This softer, subtle, subjective domain of management is what trips up most administrators and MPs to one degree or another. They key is understanding the balance between power and responsibility.

In any healthy individual or system, *power* and *responsibility* are proportionate attributes, counterbalancing each other. As we empower any staff member, we create the reasonable expectation of holding that person accountable in like measure. A lot of this rests on effective communication. It behooves both lay managers and medical leaders in group practices—especially larger groups where communication can get quite tangled—to understand the principles of effective communication and information sharing.

Here are 10 principles of communication with doctors and staff (and every other audience segment your practice has, including patients, vendors, and payers) to help you to create a more powerful and effective professional team.

1. *Communicate in a direct, timely manner.* Commit to face-to-face discussion of difficult issues, rather than "splitting" or "triangulating" (ie, complaining to others while avoiding confrontation and/or conflict). Address issues in a timely manner, rather than allowing them to fester. The courageous commitment to having what some have called "fierce conversations," with everything put on the table in person, ironically, creates an increased sense of safety/security because the process leaves no stone unturned and most often results in logical resolution of issues and greater stability. Scary, but effective.
2. *Present a united, positive front.* Always represent the best interests of the practice and its governance, even when problems are apparent and still unresolved. Just as parents do well to support each other, especially when a complaining child attempts to stir strife at the top of the family pecking order by turning one parent

against the other, don't allow anyone to play "divide and conquer" with you and your partners. Understand and respect the power of words to help or hinder any initiative that you oversee. Never publicly diminish the authority of your MP, administrator, or supervisors. This will only expose an Achilles heel at which others will predictably shoot more arrows, undermining individual performance and ultimately harming the company.

3. *Keep the jury out.* Give the benefit of the doubt regarding any negative report you hear about a person, including peers, administration, patients, or other providers. Reserve judgment until all of the required facts are understood, thereby restraining the urge to reach closure prematurely, especially under the strain of intense feelings such as anger, frustration, and worry. As you develop this aspect of emotional intelligence, you show others how to "let cooler heads prevail." There is power in rationale thinking and behavior, often requiring silence and dispassionate reflection.
4. *Uphold the chain of command.* The organizational chart defines roles and reporting relationships with an explicit chain of command structure through which power and control are to be mobilized. Strict adherence to this chain of command is essential for the support and continued empowerment of every position in the hierarchy. Therefore, ensure in every communication that no manager or supervisor is overlooked or bypassed, because doing so renders them less effective—especially in the eyes of the person(s) who succeed in nullifying their authority. For example, if someone complains to you without first having broached their complaint with their immediate supervisor, redirect them to their supervisor with the clear expectation that they will handle their situation competently. Should that not be the case, schedule a meeting of all relevant parties and discuss the matter transparently toward resolution, always supporting the supervisor in question, especially in front of the staff.
5. *Let your word be your bond.* Always mean what you say and say what you mean. Without exception, demonstrate an unwavering commitment to cultural integrity through your honesty, transparency, and authenticity. People will then listen to what you say with trust and confidence. Your impeccable honesty engenders trust, and trust produces followership and loyalty, which are basic sources of power for any practice leader. Maintain confidences, keep your promises, take responsibility when appropriate, and apologize when you're mistaken. Follow these prescriptions faithfully and people will more faithfully heed your words.
6. *Walk the power/responsibility talk.* Speak frequently about this dynamic when explaining the rationale for your decisions and actions. For example, "Because of the consistent manner in which Jane has made effective choices (ie, exercised her *power)* to succeed at projects, I recommend her for this promotion with expanded duties (ie, *responsibilities)*." Conversely, the same principle applies when communicating about negative performance or behavior: "Jane, you are being terminated (ie, being held accountable) as the result of your choice to belittle your supervisor to a vendor after being warned repeatedly and in writing that the next infraction of this sort would result in your loss of employment here."

7. *Use the power of focus.* Recognize that our focus upon people and things tends to expand, either positively or negatively, influencing how we interact with them. For example, a steady focus upon another person's faults only serves to expand our sense of their faults, creating tension and a vicious circle. We become more effective when we maintain a focus on those things that contribute most to our goals, rather than letting ourselves become distracted by lesser or counterproductive things. In your communications, therefore, create and maintain a positive outlook and focus. Help your people shift their focus in ways that support their successful actions and create a more positive work environment. For example, when a staff member is complaining about their struggles and problems, real or imagined, help them by shifting their attention toward what is working, their available resources, potential solutions, their choices, and options, rather than perpetuating the negative focus in which they have become stuck.
8. *Convey positive expectations.* There is a powerful relationship between hope and energy. Energy (motivation) comes from the core dreams that we hold deep within ourselves. The more important and realistic the dream, the more energy that is produced, thus enabling us to pursue our goals with sustained drive and commitment. The familiar concept of a "self-fulfilling prophecy" is the process of living up (or down) to expectations expressed by others. Effective managers make conscious efforts to instill hope in their people—hope about their goals, their potential, and their long-term success and fulfillment. If you genuinely believe in and express the unique strengths and untapped potential of your people, then they naturally feel the contagiousness of your positive view of them. For example, when someone says, "I just can't figure this one out," a helpful reply is, "You will, you just haven't figured it out yet."
9. *Model and require courageous action.* Too often people at work put off doing the very things that are most important for their success and happiness, simply because they are afraid of failure, discomfort, or change. Strong, resilient leaders show the habit of acting in real time to solve problems and to complete key tasks, rather than procrastinating or wishing away their problems and projects. It is this quality of reframing adversity as opportunity and maintaining faith that you will prevail in the end that separates exceptional from average leaders. Similarly, excellent managers require their staff to find the courage to follow their example in order to meet the challenges that they face. Insist that courage is not the absence of fear when challenged—that would be a superhuman expectation. Instead, courage is taking decisive action in the presence of fear, giving all of us mere mortals a green light to act (even when our knees are buckling) in order to get things accomplished.
10. *Influence change.* Expressing empathy and understanding with staff is the most important communication skill that a manager can demonstrate in order to influence the changes you desire. This begins with the willingness to listen to what others have to say and giving genuine respect to their ideas and opinions, even when they are quite different from your own. It means meeting people where they are (pacing to their tempo) before attempting to move them where you want them to go (ie, leading them). This has a profound impact upon others because it gives

them a sense of being valued and understood, two of the most important factors that determine how people feel when working under your direction. You have to connect well with others (eg, effective listening, respectful communication) to influence their thinking. By having first validated the other person's right to their opinions and feelings, even if you strongly disagree with them, you have reduced the tension that otherwise stands in the way of changing their point of view. By patiently and respectfully understanding the person, you help them to be less defensive. This builds a bridge of communication over which they are more likely to walk, and then join you where you stand.

CHAPTER 32

How Our Practice Works

An Open Letter for Lay Staff From Eye Clinic Leaders

John B. Pinto

Come gather 'round people, Wherever you roam
And admit that the waters, Around you have grown
And accept it that soon, You'll be drenched to the bone If your
time to you Is worth savin', Then you better start swimmin'
Or you'll sink like a stone, For the times they are a-changin'
—Bob Dylan

Old times in "ophthalmologyland" were once pretty fat. They were still pleasantly plump until recently. Generous fees. Little complexity. High profit margins. Lots of room for mistakes.

But the times they are a-changin'.

However, many practice administrators and owners are unwilling to face up to facts themselves, much less orient their staff to the new realities. In the years ahead, fees will stagnate and perhaps shrink, while technology costs, regulatory burdens, and general inflation will rise.

Pinto JB. *Ophthalmic Leadership: A Practical Guide for Physicians, Administrators, and Teams, Second Edition* (pp 193-196).
© 2022 SLACK Incorporated.

Great leadership obliges timely truth, shared with suitable depth and tone, with appropriate audiences. Even if your practice is doing swell, now is the time to brace staff (and yourself) for the challenges ahead.

For most practices, weathering The Great Recession has been nothing more than a warm-up drill for the next 10 years, as broad economic malaise, combined with federal and state budget gaps, oblige entitlement and payment reform.

Actually, the fees you receive may not actually be directly reduced so much as occultly debased, as Federal Reserve policies continue to reduce the inherent value of dollar-denominated payments for your work. Wage and price inflation, driven by an undisciplined printing press in Washington, in a largely fixed-fee profession like ophthalmology, will have the same practical impact on your organization's economic performance and doctor take-home pay as frank fee cuts.

That said, here's a dose of reality in the form of a draft message you can edit to fit your local circumstances and share with your staff in writing or at a future all-hands meeting. You may not think it's time to send this out today. But I can assure you that at some point in the future its message will be a vital part of overcoming the challenges which lie ahead for an administrator or physician and leading your practice in challenging times.

• • •

> To Our Staff:
>
> Your great teamwork to provide ophthalmic care since our founding in 1983 has been a valuable service to the public, a great profession for our providers, and a terrific career for all of us here at Central Eye Associates. For most of these years, we have been able to make constant small improvements, resulting in better care and caring. Despite ongoing fee cuts and rising costs, for the last 20 years our development of new services (eg, our ASC, an optical, a visiting retinal specialist) has kept all of our heads above water. Unfortunately, like every other eye care practice in America, it's getting harder here to develop new services to off-set lower fees and larger expenses.
>
> Just as the leaders of countries periodically update their citizens on the state of the things, we're writing today to update you on our performance, and share more widely than we have in the past—more widely than you will find in most eye practices—a few facts about how Central Eye Associates functions as a company.
>
> We're doing this in the belief that by knowing a bit more about how ***your*** practice ticks, you'll be able to see things better from the perspective of our physicians, you'll come up with some great ideas we can use in the future, and you'll be more understanding as we are obliged to make difficult choices about how we use our resources in the years ahead.
>
> First, a few historical facts. When our practice was founded, we were paid in real terms (after counting inflation) about 50 times what we receive today for a single cataract surgery. Rent was only $1.15 per square foot per month

… it's twice that now, and our suite is getting pretty tired and cramped. Our monthly electric bill was $53, and we pay $575 today. A great receptionist was happy earning just $8 per hour. When our practice first started performing refractive surgery, it cost about $50,000 for the needed equipment… today the start-up cost would be over $500,000.

Here's a hopefully painless economics lesson in one simple pie chart, which shows how a dollar that we spend today on overhead gets divided:

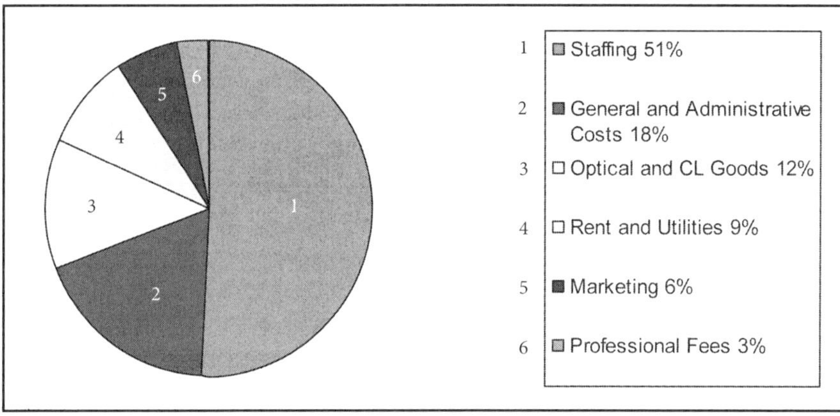

As you can see, more than half of our costs are for staffing. In the future, we're going to have to all learn together how to be more efficient and see more patients with the same staff, the same facilities, and the same provider base.

Here are a few other interesting facts to consider:

- The average patient visit generates about $160 to over $250 in net collections.
- It costs $100 or more to transit each patient, even postops.
- If we have a cancellation, we still have $100+ in overhead to cover.
- We spend about $25 in technician services for each patient visit (more when staff don't move briskly and efficiently through each work up).
- It costs us about $10 to make an appointment, look up a chart, check in a patient … and another $10 for the billing department to collect the fees from a given patient visit (and lots more than that when we enter the wrong insurance card number at the front desk).
- If we have just three cancellations or no-shows in a day, that's about $100,000 a year in lost income for the practice.

- When a patient chooses a premium IOL instead of a standard lens, we've just earned enough to pay for someone's salary for more than a week (or office rent for a day).

When a happy patient tells three friends to see our doctors, the income from those new patients over all of the years they remain in our practice can pay for a new piece of testing equipment so we can better serve our patients.

Your personal income is supported by about one and a half patient visits per day (Think about that the next time you see one of our doctors with a patient—they are earning *your* paycheck for today).

As you know, American ophthalmologists have been hit by ongoing Medicare and private insurance cuts for years. We have had to get faster and more creative every year.

We would like to reassure you that we are planning, with your help and commitment, for Central Eye to flourish for generations to come. We have six doctors and over 50 staff with the grit and the heart to make it through whatever difficulties and hard choices may face us in the future. We can be confident knowing that we are needed: In our service area we have a population of 500,000 … that's a million eyes … with an unlimited market demand to see clearly and not go blind.

We'll continue to keep you posted. Meanwhile, whenever it's in your power to turn off unused lights, schedule another patient, or urge a second pair of glasses, please do so. Thanks!

Sincerely,

Your Administrator and Board

• • •

Rewrite this letter to fit your own local circumstances. Let your people in on your forecast for the future of eye care, both the wonderful and the not so great. As Dylan urged, start swimmin' together.

CHAPTER 33

Administrative Basics

Writing Your Manager's Position Description

John B. Pinto

Famous rocket scientist Wernher von Braun quipped in 1958 to a *Chicago Sun Times* reporter, "We can lick gravity, but sometimes the paperwork is overwhelming."

Managing your ophthalmology practice is obviously not rocket science, but when done right it requires a mind-numbing array of paperwork and bureaucratic tools to get to "lift off." One of the most mundane and fundamental business tools—one too often overlooked—is the humble position description. While every staff member of the practice should have a description of their duties, I'll focus here on the position summary for your administrator. Much applies generically to the rest of the support staff, obviously.

Pinto JB. *Ophthalmic Leadership: A Practical Guide for Physicians, Administrators, and Teams, Second Edition* (pp 197-201).
© 2022 SLACK Incorporated.

A position description (otherwise known as "job description") is an abstract of one person's job in your practice. In content and detail, such descriptions lie half-way between a mere title and a full-blown how-to manual for the job.

A written position description for your practice's administrator provides several benefits:

- Before an administrator has even been hired, a position description provides the discipline needed to focus practice owners on the level of the individual they require in a new lay leader. It forces a logical match between your practice's goals and objectives and the manager's fitness for the job.
- For candidate administrators, the position description provides a helpful starting point for understanding their prospective new posting.
- Once an administrator is on board, the position description fosters clear communications between practice owners and the new manager about responsibilities and duties—it should be reviewed from time to time to assure it stays current.
- The position description is useful during periodic performance reviews ... your administrator can hardly be faulted for overlooking areas of the practice that have not been formally under their purview.
- Job descriptions affirm the administrator's supervisory authority and allows subordinate middle managers to know where reporting lines are drawn.
- The administrator's job description, taken together with the descriptions for all other staff members, assures that the hundreds of practice management details are all being covered.

The length of your administrator's position description is less important than its content and quality to deliver each of these benefits.

A position description should be a live document, drafted and then rewritten often. Unfortunately, most job descriptions are approached a little like cleaning your garage ... written in a flurry of organizational zeal and then put aside for several years. Although most administrative position descriptions start becoming obsolete almost as soon as they are prepared, they provide a useful baseline of duties and expectations that should be updated every quarter or two.

A superior administrative position description is fittingly a more elaborate document than the description for other managers or line staff in the practice. Ideally, it will include not just a dry description of practice domains and duties, but a little about the desired outcomes.

For example, it's nice to go beyond, "Responsible for supervising the practice's patient education, marketing communications, and outreach activities ..." to say something like, "... resulting in a 5% or higher annual growth rate in the number of new patients entering the practice."

For many descriptions of expected results, it's helpful to clarify a pace or timeline: "Responsible for developing a total of five new satellite offices by the end of 2009."

Although the format of your practice's position descriptions will be a matter of internal convention, and many formats work well, the outline shown in the following sample is typical and may be helpful as you proceed to tune up your own descriptions.

• • •

Position Description: Administrator

Smith Eye Center

Reports to: Dr. Smith

Core Skills and Values Inventory

- *Integrity.* A commitment to telling the truth in all circumstances, irrespective of personal consequences.
- *Communication.* The ability to communicate directly and clearly, in writing and verbally.
- *Leadership.* A demonstrated ability to build and lead a staff team, and to actively mentor and coach not only departmental leaders but providers.
- *Career commitment.* This is necessary because this is a complex and growing practice in a competitive market, and because it is realistic to expect that the practice team gauges leadership, at least in part, based on the raw time committed by the administrator to the company.
- *Product knowledge.* An intimate understanding of the various services provided by Smith Eye Center, their prices, and their profit dynamics.
- *Financial acumen.* Sufficient to evaluate, plan, and manage to agreed budgets and defined profit targets.
- *Sweating the details.* An extreme attention to operational detail and smooth daily operations is obliged in a complex and changing environment where inattention is costly.
- *A planning-oriented and big-picture management style.* The ability to not only look at the minute details of the business, but to step back and see the long-term opportunities for the practice and to prioritize in a business plan the intermediate tactics required to seize these opportunities.
- *Flexibility.* Because the final development endpoint of the practice will probably never be decided, the administrator must be flexible in their career development goals.

Core Duties

- *Broad charter.* Work with the practice owners and senior staff managers to manage an economically successful, cohesive, high quality eye care practice in the regional market. Memorialize, refine, and polish operations that are still catching up with our growth to date.
- *Financial and performance analysis and forecasting.* Coordinates, with the support of external practice accounting resources, the preparation of monthly financial statements and volume performance summary reports. Interprets these statistics verbally and in writing for monthly meetings with Dr. Smith. Participates in the preparation of various forward-looking

pro-forma forecasts of anticipated practice performance. Responsible for assuring that an appropriate cost-benefit analysis is conducted for all new projects, policies, procedure pricing, and other initiatives.

- *Profitability review and enhancement.* Develops, with each manager and doctor, individual volume performance, profitability, and cost-center goals, as well as a means of achieving these goals. Coaches doctors on where they stand compared to their revenue and volume goals. Intervenes briskly if volumes or profits lag, or if expenses accelerate beyond agreed levels.
- *Cash flow review and optimization.* Has the duty to deeply understand the myriad steps that must be followed to optimize the revenue yield from each patient encounter. Although obviously not a billing department expert, per se, develops competency to "key operator" status on the patient accounts system and has the ability to post charges, submit claims, and trace payment gaps.
- *Benchmarks review.* Memorizes the several dozen normative performance benchmarks for the practice, and knows when these are outside of normal limits. Generates monthly or quarterly performance graphs and reviews them with managers and owners.
- *Management by walking around.* Rather than just sitting behind a desk, spends significant time each week visiting all areas of the practice to check in with staff, observe operations, say hello to patients, and generally inspect the "machine."
- *Committee positions.* Chair of the Practice Management Committee composed of doctors and selected senior staff, that manages day-to-day operations. In some instances a participant and in other instances a leader, in various standing and special committee and task force efforts.
- *Ongoing market assessment.* Maintains an ongoing understanding of the practice's sources of patients (eg, alumni, referring professionals, marketing communications channels) and with third-party payers in the region.
- *Planning and development.* Participates in the preparation (and at least annual review) of the practice's strategic and business operations plan, leads the revision process for each subsequent edition.
- *Recruitment.* Involved in all provider and staff recruitment activities. Responsible, with Dr. Smith, for the final approval of all lay staff hires.
- *Supervisory authority.* Directly supervises, evaluates, and rewards/reprimands the work product of all supervisory staff in the practice. In consultation with shareholder doctors, has termination authority over all lay staff. Works to establish and revise as necessary an organization chart containing all staff members, their roles, and reporting lines in this multiservice, multilocation, regional practice.

- *Practice project and action monitoring.* Supervises the maintenance, with not less than monthly revisions, of a comprehensive "action grid," summarizing all key practice activities and projects, those responsible for their completion, and agreed deadlines. Assures that all responsible parties are meeting their deadlines. In consultation with Dr. Smith, has authority to reward and reprimand practice managers for their performance in meeting agreed goals and objectives.
- *Spending authority.* Has complete on-budget spending authority, subject to review and oversight; and has off-budget discretionary spending authority up to the limit of $5000 total impact before consulting with Dr. Smith. This spending authority will be subject to ongoing adjustment based on performance and practice circumstances.
- *Operations documentation.* Coordinates the preparation, maintenance, and periodic revisions of a practice operations manual, containing sections for each area of the practice. Participates in the periodic review of the practice's staff policy manual.
- *Clinical and business practices oversight.* Coordinates with Dr. Smith and outside advisory resources to conduct risk management. In consultation with Dr. Smith, has the ability to investigate, recommend, and carry out (upon Dr. Smith's approval) the suspension or revision of any clinical or business practices believed to be inappropriate.

• • •

In closing, an important note: It is not expected that the administrator in your practice, even the most exceptional individual, will have a 100% complete compliment of the skills and attributes suggested by the summary here.

Remember that every position description is a kind of wish list, an idealized abstract. Unless you're planning to interview robots for the job, every one of the candidates will be human. It is expected that any areas of weakness or inexperience will be realistically assessed, discussed in the open, and used as the basis for continuing education, internal delegation, or practical outsourcing.

CHAPTER 34

Compliance

Setting an Example and Sending a Message

Alan E. Reider, JD and Allison Weber Shuren, Esq

The responsibilities of the senior physician and the practice administrator span a wide range of disciplines: ethics, finance, human resources, clinical standards, and many others. Often the lead role for some of these responsibilities is delegated to others, and the physician focuses on the clinical side of the practice and the administrator focuses on overall management. While such delegation is reasonable for most functions, when it comes to compliance it is critical for both the physician and the administrator to maintain a significant presence in order to demonstrate to the staff (and, if necessary, to the government) that they are committed to the process, involved in its implementation, and have similar expectations for every member or employee of the practice. One of the greatest challenges for managers and practice owners alike is to provide leadership in the arena of

Pinto JB. *Ophthalmic Leadership: A Practical Guide for Physicians, Administrators, and Teams, Second Edition* (pp 203-208).
© 2022 SLACK Incorporated.

regulatory affairs and compliance. This is an increasingly critical area, given how high the bar is now set and how high it likely will be raised in the future.

The concept of formal compliance programs in the health care industry is not new. Ever since the National Medical Enterprises (NME) settlement in 1994, in which the government imposed a compliance program on NME as a condition of avoiding exclusion from federal healthcare programs, regulatory compliance has been a constant theme promoted by regulators as well as attorneys, advisors, and consultants. As the concept evolved, the government made it clear that compliance was not just for large health care providers like hospitals, nursing homes, or national clinical laboratories. Model compliance guidance was published for 12 different industry groups, including small physician practices.[1]

Historically, establishment of a formal compliance program has been voluntary; unless a provider was required to enter into some form of integrity agreement with the Office of the Inspector General following settlement of a government investigation, there was no requirement to develop a formal plan. However, in the health care reform legislation passed in 2010, Congress mandated that any health care provider that wishes to enroll in the Medicare or Medicaid program must have a formal compliance program in place. The effective date for this requirement was to take place once the Department of Health and Human Services published final regulations providing guidance as to what each provider must have in its plan. Remarkably, to this day no final regulations have been published. Nevertheless, proposed regulations as well as documents published over the years from the Office of the Inspector General provide adequate guidance for physician practices to understand what is expected by way of a comprehensive compliance program.

The health care reform legislation also included several new provisions designed to increase the enforcement and recovery initiatives of the government. At no time has the provider community been under more scrutiny than it is now, and as these new enforcement programs are implemented and expanded, that risk will increase. While having an effective compliance program in place cannot eliminate the risk of liability, it can reduce that risk, and may even help a practice avoid liability in the first place.

There is one other consideration to address before discussing some of the substantive elements of compliance plans. Over the past several years, the government has become increasingly aggressive in pursuing cases against individuals and, in particular, those individuals "at the top." CEOs of corporations, medical directors, and even general counsel, have found themselves to be the targets of government-enforcement actions. Over the past several years, the Office of the Inspector General has issued a number of guidance documents addressing the responsibility of management, underscoring the concept that effective compliance can only occur when an example is set at the top. This focus is based on the government enforcers' view that only when there is a commitment from the leadership of a company or of a practice, can there be an effective "culture of compliance" within a health care entity. In the case of a physician practice, the government will look to the physicians and the administrator to set the example for all of the employees to follow.

1. *See OIG Compliance Program for Individual and Small Group Practices. 65 Fed Reg 59434, October 5, 2000; also located at oig.hhs.gov.*

A Culture of Compliance: How to Get There

But how does a leader instill a culture of compliance? Unfortunately, there is no simple guide book that provides a clear direction. Furthermore, the regulations implementing the mandatory compliance program have not yet been published, making it difficult for a practice to know what steps to take in the absence of such guidance. Nevertheless, there is a significant amount of information already available that can serve as the foundation for a compliance program.[2] Further, in a recent Federal Register Notice, Health and Human Services provided a preview of the upcoming regulations that will implement the mandatory compliance program.[3]

Core Elements of Compliance

The February 2, 2011 Federal Register Notice identified the core elements necessary for an effective compliance program. As we review each of these elements, we focus on the role that should be taken by the physician and the administrator to demonstrate that a culture of compliance begins at the top and is spread throughout the practice.

Code of Conduct

Every compliance program must have a code of conduct designed to reflect the culture of the practice. Too often, physician practices that adopt compliance plans use model guidelines "off the shelf" that are purely generic in nature. The physician and administrator should be certain not only to review the code, but to tailor it to reflect the particular elements of their practice. Further, the code should be distributed to all members of the practice, and the name of the physician or physicians should be prominently displayed as endorsing all of the components of the code.

Compliance Officer

A compliance program must have a compliance officer (or compliance committee) to assure that the compliance program operates effectively. This position should not be delegated to a junior member of the practice with no apparent authority. Instead, the individual serving as compliance officer not only must have significant responsibility, but also must have access to upper level management (ie, the physician and administrator). The physician and administrator must remain accessible to the compliance officer and respond to concerns identified.

---

2. *See OIG Compliance Program for Individual and Small Group Physician Practices, Id.*
3. *See 76 Fed. Reg. 5862, 5941, February 2, 2011.*

Screening of Employees

An effective compliance program ensures that the practice does not employ any individual who has been sanctioned and is excluded from participation in the Medicare or other federal health care programs. While the physician and the administrator are not expected to perform this screening function personally, they can demonstrate their commitment by asking for and reviewing periodic reports confirming that these required screening processes have taken place.

Education and Training

A critical element of an effective compliance plan is to provide all members of the practice with regular education and training programs. These education and training programs are not limited to employees responsible for billing or other specific functions that traditionally have been hot compliance areas. Instead, programs that are relevant to all members of the practice, including the physicians and administrator, should be developed and provided on a regular basis. And during these programs, the physicians and the administrator can send an important message by sitting in the front row and participating actively. This sets a clear example from the top about the significance of these programs for all of the employees to see.

Maintain Open Lines of Communication

The role of management is critical in fulfilling this element of the compliance program. Management must make it clear that raising concerns in good faith about potential compliance violations will not be punished, but rather rewarded. We have seen too many practices where employees are intimidated from raising any potential concerns for fear of retribution.

Periodic Audits

The biggest risk facing physician practices relates to billing and coding problems. With the complex and ever-changing coding and reimbursement system, physician practices should have periodic external audits, ideally once a year. While we know of many practices that follow this rule; unfortunately, the results of those audits are not always reviewed by the physicians and, as a result, identified errors often are repeated in subsequent years. The role of the physician and the administrator is not only to engage the reviewer, but to analyze the reports that are issued and to take appropriate action in order to ensure compliance in the future.

Corrective Action

An effective compliance program must address problems once they are identified by changing conduct where appropriate, and, if necessary, taking disciplinary action against those who are responsible for compliance violations. Obviously, management must take the lead in this critical role, as without the physician and/or administrator approving such changes or such disciplinary action, they will not happen. Nevertheless, to help to assure the "culture of compliance" by setting an example from the top, physicians and the administrator should make a periodic review of all corrective actions and disciplinary actions taken as part of their routine oversight of the operation of the practice.

Real World Examples

The guidance here is not merely theoretical—many of the recommendations are based on the experience of other practices that have already taken the initiative to establish compliance programs. A few examples may serve to underscore their significance.

- A large practice promoted the need for all employees to take compliance seriously. All five principal physicians signed a letter advising their 200 employees that they looked forward to seeing them at the kickoff education and training meeting. But none of the five physicians appeared (leaving five empty seats in the front row of an auditorium where the training was held). Less than 1 year later, the practice collapsed as the result of serious financial irregularities. These physicians had sent a message to their staff that compliance training was not important enough for them to attend; what message did their staff take home about the importance of compliance generally?
- Compare the prior practice with one where the physician who headed a practice with 150 employees was the first one seated at the education and training session, participated actively by asking questions, and then advised all assembled that the compliance program was critical to everyone and that he expected everyone to participate. That program began more than 10 years ago, and the program (and the practice) continues to flourish. The practice has a compliance committee that continues to meet on a regular basis and the practice, one of the largest in the state, has not had a regulatory issue since that time. Clearly, that physician, as the leader of the practice, set an example by his conduct for all the staff to follow.
- One practice touted that since implementing its compliance program 2 years earlier, it had not had a single employee complaint about any misconduct. When the employees were interviewed, they admitted that the administrator of the practice sent the implicit message that if they raised any concerns they would be punished. Clearly, the administrator was not setting the right example to encourage open communication, a critical element in an effective compliance program.

Summary

An effective compliance program cannot operate without active participation by the physicians and the administrator, setting the standard as leaders for the staff to follow. With mandatory compliance programs to be implemented in the future, combined with the increased risks of enforcement actions to be taken against individuals, there is simply no excuse for failure to begin implementing an effective compliance program with clear demonstration of the commitment of the physicians and the administrator.

CHAPTER 35

Leading Toward the Electronic Practice

Jeff Grant

Diminishing reimbursements will make or break practices in the coming decade. While the idea of adopting an "electronic practice" to offset declining revenues probably conjures up Orwellian images of impersonal, assembly-line health care, this is far from the truth. Automation as a standard of practice can enhance patient services while solving many revenue problems today and in the coming years.

Certainly the advent and explosion of interest in electronic health records (EHRs) is causing a paradigm shift for many ophthalmologists and practice leaders. Largely due to the federal incentives for the implementation and "meaningful use of certified EHR technology," a growing percentage of practices are either implementing or considering implementing EHR.

Pinto JB. *Ophthalmic Leadership: A Practical Guide for Physicians, Administrators, and Teams, Second Edition* (pp 209-215).
© 2022 SLACK Incorporated.

Meanwhile, this EHR boom has stimulated the development of many other exciting new technologies. These related technologies that are the focus of this chapter represent innovations that all practice leaders sooner or later will need to consider.

The most forward-thinking practice leaders will embrace new technologies and set the foundation for their practice's long-term health and growth. However, it won't be enough to just buy software and services. To the contrary, selecting electronic products and services will be the easy part. The challenges are:

- Creating processes that best integrate these technologies into your practice
- Establishing an environment where these technologies are embraced
- Leading your organization through the implementation and integration of these technologies to make the difference in how effective these technologies will be

Your job as practice owner or administrator or executive is to embrace this paradigm shift and lead your organization through this transformative period. Ultimately this may well become the most important activity you engage in over the next few years.

What Will a Practice Look Like in Five to Ten Years?

While no one can say for sure, the following scenario is likely to be very close to reality.

> Patients (new or existing) log on to your website or their own secure portal. They browse available appointments and pick the one that suits them best. Of course, built-in rules make sure that only appropriate, available appointments are displayed. Patients enter or update their demographic, insurance, referral, and medical record information. A staff member quickly reviews patient-entered data, and the information is uploaded into your PM/EHR application. Upon arriving at your office, patients are identified when a finger is swiped across a reader that confirms identity, queues up various processes for your staff, notifies the staff, marks each patient as arrived, and begins the processes necessary for treatment. Insurance eligibility and benefits already have been verified for each patient, who then is escorted to a room where diagnostic testing is completed quickly. Test results are uploaded to the medical record, the patient is moved into an exam lane, and the doctor is notified on her portable device that the patient is ready in Room X and that test results need to be interpreted. After the encounter is completed, all data are entered into the EHR. Upon completion of the exam, the patient's charges for the visit are presented to the doctor for review and then posted to the patient's ledger. Any information about the patient's need to return to the clinic also is updated. Educational information is uploaded to the patient's portal, and any other staff tasks are queued automatically. The patient stops by the patient concierge desk to swipe a credit card. The receipt is uploaded to the patient's secure portal, along with the return to clinic information and a summary of the day's visit. Approximately 1 week prior to the next appointment, the portal notifies the patient according to preference (eg, email, phone calls) and the process begins again.

Does this sound like something out of a science fiction novel? Well, you might be surprised to learn that many functions described here already exist in one form or other. And we're probably only a few years away from the entire scenario becoming reality in the most progressive practices.

Time and cost savings, patient convenience, and practice efficiencies in a system like this scenario might make the difference between a practice struggling to survive and one that thrives. The conveniences built into such a practice can attract patients in droves, whereas inherent inefficiencies can have the opposite effect.

So let's delve into what you, as a practice leader, need to know and do to set up your practice for success.

Electronic Health Record

EHR finally is becoming an indispensable tool for practice efficiency and for delivering superior patient care. Leaders of private practices must be able to pick the right EHR application for their practice, manage the implementation of the EHR application, and re-engineer the myriad processes and procedures you currently have that were built for paper-based systems.

You'll need to make concrete strategic plans for extracting maximum benefits from EHR applications. The four most important EHR implementation tasks that practice leaders must focus on are:

1. Create a project implementation plan that includes a project leader, physician involvement, regular meetings, and input from staff members.
2. Ensure that your clinical staff (eg, doctors, nurses, technicians, scribes) spend the necessary time to acclimate themselves to the EHR such as by practicing data entry.
3. Deeply analyze your current processes and develop new processes that integrate new electronic tools and workflow.
4. Make no assumptions as you move through the steps of implementation. Be sure to test everything. For example, do not just assume that everyone in your clinic will like using tablets for data input into EHR (they usually won't because of weight and battery life limitations).

While the meaningful use (MU) incentives are important, focusing only on the incentives is a mistake and misses the real value of EHR. Some benefits from fully implemented EHR are:

- Increased revenue
- Potential for more patient visits
- More efficient patient flow
- Better medicine through clinical decision support (CDS), which we will discuss later in the chapter
- Sharing of protected health information with other health care providers, which can reduce adverse drug reactions, ordering of duplicate tests, etc.

The latest EHR applications include many tools that will allow practice leaders to make their practice more efficient. These applications also will make better clinicians out of your physicians. The MU measures required the software vendors to develop and include new functionality that potentially can transform the practice of medicine. Let's look at a couple of these new functions:

- *Clinical decision support (CDS).* Your EHR should provide prompts/alerts when various treatment options are due and when alternative treatments might be appropriate. These prompts could be based on your own established standards of care, the American Academy of Ophthalmology's Preferred Practice Patterns, or some combination of both. Either way, CDS should allow you to provide better, more consistent care, and help prevent mistakes that can cost the practice and your patients. A practice leader's job is to make sure providers use these tools and follow appropriate rules.
- *Clinical information exchange.* Imagine that every doctor could see every treatment a patient has received from all other providers treating the same patient. Do you think adverse drug reactions might be prevented? Do you think redundant tests and procedures could be avoided? Of course the answer is: "YES!" The capability to exchange clinical information is one of the foundations that the Health Information Technology (HIT) initiatives are based.

New Electronic Practice Technologies

One of the great accomplishments of the EHR incentive and EHR software certification program is motivation for software developers to build or incorporate some very exciting new technology. Some vendors have added functionality to their products to meet certain MU measures and taken that added functionality far beyond the requirements for MU.

Leaders of electronic practices will be required to implement many new tools and develop numerous new processes in order to optimize their practice. *Above all, don't let your practice fall behind others!* Initially these new technologies will allow the most progressive practices to lead the way. But eventually, these new technologies will become standard operating procedure for all practices.

The most exciting, paradigm-shifting, electronic practice technologies allow you to better manage patient flow, better manage patient data, and deliver better care to your patients. Here are a few.

Secure Web Portals

One of the most exciting new technologies is the use of secure web portals. These portals are basically secure websites that allow patients (and referring providers if you desire) to access certain portions of their health record. This does not mean patients actually are connecting to your server. Instead, patients have access to data uploaded by the practice to the portal's database.

A big player in the patient health portal world is Microsoft. There also are numerous smaller players. Microsoft offers a well-established patient health information portal available to the general public, as well as through EHR vendors. Another portal vendor with specialization in eyecare is Sophrona.

Many vendors have chosen to integrate with one of the established portal vendors, ie, Medflow uses Sophrona, while other vendors such as Compulink and NextGen handle their own portal needs with tools they developed themselves. Vendors with their own patient portals say they prefer to have full control over the functionality, operation, expense, and tighter integration with their EHR.

Common portal services today are patient access to exam summaries (MU measure), patient access to their medical record summary (MU measure), and patient access to educational information (MU measure). Some portals also allow you to upload letters to referring providers so that you eliminate the time, expense, and hassle of faxing or mailing letters. These referring providers have secure access to the letter, regardless of where they are when they decide to view the information.

More portal-based services are certain to develop in the coming years such as bill payment, contact lens ordering, and appointment scheduling.

Painless integration tip ... Start slowly and offer only a few portal-based services at first. This will allow your staff to build up confidence in the new technology and enable your patients to slowly grow comfortable with the services and new ways of interacting with your practice. Also, do not assume that your patient won't or can't access a service like this. Maybe ALL of your patients can't, but enough can that the service will increase your efficiency. *Do not let the exceptions guide you.*

Web-Based Patient Registration

Many practice management and EHR software vendors already offer tools that allow your patients to register and update data online. Many go several steps further by allowing the patient to enter insurance and referral details, as well as possibly the most time-saving tool—medical history information, including medications, review of systems, past family social history, surgical history, etc.

Imagine the time savings you can enjoy if your patients (even if only half of them) updated their demographic information online, eliminating the need for them to update information on paper and for your staff to enter the data manually! Going further, imagine now that these patients' medical histories were entered online and your staff simply reviewed the data before updating the electronic medical record.

In this era of eroding reimbursements, this tool alone could allow your doctors to see two or three more patients daily. If you can save only 3 minutes per patient even with half of a physician's normal schedule of 50 appointments daily, this easily would allow you to see two more patients per day. At $150 per visit, that would be nearly $100,000 of additional annual revenue for most practices!

As a practice leader, you must understand that many patients will seek out practices that invest in tools to improve the patient experience. Spending less time in the waiting room and getting through the exam in less time are tremendous patient benefits.

Your patients will notice! They also will come to expect this kind of service. Practice leaders who ignore these technologies will be placing their business at a disadvantage.

Painless integration tip ... Use email to remind patients about their upcoming appointments and include a link to your web registration pages on your website. Give preference to patients who register online. Let them know that if two people present at the very same time, the one who registered online will be seen first. As stated already, do not let exceptions guide you. There are some patients who will love this service, and you'll see the usage increase rapidly.

Automated Eligibility and Benefit Verification

In the past few years, many practice leaders have benefitted from verifying insurance eligibility and benefits (E&B) prior to the patient's arrival. They recognized that this extra effort positively impacted their revenue cycle and improved patient satisfaction by preventing unexpected out-of-pocket charges.

Normally E&B was verified by logging on to the insurance company's website and manually entering the patient identifying information, as well as manually updating the practice management software. In the last few years, we've seen more vendors offering electronic E&B services that operate from within their software and that save data directly into the appropriate fields in the software.

Even more recently, we've seen this innovation taken to yet another level where kiosks are being placed in the waiting room. This allows patients to check in on their own. At the same time, the system verifies E&B.

Painless integration tip ... Start by using the E&B verification tools included with your practice management software vendor. Make this a requirement for every patient visit. Then, look into other services—perhaps available from your practice management vendor—that allow you to place kiosks in the waiting room.

Patient Tracking and Analysis/Resource Management and Analysis

So, being the forward-thinking practice leader that you are, you've implemented EHR and begun removing paper charts from your practice. How will your staff control patient flow and know who is scheduled next for which exam room? Also, how will your doctors know which exam room they need to visit next?

Many EHR vendors offer some kind of patient-tracking module with their software. These tools provide various levels of functionality, but generally include the following at a minimum:

- Notifying your technicians that a patient has arrived and is ready to be taken into the clinic.
- Displaying where all patients are in the office at any given time.
- Providing the physician with notification about which room they need to be in next.

We are starting to see very specialized functions offered either by the EHR vendors or by third-party companies who can interface with your software. These functions allow a more complete patient flow and management of resources such as staff, rooms, doctors, and equipment. Usually, these newer offerings are much more graphical, allowing you to view flow and resource utilization at a glance.

Painless integration tip ... Don't be reluctant to integrate these new electronic tools and supplement their use with some physical device to assist with the transition. Physical devices can include a single sheet of paper with pertinent patient information or a laminated card with useful physical information. As your clinical team becomes more comfortable with a "chartless system" and electronic patient tracking, you can begin to remove the physical devices from your process. As a practice leader, your job is to incorporate the tools and extract the maximum benefit you can. That doesn't require an "all or none" approach, though. You should do whatever is necessary to move your organization in the right direction.

Summary

Your job as practice owner, manager, administrator, or executive is to evaluate the benefits of these exciting new technologies and consider when (not if) you're ready to implement them in your practice. The key will be following the suggestions detailed here concerning painless integration into your processes, educating your staff on the benefits, and educating your patients about how these new electronic technologies serve them.

The earliest adopters will encounter a few more challenges, but innovation has always been that way. As your patients experience these new technologies at other practices they visit, they'll become much more comfortable with their use. In fact, they will come to expect these technologies and services and the efficiencies provided by their use. Those practices that are the latest adopters will be seen as behind the times, outdated, and harder to work with.

In time, patients will begin to seek out electronic practices that have made an investment in and commitment to efficient, time-saving tools for themselves and those they serve.

CHAPTER 36

Leading and Managing Clinical Support Staff

Jane T. Shuman, MSM, COT, COE, OCS, OSC

There is much information written about leadership both in print and on the web. Progressive administrators read them and apply some of the principles to their work and practice. But how many of them share the information with their management team? Some do, many don't.

Much of the literature written is about the success stories of corporate leaders;, many of them are founders or CEOs of Fortune 100 companies. Yet many of the principles that made them great can be transferred to the administrative team of an ophthalmology practice. When the physicians and managers share a common vision, it becomes crucial for this philosophy to trickle down to the support staff.

Pinto JB. *Ophthalmic Leadership: A Practical Guide for Physicians, Administrators, and Teams, Second Edition* (pp 217-221).
© 2022 SLACK Incorporated.

The vision of the practice should be created by the founders and reviewed by the leadership and communicated to the staff. This is the tenet that guides the day-to-day operation of the practice; it affects all levels of staff and generally is related to the quality of care provided to the patients. The relationship of the ophthalmologist and his technicians tends to differ from his relationship with most other practice employees. They are likely to spend more time with his patients than he does; when they perform to his expectations, a dependency on that proficiency can develop. Also, they work side by side in the clinical area of the practice. This can lead to conversations, and over time, these may become less clinical in nature. It is not uncommon to see technicians begin to take advantage of this mutual respect and discuss needs (ie, time off) that are better suited for the management team.

In best practices, the organizational structure is clearly understood by physicians and staff alike: There is, and should be, a hierarchy so that all staff knows to whom they report. In the clinical area, there is usually one person that is responsible for the patient flow, technical staff, supplies, and equipment. That person's management abilities and technical skills will contribute to the effective running of the clinic.

Historically, the most skilled technician has been promoted to the lead clinical position. Current trends indicate this is not always the ideal candidate, because they may not be able to transcend above peers to become their boss. Another cause of dissatisfaction is an inability to see the "big picture" that keeps patients moving smoothly through the office.

So, then, what qualities should the lead tech possess and how do we find them? The clinical leader must have the same qualities you expect of every member of your management team. Like the others, this person must be the role model for the people that report to them, particularly as it applies to work ethics and professionalism. They must be able to provide constructive criticism, discipline when necessary, and even ensure the doctors are not demanding preferential treatment in terms of their staffing needs. Clinically, they should have a working knowledge of the skills required by their staff. This is often the first requirement that hiring practices look for.

But, by recruiting first for clinical acumen, you may be doing the practice a disservice: It is easier to teach the right person the ophthalmic skills than it is to teach someone to manage. When recruiting a clinical manager, we can learn from other industries and look for qualities that are transferrable such as successful team building, just-in-time inventories, and maintaining staff accountability. Most importantly, look for a history of providing successful customer service; after all, our patients have a choice when it comes to doctors. If they are treated at a level that does not meet their expectations, they will look for another provider.

First, create a clear job description to be shared with acceptable candidates. The duties will be fairly easy to delineate and should include the staffing of all locations appropriately, maintaining clinical supplies and equipment, and overseeing smooth, efficient patient flow. The inclusion of continuous training and education is a clinic-oriented task that is often overlooked, but is as important and the hiring and training of new staff.

As is common in other industries, many practices are turning to psychometric tests to help them determine which characteristics will be the best fit in the practice culture. This cultural fit is so important for a clinical manager because their staff must carry out the leadership team's vision. According to Mark Sanborn, "you don't need a title to be a leader." This person may actually be in your employ, having gained the respect of their peers and doctors. They, and others, should be encouraged to apply for the position but the selection process should not be limited to those already at the practice. Promotion from within has its own devilish issues to be overcome. Be aware, too, of the possibility of having them leave if someone else is hired.

If your final candidates are external ones, consider having them shadow your staff for a session or a day. Observe their interactions with other staff members, providers and most importantly, the patients. If necessary, ask open-ended questions of those that had contact with the candidates. Remember not to solicit opinions, but facts that can be used in the final decision-making process.

Once the clinical leader has been selected and become acclimated to the culture of the practice, because of the unique doctor/technician relationship, she may find it difficult to assert herself in her leadership role. Yet, it is important to "be fair and treat every employee the same," as a former boss of mine once said. This has held me in good stead through the years.

Technicians should be expected to adhere to the same rules as the rest of the staff, all of which should be found in the employee handbook. Yet they are often given more leeway than the clerical staff, for instance. One reason for the different treatment is the relationship with the provider, another is the national shortage of experienced technicians, and often seen is the third reason, a reluctance to change.

The qualities that allow a technician to excel often include the following characteristics:

- A desire to help people maintain good vision and their independence
- An attention to detail
- A comprehension of the ocular system
- A self-confidence in their abilities to provide the physician with the information necessary to make an accurate diagnosis and treatment plan
- Many years of experience in the field often the same practice.

Ironically, many of these are the very qualities that frustrate their supervisor or doctors. As the Baby Boomers reach retirement age, when eye diseases become more prevalent, practices are meeting the increase in demand by streamlining their processes and encouraging their technicians to meet the productivity benchmarks. Along with the demand for increased productivity is the push to provide superior customer service, knowing today's patients have their choice of eye doctors. The increasing number of websites that post consumer opinions now include providers of medical care … social networking sites spread positive and negative experiences like wildfire.

Taking the mission of customer service to heart, many technicians interpret that as an opportunity to spend time with the patient, even if the conversation is not focused on the reason for the visit. They express difficulty keeping the patient on track, when a slight touch on the shoulder and a reminder why they are here will usually do the trick.

Alternatively, there may not be clear expectations of what work-up components are related to the chief complaint and they consequently either provide the doctor with too many components or not enough. Either case will be a cause for concern, warranting unnecessary time either in the original work-up or by calling someone in to perform the workup components that were missing from the original work-up.

One way to improve the likelihood of providing the ophthalmologist with the appropriate work-ups is to develop a written work-up protocol by appointment type and/or diagnosis. Whenever possible, there should be consistency among providers within a practice that will reduce the frequency of errors. Yet, when tests are performed incorrectly or not at all, someone must circle back to the work-up tech and provide constructive criticism. Without that, the technician is likely to assume they performed correctly and will continue to do so, frustrating the doctor(s) even further.

Who is the logical person to communicate the errors to the techs? If there is a clinical manager, this task falls to them, but someone must inform them with the paper chart in hand or referring to the electronic visit note. Even in best practices, this is where communication often fails; the practice is busy, people may forget, or the doctor may not want to make waves because "it wasn't a big deal" or "did not harm the patient." But, when the same tech repeats that error time and time again, they may begin to question their competency and show preferential treatment to other members of the clinical team. Over time, this reinforces the close relationship between that doctor and certain techs, and alienates the others.

Clinical staff must be accountable for their actions, just like the other office staff. In order to track their responsibilities, the job description should be clear, just as it was for the manager. Although the primary responsibility is to provide direct patient care, a common complaint is that the techs are not occupied between patients or when the physicians are on vacation. Duties (daily and otherwise) should include the following:

- Scribe as necessary
- Direct patients through the office
- Diagnostic testing as appropriate
- Triage patient phone calls
- Refill prescriptions
- Clean and stock exam rooms
- Skills development
- Instrument calibration and minor maintenance
- Maintenance of clinical inventories

Many of these tasks are dependent on having patients in the office. A way to minimize the belief that they are not needed when the doctor is away is to include duties that are typically more clerical in nature. These include:

- Booking appointments
- Purging medical records
- Scanning documents into the electronic medical record
- Working recalls

Not only will this keep the clinical staff busy during quiet times, but it provides the benefit of insight as to the "other," yet equally important side of the practice. Techs are accustomed to knowing what they will face when they call in each patient. The plan has been outlined for them in the last chart note; they have information to reference, even for new patients that have completed history forms. In sharp contrast is the unknown on the other end of the phone and the patients waiting longer than expected, directing their displeasure to the front desk staff.

To complete this circle of mutual understanding, the clinical manager should invite the clerical staff to observe what happens behind closed doors when the tech is involved in patient care. The expression that "a picture is worth a thousand words" is quite applicable here: Without having the first-hand observation, they may wonder what takes them so long.

The person that supervises the technical staff must not be afraid to uphold the rules that others in the practice must also abide by and begin disciplinary action when necessary. The staff member that may challenge this structure the most may actually be the "sacred cow" on the tech team. Generally speaking, they have been with the practice, or one of the doctors, for many years. Some may have been a team since the doctor was first in practice ... medicine has changed dramatically in that same time frame. They may resent taking direction and may push back on the suggested changes.

When necessary, the final outcome of the disciplinary process may be a termination of their employment. This generally serves as a wake-up call to the others that no one is safe and that the parameters that are outlined in the employee manual will be upheld. Often the person that needs convincing of the logic of this decision is the ophthalmologist. This move constitutes a Change, with a capital C.

No one embraces change; it takes people out of their comfort zones and until the new situation has been adjusted to, there may be some awkwardness during the learning curve. Yet, in the current difficult economic times, there are many changes to which doctors, management, staff, and patients will have to adjust. Reimbursements are declining: In order to maintain the same revenue stream, we need to see more patients without increasing our costs. To increase the revenue, we need to see even more patients, often necessitating more diagnostic tests and surgeries requiring the techs that are change resisters to work *smarter,* not necessarily *harder.* If they do not have a strong leader, they are likely to dig in their heels instead.

Combine with this the transition to an electronic medical record that will change almost every aspect of the familiar workflow. The clinical leader and their staff must be able to keep pace with the patient flow and system changes. Otherwise, the patient satisfaction rate may suffer.

We have examined the qualities of technicians and potential pitfalls when providing them with structure. We have looked at the clinical leader and the relationships of all of them with the doctors. However, it is important that we not lose sight of the true leaders in the practice: the patients. Without them, even the most successful practice will fail.

CHAPTER 37

Questions That Can Improve Your Bottom Line

John B. Pinto

"Animal, vegetable, or mineral?" The children's game of 20 questions comes in a grown-up ophthalmologist's version that can boost your practice's strategic sharpness, operations, and profits.

As a clinician, you long ago developed, refined, and memorized a question set to help you understand your patient's eye health. You do not ask every patient every question. But by the end of a typical clinic day, if we were to take an inventory, we'd see a score of questions that you've asked over and over again.

The clinical question set you use today is probably a lot shorter than the questions you used in the first year you practiced—you've learned what can be left out and what answers can allow a shortcut to the end of the exam. The most

Pinto JB. *Ophthalmic Leadership: A Practical Guide for Physicians, Administrators, and Teams, Second Edition* (pp 223-226).
© 2022 SLACK Incorporated.

thoughtful doctors refine and personalize their clinical question sets to the last day of active practice.

You pose some of these questions to the patients directly, or to their family members in the exam room. Some of the questions are posed to the tissue you observe through a slit lamp or to the lab results in your hands. Some of the questions are asked of an internal colleague down the hall or a subspecialist consultant. Of course, some of the questions are muttered to yourself, when a real puzzler arises.

The same game of "20 questions" can be applied to the management side of your practice. Here's a starting point, with questions you can refine and apply daily, weekly, and in some cases monthly or annually in your practice. Some questions are micro, some macro. Some questions should be posed directly to management staff. Some should be posed to rank-and-file staffers. Some of the answers you get will speak for themselves and some should be cross-checked with outside experts.

Pinto's Questions

1. *Do we know what we want to do?* Too often, surgeons show up for work with goals that are no more defined than, "Let's make it through the day." The start is understanding your personal goals deeply, and having these drive a formal strategic business plan. In the wise words of Henry David Thoreau, "Go confidently with your dreams. Live the life you have imagined."
2. *How cohesive is our practice team?* Does your practice have sufficient organizational "connective tissue" so that the lofty goals held by the doctor-owners are being translated completely into workaday action?
3. *Do we know what dimensions of our practice are growing, shrinking or staying the same?* Practice financial data are often too late, too scant, too short-term, or not sufficiently segmented to back up your hunches. Bookkeeping controls must be in synch with the scale and financial challenges of your practice.
4. *Do we have control over the volume of patient visits and the mix and volume of surgical cases in our practice?* Rather than just taking what comes through the door, you should establish specific volume performance goals for the year, describing the number of new and total patients and mix of services you want to provide. You should then compare these figures monthly to actual performance, implementing whatever marketing actions are needed to meet your goals.
5. *Are there costs we could reduce without adversely impacting the quality of care we provide?* For example, replacing in-house patient transport vans with on-call taxis might still allow the desired end of serving indigent patients, but at a lower cost and with greater flexibility.
6. *Would these cost containment efforts backfire and actually harm profitability?* For example, by reducing marketing costs $50,000 a year, you might reduce revenue by $100,000. By dismissing two technicians, patient waiting time may climb to the point of reducing alumni referrals.

7. *Are there steps we could take to improve the quality of our patient care without adversely impacting profitability?* Remember that quality is not just clinical outcomes, but patient *perceptions*. For example, handing every patient an inexpensive printed fact sheet describing their chief complaint and your treatment approaches would save some of the cost of having staff spend extra time educating each patient, and would potentially improve patient compliance for better care. Everyone wins.
8. *When will we post charges, submit claims, and receive payment for the services we're providing to patients today?* Too often, doctors concentrate on the over-90-day account column when the real problem is far earlier in the chain of events (ie, a bottleneck in the insurance department), generating a delay in claims submissions. Ask staff at the front lines about the time lag from service to posting to submission, and what happens when a Medicare check hits the door.
9. *How many hours do our staff work every day, and how many hours are they paid for?* Practices, as they grow, can carry forward informal and sometimes even overpermissive wage and hour policies. This laxity can generate several negatives. Selected staff will abuse the system, claiming payment for extra time they didn't work each day. This costs the practice real dollars, and worse, leads to lower morale among the nonabusers. Overtime can get out of control. And valid claims can be made against the practice for violating labor laws.
10. *Could we have seen more patients in the clinic today or performed more surgical cases?* Most surgeons end their work day with a cushion of unsold "inventory." It may not bother you that a few no-shows leave you with time to read the paper. But remember that marginal, incremental revenue represent the bulk of your profits, since fixed costs are already covered. Just three missed exams a day in a typical solo practice can trim $100,000 from your annual income.
11. *If we ended the day providing less care—doing less work—than was possible, what could we do to improve?* Giving yourself a five-figure annual raise could be as simple as adding one or two slots to the appointment template or calling patients 24 to 48 hours ahead of their appointment to reduce no-shows.
12. *If we saw all the patients or performed all the cases we were capable of, what's holding us back from doing more?* If growth is a goal, look for opportunities to increase everyone's productivity. Potential answers lie in back-office technology, increased tech training, or increased physician delegation of care to optometrists. Note that you may not want more patients packed into the day, but an extra hour to spend with your family. Knowing your goals is the start of achieving them.
13. *Are we extracting a full measure of value from every staff resource in the practice?* Look down the clinic hallway. Are techs just standing around waiting for a doctor to emerge, or are they calling to remind the next day's patients of their appointment? Now look at the front desk. Are receptionists hanging out waiting for the next patient to arrive, or are they prepping the next day's charts? You wouldn't put your investment portfolio in an interest-free checking account—why would you let a $15-an-hour member of your staff not *continuously* earn their keep?

14. *Are we extracting full value from every* ***other*** *resource in the practice?* Satellite office or surgical facilities left vacant most of the week were affordable in an era of $1500 cataracts. Today, all offices should be open full-time, and an increasing number of practices are adding evening and weekend hours to extract a full measure of value from fixed asset costs.
15. *Are we even in the right business?* Have we gone too far in turning a cataract practice into a LASIK practice now that fees for refractive surgery are falling and volume growth is stagnating in some markets? Have we considered ourselves a surgical practice only and missed optical dispensing opportunities?
16. *What's our exit plan?* Smaller practices have an easy answer: Sell to another practice in the community or bring a successor surgeon in a few months before retirement. Large and "mega" practices have a more complex challenge. Since the demise of corporate management companies and hospitals backpedaling from '90's merger mania, divestiture options have narrowed. For these large practices, succession planning should be nailed down at least 5 years before the retirement of the most dominant provider.

• • •

Summary

In the heat of daily battle, few surgeons and few managers take the time to ask these questions, much less act on the answers. Your practice—in both clinical and business dimensions—is the most important "patient" you care for. It's certainly the most demanding. Learning to ask the right questions every day will improve your organization's treatment plan and prognosis.

CHAPTER 38

Contingency Planning in a Less-Certain Environment

John B. Pinto

As this book goes to press, America's ophthalmologists and eye care administrators are in Medicare limbo ... not to mention double-dip great recession limbo, COVID-19 limbo, peak oil limbo, global warming limbo, world economic meltdown limbo.

It's hard to tell if this is an especially spooky era we live in, or if the 24/7 news and information cycle we all live in just makes it seem that way.

All we can know for certain is that these times *feel* profoundly uncertain. And its simply not very healthy to feel durably uncertain and worry the day away, without doing something to at least try to plan for, and mitigate, all of the nasty possibilities.

Pinto JB. *Ophthalmic Leadership: A Practical Guide for Physicians, Administrators, and Teams, Second Edition* (pp 227-230).
© 2022 SLACK Incorporated.

At the level of your personal and business financial life, this is rather easy to do. It is merely a matter of writing down a list of the looming events you most fear, and then writing out a contingency narrative for what you would do to solve each problem.

Here is a list of the most common, generic anxieties I hear when making my consulting rounds throughout the country, along with a few generalized mitigation strategies for each one.

• • •

- *Long-slated Medicare fee reductions will actually stick next time, and our doctors will take a massive pay cut.* This is certainly the biggest, nastiest monster in the closet for most eye surgeons. The average ophthalmology practice derives 60% of its cash flow from Medicare. In addition, most private payers index their payments to Medicare fees. First of all, an abrupt double-digit cut of this magnitude is unlikely (in my view) to be imposed, absent an abrupt national emergency. Too many powerful forces are aligned against this kind of shock therapy for America's entitlement overdrafts. But it could happen. Here are some practical buffers to ease your mind:
    - Build rainy day reserves, so that if you experienced an abrupt cut in fees, you would have several monthly of operating expenses in the bank that you can call on as a buffer fund to give you the time to figure out what to do next.
    - Diversify, to the extent feasible, and become less Medicare-dependent.
    - Make sure you are dispensing optical goods, which typically boosts profits 10% ... it could be 15% if a severe Medicare fee reduction was applied.
    - Shift as many patients as you can to associate, optometric providers, allowing doctor-owners to focus care on higher-yield secondary and tertiary care.
    - Generate a financial "what-if?" pro forma showing the impact of a 21% fee cut on your top line, and the steps you would reasonably take to boost marginal revenues while trimming costs.
    - Sit back and realize that if something as massive as a double-digit Medicare fee cut came to pass across the board, that every lay staff member, most vendors, and some landlords would be constrained to align their payment demands with your constrained circumstances ... in the typical settings even across the board staff wage reductions would be grudgingly accepted.
- *I won't have enough to retire on and live the way I had planned.* This ranks just below Medicare fee cuts as the greatest fear of mid-career surgeons. Here are some coping strategies.
    - Realize that there are only three key dependent variables you have to work with: when you retire, your retirement savings, and the lifestyle you aspire to after you retire. You can retire later, save more aggressively, or live more frugally. Taken together, that adds up to a lot of control.
    - Obviously, each one of these three variables are under your direct, personal control.
    - By controlling one or more variables effectively, you're in the clear and your comfortable retirement will be ensured.

  - Keep in mind that most 30-something, 40-something, and 50-something ophthalmologists have dreams of early retirement, but ultimately end up retiring much later than they planned, not because they were forced to, but because in their 50s, 60s, or 70s they were still not ready to leave the profession. This kind of work is simply way too much fun to retire from.
- *We'll could lose a key staff member, who is the only one who knows how things run here.* If you feel in the least way exposed to this issue, which could have as easily been the case a generation ago as today, you should work on mitigation efforts that are pretty easy.
  - In the smallest of solo practices, the doctor-owner needs to know how every nuance of the practice works ... they should know how to post a charge, submit a claim, handle credentialing, or generate and read the financial reports.
  - The most common exposure is in smaller practices with just one beleaguered billing guru. In these settings, the office manager—at the very least—should be able to step in at a moment's notice to preserve cash flow.
- *We could lose a key doctor who generates a significant percentage of practice income.* In smaller practices, an individual doctor's prospective departure, disability, or death is always a nail-biter.
  - The first line of defense is to build in redundancy ... if your practice is critically dependent on a high-earning retinal surgeon, have a Plan B to bring in a guest doctor if you lose your core retinologist.
  - In two-doctor partnerships, disability and life insurance policies should be taken out to hedge against low-odds events.
  - Shareholder agreements should be crafted with noncompete and long notice period recitals to buy time to respond to a doctor's defection.
  - The practice administrator and accountant should have tucked away a contingency pro forma showing how the practice could still land on its feet if it lost a key producer.
- *Our local hospital is going to "own" access to premium dollars and access to patients in our market before long.* This throwback concern from the 1990s is raising its head again with the emergence of nascent private equity-owned practices.
  - Ultimately, you should realize that unless you have a pure self-pay practice, your customer is not the patients, but the payers and other institutions that control the premium dollar.
  - If your local institution is in a position to control your access to patients, you can pout or you can insinuate yourself into that institution ... this may either oblige that your practice merge with the hospital or dominant multispecialty medical group, or you may be able to play on the fringes, at least for the time being.
  - If the world moves back to a prepaid environment, the winners will be those efficient practices that can turn a patient visit for the lowest possible cost.

  - Your ultimate recourse and mitigation strategy is to leave the market and find a freer environment; senior corporate executives and military officers relocate every few years—the same may be obliged of you if you want to optimize your earnings and independence.
- *Because of fast-rising national debt, the value of the dollar will fall ... our practice costs will rise, while Medicare fees won't keep up with the resulting inflation and we'll be under water. My retirement savings are doomed.* As the old man used to say, there are *problems* we solve and *issues* we have to learn how to live with. The destiny of the dollar, Middle East peace accords, rising seas, or nuclear proliferation are beyond our individual control. If (or when) the dollar tanks, everyone will be in the same boat. But if this happens, I can't think of too many professions in a better position than eye care to survive the storm. Just keep reminding yourself that there are 650 million eyeballs in America and a nearly unlimited market demand for not going blind. As a nation we're making fewer than 1% more eye surgeons a year, at the same time that the demand for ophthalmic services is growing about 5% per year with the Baby Boomers streaming into retirement. As Bob Marley wrote in his song made popular by Bobby McFerrin and President Reagan, "Don't worry, be happy."

CHAPTER 39

Collaboration

The Key to Better Management Decisions

John B. Pinto

Practicing ophthalmology, in today's formidable environment, obliges the juxtaposition of two quite different and often conflicting personalities and leadership styles: the naturally independent style of surgeons and the necessarily collaborative style of business managers.

When faced with a problem, the inclination of most surgeons is to say, "Let *me* operate." The manager with a problem is more likely to say, "Let *us* call a meeting."

What works best, autonomy or collaboration? Both styles have their place, and both can lead to tremendous problems in your practice when misapplied. A surgeon obviously can't operate by committee, any more than a manager can act autonomously.

Pinto JB. *Ophthalmic Leadership: A Practical Guide for Physicians, Administrators, and Teams, Second Edition* (pp 231-234).
© 2022 SLACK Incorporated.

But as practices get larger, and both the medical and commercial dimensions of modern practice become more complex, it's important to steer toward more and more collaboration at all levels.

Improved collaboration can be achieved with effort in just four practical areas: channels, communication, open sharing, and delegation. Let's explore each of these in turn.

Channels

The unfortunate assumption of many staff in the typical ophthalmology practice is that they're to be seen and not heard. As a result, many support staff won't tell you what they think unless they're directly asked. Not much collaboration will happen until you open up channels, and this has to be more than setting up a suggestion box. You won't get great input until you ask for it. Here are some examples of practical, underused channels:

- If you're the administrator or managing partner of your practice, sit down for coffee or lunch with two or three lay staff at a time to informally talk shop. Spend 90% of your time listening. The channels you open with the first few meetings will make these same staff more comfortable approaching you when problems or opportunities arise … even before you ask.
- Meet at least quarterly with associate providers. Review their performance statistics and draw them out about their career goals.
- It can be especially useful to open channels with staff who are about to leave your practice on good terms. Such staff are often willing to be more candid than staff who remain behind about the problems they see.

Communication

This needs to take place at every level of your practice and, with increasing practice scale, needs to steer toward the formality of written rather than oral communication.

- Meetings have always been the bane of medical organizations. But meetings are an irreducible obligation in the best of practices. As a rule of thumb, budget each week an average of at least 1 hour of doctor time and 90 minutes of nonsupervisory lay staff spent in meetings. These figures more than double for managers and MPs. If you're spending any less time than this, you are probably not communicating and connecting enough to keep up the pace of collaboration.
- In the typical mid-sized practice, job descriptions, policy documents, and procedure manuals should run to hundreds of pages. It's grueling to create the first draft of these reference materials, but much easier to collaborate on procedures and constantly improve them if these are formally written down.
- As a surgeon-owner, even if you have already made a decision, sometimes it's important to ask others for their opinion. This can be done with a few informal hallway conversations, or more formally as a group meeting or written survey.

- In larger practices, when a new policy has been made, it's helpful to post it in writing for a comment period. Let's say you've just decided that half of all staff vacation time should be scheduled during doctor downtime. Even if you're firmly committed to this new policy, giving staff the courtesy of input can take the sting out of it—and you may actually receive suggestions that improve the new policy.

Open Sharing

When I conduct surveys of client staff, their greatest frustration is rarely centered on wages or work conditions—lay staff most commonly complain that they don't get enough feedback and information, especially from practice owners. It's incredibly helpful to let your entire staff know about your future plans for the practice and your reasons behind office priorities and policies. When the going gets tough you don't have to be "Dr. Sunshine" when collaborating in this way. Be candid about difficulties in the practice … the more brains you plug into each problem, the better the solutions will be.

Delegation

Collaboration means sharing. And sharing—in a business context—often means delegation:

- Practice board meetings commonly bog down with minutia. Push decisions as far down the organization chart as you can.
- Doctors should not be making decisions that can be handled by the administrator. Adept administrators do not make decisions than can be handled by department heads.
- When a decision involves more than one practice department, choose staff from each impacted area of your practice to weigh in on the matter.

• • •

One particularly efficient process to foster collaboration is called nominal group technique (NGT). In just a few minutes several staff members or doctors in a group meeting (up to about 20 people) can dissect problems, weigh numerous solutions, and democratically arrive at a consensus. Although there are several variants on NGT, here's a four-step process I think you'll find effective in achieving "groupthink."

Choose a moderator and hand out pens and paper to the group. Read a clear statement of the problem at hand. For example: "We have agreed that a complete new patient exam should not take more than 65 minutes. However, based on our latest time study, the average time is 83 minutes, and only a third of our patients are checking out within our agreed 65-minute deadline. How can we solve this problem and improve clinic flow?"

Announce that everyone has 5 minutes to privately brainstorm all the possible solutions, writing their ideas down along the way on the paper they have been given (these are not to be handed in).

When the 5 minutes are up, call time. Then go around the room and ask every member of the group to describe *one* of their solutions. As this is done, no one should comment or shoot down any of the ideas. Go around the room as many times as it takes to get everyone's ideas expressed. As each participant describes their ideas, a scribe should write these down (and number each) on a flip chart or white board.

It's not unusual to get dozens of possible solutions up on the board. Next, vote as a group on the best ideas. Ask the group to write down the numbers corresponding with the best three solutions on the board. Then go around the room and get everyone's votes—the scribe records these.

If the moderator moves things along briskly, NGT can generate a collaborative, ranked-order list of great solutions to even the toughest problems in under 30 minutes. You can apply the NGT process or a more orthodox, open group discussion to refine each of your top solutions.

• • •

Groupthink is definitely the way to go. But don't go overboard. It's easy for everyone to fall in line behind the emerging trend of the group, even if that trend is wrong. In the midst of collaboration and teamwork, there is still a vital role for members of a group to speak up and go against the popular tide. Researchers have found that the most effective way to avoid this herd mentality from taking over during group meetings is to make sure that the group is as diverse as possible. To this end, a meeting on the scheduling template should include technicians, receptionists, and managers—not just doctors. A meeting on budgeting for the next year should include not just practice insiders, but the practice's outside finance and accounting counsel.

CHAPTER 40

Ophthalmic Practice Motivation

A New Inventory Tool for Staff and Providers

John B. Pinto and Craig N. Piso, PhD

Motivation (mōtə'vāSHən) ... noun, The reason or reasons one has for acting or behaving in a particular way; the general desire or willingness of someone to do something.
—The Oxford English Dictionary

Motivation is the drive we all recognize in those we most admire and try to emulate in our own lives.

Since our earliest days, as the children of our parents, the students of our teachers, and the employees of our bosses, most of us try to excel.

For the most fortunate and accomplishing people, your source of motivation commonly shifts from an external locus (eg, parents, teachers, bosses) to an internal source. As we grow up, we naturally we want to accomplish great things for *ourselves.*

Pinto JB. *Ophthalmic Leadership: A Practical Guide for Physicians, Administrators, and Teams, Second Edition* (pp 235-238).
© 2022 SLACK Incorporated.

Being motivated enables us to take action and get things done, rather than feeling depressed, bored, or stuck. Motivation energizes our feelings, thoughts, and plans … both personal and professional. Without motivation, we stagnate, burn out, and fail.

As you think back on your own personal experience, you will probably recognize that you have been the most highly energized when you experienced the two core components of motivation:

1. A sense of the *importance* of your goals…
2. And a sense of *confidence* in your ability to achieve them.

Motivation is always a question of balance. Too *little* motivation and you won't make plans, much less accomplish them. Too *much* motivation—or motivation energized solely by greed or jealousy or insecurity—will lead to obsession, dissatisfaction, and failure. Whether you are an eye surgeon or work for one, finding the right motivational balance will advance both your individual career and the success of your practice.

Ophthalmic practices become most successful when led by highly motivated doctors and senior lay staff who share a passion for an important and attainable clinical and business outcome. This "motivation inventory" has been developed to assist you (and us!) in understanding and potentially enhancing your motivation.

We would urge you to use this inventory internally to stimulate helpful conversations and to facilitate strategic planning.

• • •

Please follow the instructions below and complete all three sections.

Your current position (eg, Administrator, Dept Head, MD, OD): ________________

Your current age: ________________

How long have you working in this practice (in any position): ________________

Practice size (current number of MD/DO providers): ________________

Part One

Following is a list of short statements. Next to each statement, please enter a number from 1 to 5:

5 = I strongly agree with this statement.

4 = I agree with this statement.

3 = I am neutral ... I neither agree nor disagree with this statement.

2 = I disagree with this statement.

1 = I strongly disagree with this statement.

I feel a sense of drive and energy about how I'm living my overall life.	
I am the "captain of my ship," directing and controlling the course my life is taking.	
I am hopeful and optimistic that I will reach the most important goals for my life.	
I am almost never the victim of circumstances and forces beyond my control.	
I have a clear vision of my successful future life.	
I know what to do today to achieve the goals I have set for myself.	
I recognize and am grateful when good things happen to me.	
I persistently "go the extra mile" for my goals, even after I experience setbacks and failures.	
I possess the confidence to take those risks needed to reach my goals.	
I am usually ready with "Plan B" actions when I encounter unforeseen obstacles or setbacks.	
I ask for help and team up with others to work toward making my dreams into reality.	
I view any failure or setback as a signal to keep trying.	
I am largely motivated by my own internal goals, not driven by other people.	
I am motivated by a purpose greater than myself.	
Please add up your Part One score and enter here	

Part Two

Please rate overall your enthusiasm on a 1 to 5 scale ... "1" is low, "5" is high: In the past few weeks, my enthusiasm for...

... my overall career has been a	
... learning new things has been a	
... reaching out to other people has been a	
... taking on new challenges has been a	
... working harder/smarter has been a	
... the things I normally would enjoy has been	
Please add up your Part Two score here	

Now add up your total score for Parts One and Two and enter here	

The maximum score is 100 points. There is no minimum "passing" score that we would impose on you. Instead, ask yourself if you think your relative score is in line with the drive *you* think you need to accomplish your professional goals in the practice.

Part Three

If tomorrow you could change any three things about your circumstances, your education and skills, your interests, or your motivation; these three things would be:

1)

2)

3)

Any other comments?

• • •

In addition to your individual score, you may find it interesting to:

- Use this inventory as a board or management committee group exercise to identify opportunities to elevate the collective motivation of the group to meet lofty goals (or, conversely, to deflate the goals somewhat to fit the lower motivations of the group).
- Use this inventory to examine and discuss any concerns you may have about a provider's or staff member's career motivation, or to shed a light on recent performance gaps.
- Use this inventory to better understand the motivation of a candidate for promotion.

Motivation, for all of its critical importance to your practice, is tricky to quantify. The most gifted administrators and practice owners are able to intuitively understand the motivations of their people, and harness these to further their ambitions for the company.

We hope that this somewhat more objective tool will help you better gauge how you and your staff measure up, and will lead to spirited internal discussions.

CHAPTER 41

How to Find and Reform or Eliminate the Weakest Members of Your Practice Team

John B. Pinto

In the words of that dearly departed ophthalmic management consultant, my old pal Bill Borover, "There are only three kinds of staff members and doctors: 'plus,' 'minus,' and 'plano.'" Indeed, every practice manager and physician-owner today has to be extra skilled at "refracting" the quality of their staff. As ophthalmic management continues to become more challenging, just one negative or low-performing member of the team can be both directly costly to the business and indirectly corrosive to staff morale.

My experience visiting hundreds of otherwise great practices points out a high level of resistance by some doctors and managers to reforming or removing these weak links in their business. Sit back and think if you've been harboring any of the following in your practice:

Pinto JB. *Ophthalmic Leadership: A Practical Guide for Physicians, Administrators, and Teams, Second Edition* (pp 239-241).
© 2022 SLACK Incorporated.

- The doctor in a group practice who holds themself apart from the rest of the team and refuses to follow protocols agreed to by every other provider.
- The tech who is sweet as pie to "their" doctor, but caustic with the rest of staff.
- The billing clerk who makes repetitive errors and passes on mounds of rework to their colleagues to clean up.
- The marketing and outreach coordinator who is too independent to be accountable for their whereabouts and productivity in the course of a work week.
- The surgery center manager who hides behind a smokescreen of regulatory compliance or quality assurance to resist efforts to reduce operating costs and increase efficiency.
- The administrator who is more concerned with rescuing their career than growing the volume and quality of the practice.
- The optician who long ago stopped their enjoyment of working with the public, and is now just going through the motions.
- The outside accountant who is kept on retainer not so much for their competency, but out of habit and because they have become a personal friend of the doctor.

When lecturing to groups I commonly ask the question: "How many of you have at least one person in your practice today who shouldn't be there?" Almost every hand goes up. When I ask the follow-up question, "How long have you felt this way?", the typical response back is counted in years, not months.

This resistance to reform or terminate weak players has many causes, the foremost of which is a reluctance to be confrontational or to rock the boat. Managers and doctors especially hate the thought of any near-term financial hiccups. The typical manager will say, "Dr. Nasty has always been that way, but we wouldn't dare let him go—he's responsible for covering a quarter of our overhead." Obviously, this same unpleasant doctor may in the long run be the cause of high staff turnover rates as well as the defection of patients from the practice.

Here's a simple set of screening questions you can use to assess your personal tolerance for and response to underperformers. Answer these honestly, and you'll be halfway to a stronger, happier practice.

1. Do you have a clear "line in the sand" when it comes to performance and behavioral expectations or are you inconsistent, applying different standards to various staff? Do you have any pet staff or doctors who receive extra gentle treatment because their productivity is high or they are deemed the only people who know how to perform key tasks? Do these people know they're getting a free pass and are they acting out accordingly?
2. Are you clear about communicating expectations and do you let staff know when they have crossed the line? Do your staff know where this line lies and respect it, or play games seeing how long they can misbehave? Remember, staff respond best to supervisors who are very tough, but fair.
3. Has your practice developed to the point of having middle managers? Have these managers embraced the practice's standards or do they work together as a group—a kind of unspoken trade guild within the practice—aligned against the interests of the doctors and patients all to make their jobs more pleasant? If so, what have

you done to bring this group around to seeing that by serving the patients well, everyone wins?

4. Have you fostered a "consequential environment," one where violations of practice expectations regarding policy (eg, arriving late to work, poor rapport with fellow workers, shoddy or inconsistent output) have a consequence? Or are you unconsciously rewarding the misbehavior of a few offenders, while killing the moral of productive staff who see their peers getting away with breaking the rules?
5. If you are an administrator or office manager, do the doctors back you up in disciplining staff, or have they made some staff untouchable? Have you been granted both the responsibility and the authority to take corrective action? Do you then apply the rules fairly to everyone or shield one or more personal friends?
6. If you are a doctor, do you grant yourself special allowances without regard for the impact your behavior has on others? (Especially for things like late arrival that hold up the rest of the team.) Or do you admit your errors and missteps openly in group staff meetings and work to improve your contributions to the team?
7. If you are the practice's MP, have you exerted your leadership on the toughest part of the job—counseling and censuring errant peers? Or do you let errors and omissions slide for the sake of harmony? A mollycoddling approach in this area is false economy, especially when dealing with younger associate doctors … experience shows it's better to come down rather directly with young doctors. If they can't respond to the imposition of group standards as an associate, it's better that they are not allowed to progress to partnership.
8. Is it easy or hard for you to decide what the consequences should be for staff and provider misbehavior? In larger practices, these should be spelled out in writing and often take the form of progressive discipline, including such things as fines for chronic tardiness.
9. Are your desires for the practice aligned with incentives for staff and doctors? If you want a markedly busier practice, make sure that financial incentives are in place for both selected lay staff and for providers. If you are trying to trim costs, be sure to reward staff who come forward with ideas that trim costs while leaving the quality of care intact.
10. Are you honest about the cost-benefit of keeping inappropriate staff on the payroll? All too many managers, especially those working in adverse labor markets and facing the chore of finding a new clerk or tech, take the easy way out and decide to live with weaknesses that are costing the practice dearly in the long run.

Far too many practices wait for annual reviews to take corrective action. In the best practices, performance standards are clear and public, and vigilance is applied daily. Great performers are rewarded lavishly and publicly, while weak links are gently shown the way to the door.

As the children's ditty goes, every party has a pooper … and nearly every practice has one, too. No matter how strong your team, there is someone in your practice today who is the weakest link. One of the most important tasks you have as a manager or owner is to discriminate between those deserving removal and those deserving extra attention and loving, patient reform.

CHAPTER 42

Leadership Decisions Inspired by Behavioral Economics

Erik F. Kruger, MD

It's Friday and, as usual, you've left the office a little later than expected. It's now 6:42 PM. You've arrived at a friend's cocktail party and are enjoying a martini (three green olives stuffed with bleu cheese, please). Dan, a research scientist in psychology who studies decision making under conditions of uncertainty, has engaged you in what at first appeared to be idle chatter but has become quite a bit more intriguing. A waitress walks by with a plate of hors d'ouevres, and as you reach for another mini-frank wrapped in phyllo dough, Dan tells you about Linda.

Linda is 31 years old, single, outspoken, and very bright. She majored in philosophy. As a student, she was deeply concerned with issues of discrimination and social justice, and participated in antinuclear demonstrations.

Pinto JB. *Ophthalmic Leadership: A Practical Guide for Physicians, Administrators, and Teams, Second Edition* (pp 243-252).
© 2022 SLACK Incorporated.

He asks you what you think is more likely. (1) Linda is a bank teller or (2) Linda is a bank teller and is active in the feminist movement.

When this scenario is presented, 85% of respondents will choose the second option. Most "feel" that the second option "seems" to be the more likely choice given the narrative vignette about Linda, though most are not exactly sure how they came to that conclusion.

Intuition aside, it is impossible for the probability of the conjunction of two events, Linda being a bank teller *and* active in the feminist movement, to be more likely than either one of these events occurring independently. The correct answer therefore is the first option. "Linda is a bank teller" is more likely.

How are we led astray from the truth by a flawed sense of what "seems" correct? The answer lies in heuristics, biases, and the field of behavioral economics.

• • •

Heuristics are mental shortcuts that we use to assist in our decision making under conditions of uncertainty. These rules of thumb have evolved over eons to be fast and efficient at reducing the complex tasks of probability estimation and value prediction to more simplistic judgmental operations. In general, they serve our needs well. Nonetheless, when the right circumstances are present, they leave us vulnerable to biases that can significantly affect the quality of our decisions.

The management at Disney accurately distilled the essence of leadership when they said that as leaders we are entrusted with "telling the great story" of our organizations. We are responsible for transmitting the values of the company, guiding strategy, and inspiring passion and interest. We are accountable for the oversight of legions of financial data upon which rest the organizational decisions of tomorrow. We pride ourselves on our ability to amass data from disparate sources and cull from the data a logical course of action that inures maximally to the benefit of the groups that we lead.

Though we would like to think that our mental processing is orderly and logical, most of the time we are left to carry out our most difficult decision-making tasks under conditions of great uncertainty. Furthermore, the complexity of our decisions and the time pressures that we face only exacerbate the difficulty of navigating this multifaceted slalom. Under these circumstances, we tend to default toward the use of heuristics to facilitate our decision making. In turn, we are prone to the biases that these heuristics can engender. They creep into our decisions undetected and, as the behavioral economist Richard Thaler says, they "nudge" us away from rational thought. Our experience with Linda is typical.

The field of behavioral economics developed around the work of Daniel Kahneman and Amos Tversky. Kahneman and Tversky were psychologists evaluating decision making under conditions of uncertainty. The broad applicability of their findings resulted in a Nobel Prize in economics and profoundly influenced a multitude of disciplines including medicine, psychology, cognitive science, and business management. A full discussion of behavioral economics is beyond the scope of this chapter. However, with respect to its influence on leadership decisions, much of the fundamental work is pertinent.

In this chapter we will survey some of the fundamental principles of behavioral economics. We will see how these principles quietly influence our thoughts, alter our assessments of ourselves and those we work with, and invisibly alter our judgements. By reviewing relevant experimental research as well as real life situations, it will begin to become apparent that the addition of this knowledge base to our strategic armamentarium may allow us to be more astute in our understanding of the hidden forces that motivate our decisions, and in turn assist in our ability to produce more rational and robust decisions for our organizations.

Representativeness

We use the representativeness heuristic when we are asked to think about the likelihood that a certain item belongs to a specific class of items, that a given event originates from a particular process, or that a particular process will produce a given event.

Looking at questions such as these, we tend to be pragmatic. We might ask ourselves to what extent does item "A" resemble class of items "B." Resemblance in this context includes features such as physical characteristics, personality, timing, etc. The greater the resemblance we perceive between item "A" and class "B" for example, the higher the estimate we will give that "A" originates from "B." The lower the resemblance, the lower the estimate that "A" originates from "B." The fundamental flaw in the representativeness heuristic is that we assume conjunction of similarity and probability. This is often not the case. As we shall see, biases arise in our decision making because there are factors that affect probability, sometimes quite significantly, that have no equivalent effect on similarity.

An example of one such bias-producing variable that affects probability, but not similarity, is base-rate frequency. Base-rate can be thought of as the overall frequency of "X" in the group from which we are sampling. In an intriguing experiment, participants were told of a group of 100 people, 30 engineers and 70 lawyers.[1] Next, they were given a narrative vignette that described a given person in the group, and they were asked to decide the probability that the person was an engineer. The majority of people chose based on how well the vignette fit their impression of an engineer or a lawyer with little regard to the underlying base-rate probability of 30% engineers in the population. In a second condition of the same experiment, the base-rate frequencies were reversed and participants were told that the population from which the vignettes were drawn was 70% engineers and 30% lawyers. With the right vignettes, participants still provided responses that neglected the base-rate frequency and gave estimates of "engineer probability" that were similar to or the same as those in the first set of conditions.

What is happening here? In the absence of representativeness data, participants will correctly deploy the base-rate frequency data and assign a probability of 0.3 that a given person is an engineer in the first experimental condition and 0.7 in the second condition. However, if representativeness data are provided by the narrative description, and in turn participants have a "feel" for the person, the information in the narrative will trump the base-rate frequency data and be used to estimate probability. With the right experimental conditions, participants will not report any probability difference in the likelihood that a given person is an engineer between the two experimental conditions. So as not to be swayed too far by our "impressions," base-rate frequency should be in our thoughts when we make decisions that relate to people and events.

Another potential bias of representativeness is the sample size of the population. No matter how our intuition lobbies the opposite, groups that are larger in number are probabilistically less likely to show variability and stray from the mean for a given "one-time" sampling than groups with smaller numbers.

Imagine you are the practice administrator at AwesomeCare, a group of eye doctors with a long history of service to the community. On any given day, you expect an average of 5% of patients to arrive without their insurance information. Should you expect 30% of patients to arrive without their insurance information more commonly on a day when there are 100 patients being seen or on a day when there are 20 patients being seen?

Strange as it may initially seem, we would expect a day when 30% arrive without their insurance information to occur more commonly when there are only 20 patients being seen than on a day when there are 100 patients being seen. Though these days may seem "light" in terms of patient numbers, there is actually a greater likelihood of extreme variances occurring on these "light" days. With respect to staffing needs, they may turn out to not be so "light."

This is counterintuitive for many of us and is based on the "law of large numbers" from probability theory. Managers responsible for processes often fail to account for sample size bias and may search through a plethora of causes in their quest to identify what produced an extreme process deviation. Unless they are actively sought out, inaccuracies introduced by sample size bias often go undetected. AwesomeCare may be able to scale back staffing on lightly scheduled days, but quite possibly not as much as they might initially think from an isolated analysis of patient volume.

A third bias that can influence our thinking when we use the representativeness heuristic is that of chance itself. Results that occur by chance in a large, global population are usually not the same as results that occur in a smaller, local population drawn from that global population. Each of the parts of the whole need not represent the essential features of the whole. Failure to recognize this and to account for it can once again lead to weaknesses in our logic.

The "gambler's fallacy" is an example of such an error and is rooted in the misinterpretation of a local population for a global one. If one plays roulette and has seen a long run of "red" occur, it palpably feels as if the likelihood of "black" coming up is increased … one may feel that black is "due." Black is, in fact, not "due." Chance deviations within a small sample that stray from the characteristics of a larger population do not self-correct themselves back toward an equilibrium in that local sample. Though black is not "due" for our gambler, we can assume that, given the multitude of other players sitting at a multitude of other roulette wheels in the casino, black will come up in a way throughout the casino that dilutes this particular run of reds that our gambler has seen. In the end, the casino can rely on 50% red and 50% black. Unfortunately for our gambler, he cannot rely on the same.

At AwesomeCare, the clinic manager Mr. Ken Doo noted that the last 25 older patients took on average an extra 5 minutes each to check in. Does this group of older patients reliably represent older patients in general? Should he change the check-in process to accommodate this extra time requirement or monitor to see if this was a small sample straying from the characteristics of a larger population? With respect to our organizations, its systems, and our attendant decisions that relate to groups of data, we need to first identify if we are looking at the global population or a smaller local population drawn from that global group. Next, if we are looking at a local group, we need to know that if that group is large enough from which to draw reasonable conclusions with respect to the known characteristics of the global group. With this information at hand, we are primed to move toward greater fidelity in our decisions.

Regression to the mean is the next bias we might observe when we use the representativeness heuristic. Imagine that AwesomeCare has recently opened two new optical retail stores. Brenda, the manager of "Lenstacular" gives you data that show phenomenal revenue growth for the month. You are overjoyed and heap praise upon her. The following month, the revenue at Lenstacular is down some from her last report. Meanwhile, revenue at your other retail outlet, "Spex," is suddenly and significantly lower. You chastise Ty, the store manager. The following month revenues at Spex are seen to move back toward expected norms. What do you conclude? Is it that we should be more parsimonious with praise for our managers because praise only leads to subsequent slacking and we should reprimand poor management because it leads to rapid improvement? Possibly. That said, irrespective of all other possibilities, there is a fair chance that if nothing was said to either of the managers that we would have seen the same revenue movement that we did for each of the two stores. We may simply be witnessing movement back toward the average … regression to the mean.

While some managers do begin to slack after they have "wowed" their boss and some do improve long term when they fear for their jobs, irrespective of what Brenda and Ty can control, the chaotic scrum of variables that leads to revenue for a given month in a retail environment may just be responding to the elastic pull of regression to the mean. Doubtless, the reason we hire quality managers is that we expect in the long run they can have a positive effect on the mean itself. That said, over the short run it can be difficult for us to say with veracity what effect our influence has on them, and what their influence has on the people and data they manage. The subjects of reward, punishment, and motivation are of course complex and full of the unexpected. That said, the principles of regression toward the mean should be recalled when we formulate decisions that relate to our people and our processes.

A final thought experiment helps elucidate how all of the biases introduced by representativeness can summate. Imagine that one of the best cataract surgeons at AwesomeCare, Dr. Lux, has not had a case of postcataract surgery endophthalmitis, a serious eye infection that can occur after eye surgery, in over 10,000 surgeries. The incidence of postsurgery endophthalmitis in the general population at large is about one case per 5000 surgeries, so it seems Dr. Lux is doing pretty well. He is shocked and dismayed when he sees his second postcataract surgery endophthalmitis case in the office only 20 surgeries after the his first case of endophthalmitis. An "all hands on deck" search for the etiologic cause for this sudden increase in frequency assignable to his technique or to the systems and processes at the surgery center where he operates is completed and is unrevealing. Dr. Lux is a good doctor with a strong concern for his patient's welfare. At an office board meeting, he cites the data of a colleague, Dr. Super, who uses the antibiotic Cephakillall in the eye at the time of surgery and has not had an endophthalmitis case in over 20,000 procedures. Dr. Lux requests that Cephakillall now too be used in the eye during his surgeries at considerable additional expense to the organization and potentially contributing to the risk of Cephakillall-resistant bacteria in the general population. Given the recent events and Dr. Lux's pleas, and with the best interest of their patients at heart, the board approves his request. After 1 year, with the addition of Cephakillall at the time of surgery, Dr. Lux has not seen another endophthalmitis case. He is pleased with his "innovation" and the rational decision making of his organization.

Given the underlying probability of endophthalmitis in the general population, should we be concerned about a run of two cases in a short time span? Though there should always of course be concern with respect to the patient's health, we should not expect this small local sample drawn from a much larger global population to maintain all of the characteristics of that larger population with respect to the incidence of endophthalmitis. A chance run of two cases over a short time is certainly possible and "bound to occur" without any required explanation. We would expect this run to be diluted out in the larger global population, as was the case with our gambler at the roulette table.

Is the use of Cephakillall by Dr. Lux effective in lowering the rate of endophthalmitis? Maybe it is and maybe it is not. Once again, the sample size may not be large enough to know if there is a real difference between his local rate of endophthalmitis and that seen in the global population of cataract surgeries in general. Controlled clinical trials seek to ensure that an ability to detect a difference between the local sample in the trial and the global population as a whole is built into the study design of the trial. Like the sirens of Greek mythology calling out to Ulysses, the seductive nature of anecdotal evidence in a local sample can lure us away from rationality unless we too steady ourselves against it in our decision making.

Should our cataract surgeon be pleased with his ensuing results after adding Cephakillall? Though the "improvement" in his incidence of endophthalmitis may be due to the Cephakillall, it also might be explained by other possibilities that have nothing to do with his intervention, such as regression to the mean. Regression to the mean alone would predict that after an extreme variation from the population average, we would expect movement back toward the mean without any outside forces intervening. Therefore, it's quite possible that even without the addition of Cephakillall he would not have had an endophthalmitis case for many more years.

Availability

Another heuristic that we use to assess the probability of an event, or the frequency of some class, is availability … the ease that like instances or occurrences can be brought to mind. Instances of larger class are recalled easier and more rapidly than those of smaller class. In general, we are served well by this oversimplification. If we try to estimate the likelihood that a person is a member of a given group, we may think of groups that have similar characteristics as the person under consideration. With broad generality, this person is more likely to be a member of a large, similar group that has characteristics that are similar to theirs. Recall Linda the bank teller.

With availability, our estimation of the size or frequency of a class is biased by how "retrievable" like members of the class are ... how easily they can be brought to mind. Retrievability is in turn determined by temporal proximity and salience ... how recently was something experienced and how much of an impact did it have on us. The subjective probability that a given person will provide, for instance, of the likelihood of an auto accident is correlated with the recentness that they have seen an auto accident on the road. This is temporal proximity. The impact of having been in an auto accident themselves would also typically alter subsequent estimates of the probability of auto accidents. This is salience. Taken in combination, those who were themselves in an auto accident last week will give dramatically different estimates of the likelihood of an auto accident from those who can remember reading about an auto accident in a newspaper 6 months ago. Retrievability affects what is available, and what is available affects our decisions.

Consider that the board of directors of AwesomeCare, has asked you to consider the factors involved in the construction of a new ambulatory surgical center. Organizational needs dictate that this center be in the proposed location to maintain a competitive edge against another local medical group, BollocksCare. Your thoughts turn to the various difficulties that may be encountered during the project. You think about the likely problems: cost overruns, effects on the revenue of your current operation, contractor tardiness, the list goes on ... a veritable bevy of very real concerns. But somehow, you can't get rain out of your head.

It seems that recently a once in a lifetime series of weather events nearly produced flooding of a local river in the area you are thinking about building. It did in fact produce flooding in the adjacent town, but not where you are proposing to build. You have been assured that this will never actually occur at your chosen site, as it did not this time, because of a state of the art levee system that is in place. You have consulted with your own "flood" of engineers, meteorologists, and city planners who have all deemed that a flood in the proposed area cannot occur. That said, mental images of buildings partially submerged underwater in the adjacent town during the recent flood permeate your brain. Despite your prudent, meticulous analysis and it's favorable results for going ahead, those images keep "popping up" and distract you from a detailed analysis of the other more abstract, but very real, potential problems.

The temporal proximity and salience of the recent flood in the neighboring town makes this highly unlikely event prone to the retrievability bias and in turn it is highly available to you in your planning. It may be so available that in your overweighting of this event you underestimate the import of the more real threats. Knowing in advance that we are prone to the biases associated with availability can help facilitate their attenuation. We would do well to add "biases in our problem list" to the problem list itself.

Anchoring and Adjustment

The final bias prone heuristic that we will explore is that of adjustment and anchoring. Tversky modestly said of anchoring, that he was not describing anything that "advertisers and used car salesman" did not already know.

In making estimates of probability, we set our mental thermostats, or anchor, at some start point and adjust up or down. The value of the start point may be suggested by the nature of the issue at hand or it may be derived from a partial computation. In either case, adjustments from that initial anchor are typically insufficient. Given these insufficient adjustments, different starting points will yield different estimates of probability with a bias toward the value of the starting point. Influence the mental set point for an estimate of probability and you will influence the final estimate of that probability. Alternatively, if someone influences your anchor regarding an estimate of probability, you too will likely generate biased probability estimates. All of this can produce some very strange effects.

If participants are asked for the last four digits of their social security number and are then immediately asked to estimate the number of doctors in New York City, on average, those with "larger" social security numbers tend to give estimates that are larger than those with "lower" social security numbers ... repeatedly and predictably. What do the digits of a social security number and doctors in New York have in common? Nothing. Despite the total irrelevance of our social security number to the doctor count, our mental shortcuts are primed and anchor to this figure. When we then try to estimate how many doctors there might be we are erroneously tethered to the social security number figure as an anchor and adjust inadequately from there.

Biases of adjustment can also be seen in conjunctive and disjunctive events. A study by Bar-Hillel[2] highlights these types of adjustment biases. In Bar-Hillel's study, the following assumptions are made regarding three bags of marbles:

1. Bag A is 50% red marbles and 50% white marbles.
2. Bag B is 90% red marbles and 10% white marbles.
3. Bag C is 90% white marbles and 10% red marbles.

Participants were asked, "Is it more likely to: (a) Draw a red marble from bag A? (b) Draw a red marble seven times in a row from bag B? (c) Draw a red marble once in seven tries from Bag C?"

Drawing red on a given try from a bag that is mostly red, such as Bag B, is quite likely. However, doing it seven times is less likely. Much less likely. This is a good example of a conjunctive event, and the overall probability of a conjunctive event is less than the individual probabilities that form it. Once is likely. Seven times in a row, and the probability plummets. Most of the time we fail to adjust accordingly from our initial impression of the high probability and will overestimate the likelihood of these conjunctive events.

Drawing a red marble one time from Bag C, which is mostly white marbles, would seem to be unlikely and it is. But try seven times and the likelihood goes way up. This is a disjunctive event. The probability of a disjunctive event is greater than the individual probabilities that form it. Here, the probability of drawing red on one try is indeed unlikely. But given seven tries it becomes more likely than not. This time we fail to adjust appropriately in the other direction. Our initial impression of a low probability rules the day, we fail to adjust up, and we will tend to underestimate the probability of the event.

Despite our intuition, drawing a red marble once out of seven tries from a bag that is mostly white marbles is actually the most likely of the examples, and drawing the red marble seven times from a bag that is mostly red is the least likely of the three. Most research participants, and probably most of us, underestimate the likelihood of the disjunctive event and overestimate the likelihood of the conjunctive event.

Consider that the launch of a new product or service has a conjunctive character. Imagine that after 20 years of only treating adult disease, AwesomeCare decides to hire a new pediatric specialist, Dr. Rainbows N. Puppydogs.

Assuredly, there are many new factors to consider: coordinating appointments with school schedules and parent's needs, entertaining bored children in the waiting room, obtaining pediatric exam equipment, and many more small but manageable problems. Individually these all seem easy to accomplish, with a low likelihood of failure. You have therefore assured the board that there should be no problems when Dr. Puppydogs starts next week. But there are problems. The dancing clown DVDs for the waiting room did not arrive on time. Chaos ensues. Children are running around screaming, and the adult long-time patients are rescheduling and fleeing the premises.

Each step in the new process may be fairly straightforward and indeed quite likely, be it the timely arrival of the dancing clown DVDs you ordered for the waiting room or the drawing of a red marble from a bag that is 90% red, though with enough steps the probability of overall success drops as it did with the marbles. Though most of us have some intuitive sense of the forces at work that can tend to disrupt a multistep project, we tend to grossly underestimate their significance. Unless we take their conjunctive character into account, we are vulnerable to flawed decisions—with respect to our projects and processes.

Disjunctive events can be unsettling to our decisions as well. In many complex systems, the risk of any one elementary unit failing may be quite low. Though there may be many "moving parts," the likelihood of failure of any one moving part is extremely low so we assume the likelihood of overall failure is low.

Imagine that the billing department at AwesomeCare has four dedicated associates, assiduously plodding through the office's billing claims. Their computers almost always function seamlessly. The network connection to the third party payer tends to run smoothly and efficiently. Typically adequate staffing at the third-party payer facilitates timely processing of claims. The postal service delivering the daily checks in time for payroll at AwesomeCare almost never has a breakdown of the conveyor belt at their main mail sorting facility. Though each step has the small possibility of failure, we tend to neglect these small possibilities for the din of the overall process humming away steadily. But each step must function well each and every business day, day after day and week after week. Given these parameters, the total risk of failure may be quite a bit higher than is first apparent. A breakdown in that mail sorting conveyor belt, or drawing a red marble from a bag that is mostly white marbles, actually occurs with greater regularity than we would imagine given sufficient repetitions of the process. If we are not factoring in the peculiarities of disjunctive events into our decision making, we are most likely going to underestimate the shortcomings embedded in our decisions. Infrequent rare events that can derail a process occur more than one would expect from the nature of the individual steps. We can of course never entirely eliminate the "unforeseen unforeseens" from our business processes. However, proactively accounting for anchoring and adjustment biases that are inherent in disjunctive events can assuage their effects on our leadership decisions.

It's enough to make you lose your marbles. Most of the biases associated with heuristics are not intuitively obvious and that is just the point. Kahneman and Tversky have pointed out that it is not surprising that we continue to use the aforementioned heuristics ... they serve us well most of the time. What is surprising is that we do not notice the statistical principles that engender bias when these heuristics are used. Most likely, it is an issue of attentiveness, or the lack thereof. There is more variation in the average word length between this line of text and the last line you just read than there is between the average word length on this page and that on the last page. You didn't notice that? Not to worry, you're not alone. But if you were prone to noticing that sort of thing, you might have picked up on the relationship between sample size and variability that was touched upon earlier in the discussion of representativeness without any explanation required. Because we do not usually "attend" to things like average word length on a page, even though the truth is "right there," we miss the opportunity to account a priori for the biases that emanate from our otherwise useful heuristics.

An understanding of these ideas and many of the other principles of behavioral economics affords us the opportunity to mitigate against some of the factors that can contribute to flaws in our logic. With more robust logic and a greater understanding of how we make the important decisions that we do, we are poised to produce empowered decisions of higher quality and to in turn become more efficacious leaders for our organizations.

References

1. Kahneman D, Tversky A. On the psychology of prediction. *Psychological Review,* 1973;80(4):237-251. doi:10.1037/h0034747
2. Bar-Hillel M. On the subjective probability of compound events. *Organizational Behavior and Human Performance,* 1973;9(3):396-406. doi:10.1016/0030-5073(73)90061-5

CHAPTER 43

Ten Simple Steps for a Successful Practice

John B. Pinto

I hear the same envious refrain nearly every day. Doctors and managers with faltering practices look longingly at their more successful colleagues and ask, "Why isn't our practice as prosperous as theirs?" The two-fold answer is remarkably simple.

Some of the most successful practices are that way because they're located in charmed locations. I have one client in the Southeast, who is the only eye surgeon for a service area with more than 80,000 people. The average ophthalmologist in America competes in a market that only yields about 20,000 people per eye surgeon. Attractive markets like Denver only have about 10,000 people per eye surgeon.

Pinto JB. *Ophthalmic Leadership: A Practical Guide for Physicians, Administrators, and Teams, Second Edition* (pp 253-255).
© 2022 SLACK Incorporated.

Good fortune takes other forms. I have a client in the Pacific Northwest whose market is a retirement haven containing more than 25% seniors—the typical market has only half this senior population. Some surgeons work in markets so rural that staffing and facility costs are a fraction of what their urban cousins pay.

What about those practices whose locations aren't so fortunate? Every other flourishing ophthalmologist I know has had to get there the old-fashioned way—they've worked hard and survived the pitfalls that can undermine success in the increasingly complex and demanding business side of eye care. What was once a very forgiving enterprise that could be run loosely with great success is now a business like most others, with steep penalties for neglect. Regulatory and payer burdens are multiplying. And practice expenses are rising each year in an essentially fixed or falling fee environment.

Only the most fortunate surgeons can work in "easy" markets. For the rest, I've compiled a short priority list of simple steps than can help to assure you control over your business affairs and ultimate commercial success, even in the most demanding markets.

1. *Make great decisions.* It sounds easy, but it's not. After making sure that your decision is ethical and legal, most decisions should boil down to one simple test: Which is more profitable, Option A or Option B? Gather the facts, and let the facts make your decisions.
2. *Don't make business decisions by yourself.* Engaging every individual likely to be impacted by your decision is good politics. Getting the counsel of people smarter or more experienced than you are on the subject is plain common sense. The sharpest clinical minds are often frustratingly dull when applied to business affairs.
3. *Strive daily to increase profitability without reducing quality, and to increase quality without decreasing profits.* In mature practices, large profit and quality gains are rare. But even the most developed and refined practice can make small, incremental improvements.
4. *Leave your options open.* Think twice before abandoning patient services, closing down an office, or dismissing a key staff member because of some perceived slight. Even if you do not dispense glasses today, leave room in your new office facility for a dispensary adjoining the reception area. Take an introductory LASIK course to stay current, even if you never plan to perform refractive surgery.
5. *Get and stay diversified.* Sharply falling refractive surgery profitability is just the latest in a long list of hard lessons in the business of ophthalmology. For safety, no single patient service and no single payer (with the possible exception of Medicare) should represent more than a third of your cash flow.
6. *End each year with more and better relationships than you started out with.* Be balanced in your relationship building, including patients, payers, staff, local institutions, venders, lenders, and fellow doctors.
7. *Be disciplined.* Most practices that get into trouble do so because their lead doctors are undisciplined in one way or another. They set performance standards for staff that they are unwilling to keep themselves. In any area where you have a history of being poorly self-disciplined (eg, financial, exercise, dietary) hire an outside source of discipline.

8. *Work harder, after you have exhausted all opportunities to work smarter.* The most financially successful surgeons I know in the world are "B" students who did exceptionally well because they simply work harder than their peers.
9. *Seize opportunity.* The most successful people in business are rash and opportunistic. If you think there are no more opportunities left in eye care, you're not looking hard enough. And if the opportunities you *can* see aren't appealing, it may be time to find a new profession. When opportunity knocks, take the hinges off the door. Most importantly, have sufficient personal and business capital reserves on hand to be able to accept reasonable risks.
10. *Pro-forma every major business decision.* Using your current income statement as a baseline, review the impact of adding a new satellite, a new doctor, or a new patient service to your practice. Have the intellectual integrity to believe the numbers rather than relying on hunches and guestimates. At the same time, trust your instinct. A bad feeling about a potential project should trump even the rosiest financial projections.

Section IV

Leading Through Change and Transition

CHAPTER 44

Confessions of a Reluctant Managing Partner

Paul S. Imperia, MD

I hate John B. Pinto. I also hate to be wrong. These two facts are related.

Over the 20+ years I have known John and he has consulted with our practice, there have been many instances of him making recommendations that have felt uncomfortable, unnecessary, or unrealistic. In hindsight, most of these recommendations, I hate to admit, were exactly what we should have done, what we ended up doing, and what we would have benefitted from by doing earlier. John's advice to create an MP position in our practice was one such recommendation. We put it off for 15 years and now wonder how we functioned without it. John, I hate you ... again. (Actually, John is also a personal friend whom I have fly-fished with in Oregon, Colorado, and the Pacific Islands).

Pinto JB. *Ophthalmic Leadership: A Practical Guide for Physicians, Administrators, and Teams, Second Edition* (pp 259-264).
© 2022 SLACK Incorporated.

This chapter is oriented to (1) practices who do not have an MP and might be skeptical of the need for the position and (2) doctors who are contemplating becoming an MP and are wondering what's involved. I'd like to outline the history leading up to our decision to have an MP, what kept us from doing it sooner, a general job description, and what the impact has been on our practice and my work life. In short, I believe any practice can benefit from the position and regarding the job, like most things in life, nothing good comes easy.

When I joined Medical Eye Center in 1991, we had four ophthalmologists, three of the four joining the practice within 5 years of one another. The senior partner, in his 60s, had been managing the practice for many years, had built a very successful organization, and continued in the managing position. Our front office manager acted as practice administrator and we had manager positions in the optical and technician departments. Like many smaller practices of the era, and perhaps still today, the senior partner was the de facto MP. There was no working board of directors. The senior partner might or might not seek the council of the junior partners. The junior partners certainly had a say, but it was understood by everyone that the senior partner had ultimate say and veto power.

This scenario can work well, depending on the practice and people involved. However, I would advise that the senior partner is not necessarily the person most suited to the job. Having a formal election, term of office, specific job description, and decision-making structure based on a board of directors composed of practice owners is preferable and, I think, necessary as a practice grows. Upon our senior partner's retirement, the next most senior doc expressed an interest in the position. It seemed like the natural law of hierarchy and everyone went along without much discussion as to expectations and structure. For a variety of reasons, including the lack of that formal structure discussion, that partner did not work out as an MP and eventually parted ways with the practice.

That left me, my other same-age partner, and our administrator to run the practice. We decided we did not want nor need the MP position. This derived from a few false assumptions and our practice situation and culture at the time.

We assumed that a practice our size did not warrant nor need an MP. We could effectively make decisions and develop strategy amongst the three of us. What we failed to appreciate was that, even with just two owners, there was no go-to person to help the administrator and staff carry out those decisions and strategy on a day-to-day basis. This would lead to management often working with assumptions of what they thought the partners wanted. A drift in their direction compared to the direction we thought they were going would result. I would therefore encourage even the smallest of practices to adopt the MP position.

Another assumption driving our decision making regarding leadership structure was our perception of what the position entailed. We imagined that the MP would have significant decision-making power that might be used for self-benefit. A contributing factor to our unwillingness to single out one partner was our compensation formula at the time. We were 100% "eat what you kill" with an overhead allocation method that, in retrospect, led to an undesirable amount of internal competition and conflict. We did not want one partner to be more powerful or influential than the other. Our compensation formula is still partially production-based, however, we don't try to figure out who to tag with what overhead and we share a portion of income equally. This has led to a more cooperative spirit amongst the partnership. However, at the time, egalitarianism and looking to the CEO to make sensitive decisions and arbitrate conflict seemed the safe path.

Our false assumption was that the MP has individual decision-making powers. In my mind, one of the most important things to understand about the MP job description is that the MP functions at the pleasure of the board of directors, ie, the practice owners. They carry out the board's strategic plan within all aspects of the practice and should not have the power to make any major decisions individually. An MP that deviates from that mandate, I would imagine, will have a short-lived tenure. There will be many daily operational issues and strategic details that you will be called upon to decide without board input. However, your decisions will be driven by the board's broad mandate. Besides making the other partners feel safe, this structure provides security for the MP. It helps, when having difficult discussions with staff or associates, to remind yourself and the person across the table, that this is not personal—you are only carrying out the board's wishes. There is also security in not being required to make solo major decisions without board input, which could later be judged harshly.

Back to our history. We functioned without an MP for the next 17 years. During that time, we hired a business school-trained administrator and CEO, added an ASC and ASC director, developed a very successful refractive surgery practice, established four satellite offices, hired two optometrists, developed a comanagement program, bought a retiring physicians practice, hired an in-house accountant, built a new 30,000 square foot building, and hired three younger fellowship-trained ophthalmologists in plastics, cornea, and retina. We did much of this during the worst economic downturn in our lifetimes and, sometimes with difficulty, kept our heads above water. So, you obviously can function without an MP and succeed. However, the strain on our staff and organization of not having adequate MD involvement in daily operations, and the frustration of the owners in not feeling in control of our own practice, grew and grew as we grew and grew. This lack of leadership was not so evident during good economic times, but became more so during the more recent challenging period.

Our "governance" model during this time was to basically give our CEO a broad idea of what we wanted and expect him and the management staff to carry out our vision. My partner and I worked hard in our own clinical practices, brought our grievances to management when things weren't working, and stayed out of most operational issues. We used our CEO to make recommendations and be the judge and arbiter on any potential issues of fairness or conflict in regard to compensation and utilization of resources. We were relatively uninvolved in many aspects of the organization, especially given our growth, size, and complexity.

This model was not without some upsides. There were fewer distractions from clinical practice. The two partners felt equal in decision making and significance. There was some conflict avoidance in the form of delegating delicate interpartner decisions to the CEO. The CEO and management team felt and were powerful. Ignorance was sometimes temporary bliss.

The downsides were several. Interpersonal partner conflicts could become much worse when expecting someone else to manage them. There is no substitute for open and accountable communication amongst the partners, which we have spent many years developing to reach a good level of trust and cooperation. Every partnership has difficult decisions, especially around money. A CEO can help moderate these discussions and supply reference data, but it is unrealistic to expect the CEO to act as judge. A board of directors and an MP lends structure to these sensitive discussions and lessens the chance for personal conflict.

Another downside was the phenomenon of mission drift. The management team would hear the partners' broad vision plan. However, what they heard was sometimes different than what the partners intended. Partner directives were sometimes soft on detail. The two partners might have somewhat different opinions and/or priorities, leaving the CEO to sort out a consensus direction. Time and energy were lost in redirection efforts, causing frustration for partners and managers alike. There was no one partner to go to for constant operational issues. This left managers with direction that was either absent or inconsistent. Since no one partner was tasked with managing nor given the authority to make operational decisions, partners could be become complacent or not accountable (I'm including myself here). We didn't know our practice well enough and had the increasing feeling of losing control over it.

We grew, added more doctors, more programs, a new building, and had to face a multitude of management decisions brought about by the economic downturn. It became more obvious that we needed one partner to be reporting to the Board, directing the strategic plan, and involved in the daily management of the practice. We were still hesitant because of all our history, misconceptions, and false assumptions. However, there were rumblings that John Pinto would be bringing up the topic at his next visit…

Before contemplating the position, I called my cornea fellowship mate, whom I knew had been the MP at a practice similar to ours. It was sobering. He described a job that required a significant amount of his time with little compensation. Most of his partners appreciated his efforts, but thanks were not commensurate with effort or accomplishment. The job involved having difficult conversations with managers and doctors. It required a lot of attention to detail, follow-through, and unheralded behind the scenes work.

I asked him why, after 12 years in the position, he continued? His answer was candid and illuminating. Despite the meager compensation and rare pats on the head, he took satisfaction from following through on projects that he knew benefitted the practice and wouldn't happen otherwise. He enjoyed earning the trust of his peers by presenting well thought out projects and assessments. The partnership trusted him because he tended not to be defensive, invited feedback, and kept agreements. He was not afraid of conflict or change, and tended to be direct and open and comfortable having difficult conversations. He liked to lead by example. He was not a conversationalist, but his peers told him he was a good communicator. He described himself as a high control, detail-oriented person, maybe a bit more OCD than the average ophthalmologist (which would place him pretty high on the scale). All of this was sounding strangely familiar. Many of his descriptors resonated with me, not always in a flattering or comfortable way. Finally, he said, nobody else wanted the job.

When Pinto visited our practice this last time and again brought up the MP position, we finally agreed we needed one. Then came the process of deciding who. In typical fashion, we let our CEO open the discussion and voice his preference. He named me primarily because of a significant amount of work we had done long-term together on developing the refractive surgery program. My partners were supportive, and I decided to give it a try.

So how has this played out for the organization and me personally so far?

As I write this, I am only 6 months into my 2-year term. There is unanimous agreement that we are far better off with the position than without it. Although it would be nice to assume this is because of my stellar management skills, in reality, I believe, it is largely just the creation of the position.

I have been very careful to avoid any personal agendas. Initially I would run everything by the board. I quickly found this to be exhausting and impractical. I am getting better at making day-to-day decisions that I'm confident are consistent with the board's wishes. I reserve going to the board for the bigger strategic and financial decisions.

I generally dislike meetings. My meeting schedule has multiplied to include weekly meetings with the CEO, monthly meetings with the management team, monthly board meetings, attending the monthly departmental meetings, and attending an annual conference for MPs. Meetings, ironically, have become easier for me to tolerate. I believe this is due to now having the license to represent the partnership and be engaged and directive.

Attending these meetings, most of which have not had a partner in attendance for many years, has been enlightening. I have become aware of operational issues that the staff has been struggling with that can be "unstuck" with some simple MD perspective and involvement. I have encountered many instances of doing things a certain way under the assumption that it is the way the partners want it done, with no relation to what any of the partners actually want. Many times I'll make a suggestion, and the staff will be somewhat awestruck with a "We can do that?' expression, assuming the doctors would never go for it. Managing your managers is one of the most important aspects of this job that pays significant dividends.

Managers enjoy having one partner that they know they can go to, without repercussions from the other partners. The managers save time, energy, frustration, and money by seeking and getting clear, detailed answers and direction. The CEO feels safer, more productive, and less out on a limb having this management partnership, especially when it comes to developing new doctors and programs.

I definitely have less time to answer email, read journals, make phone calls, surf the net, etc. My days, rarely slow in the past, now seem constantly full. I am hoping this is related to learning the job. Despite the increased time and energy commitment, I am very satisfied to feel like I am making a difference. I feel more connected and engaged in my practice, which increases my job satisfaction and is energizing. My personal productivity has increased since I feel like I need to set an example. My practice has become the test lab for many new programs and initiatives, which is invigorating for me and my team.

If you are in a practice of any size, my opinion is that you would benefit from having an MP. If you are someone contemplating taking on this responsibility, if you are high control, detail-oriented, open, direct, and organized, and you look around the room and everyone is taking a step back and looking at you … you're probably the one.

CHAPTER 45

Strengths and Limitations of the "MD-as-Administrator" Model

John Campbell, MD

Note: This chapter and the chapter that immediately follows should be read together. They frame up the thoughtful perspectives of the outgoing and incoming MPs of a highly successful California practice that, despite decades of success, is still undergoing growing pains ... as all practices do. —John B. Pinto

My practice in Marin County, California, has roots going back to 1946. Fresh out of residency in 1979, I joined the two founding partners. We had three office workers. Today, the practice has become "MarinEyes," three MDs, two ODs, and 26 other full-time employees. With two locations, a surgery center and laser center, we are presently recruiting our first professional administrator. It's long overdue. I am here to tell you about the joys and the frustrations I have experienced in

Pinto JB. *Ophthalmic Leadership: A Practical Guide for Physicians, Administrators, and Teams, Second Edition* (pp 265-271).
© 2022 SLACK Incorporated.

my 31 years as the physician/administrator of MarinEyes and how I decided to move to a new model of a professionally administered practice.

The AAO has provided us with a useful set of white papers on ophthalmology practice models. The models are physician-only, physician with technicians, and the physician with optometrists. The emphasis is on the clinical team as the distinguishing comparator between models. These are operational models.

I have experienced all three of the Academy's operational models as a physician-administrator. I find the models useful; however, I'm going to discuss practice structure from an administrative perspective rather than from a clinical/operational point of view. Let's review two examples of the physician-administered practice model.

Case Study 1: Dr. Richard Lee's AAO Model Practice

The most obvious advantage of having an MD-owner as administrator of their practice is saving the salary expense. Dr. Richard Lee describes this beautifully in his AAO white paper. It should be noted that Dr. Lee is an astute businessman as well as a fine practitioner. Simplicity is the key element in his model of an ophthalmology office with minimal staffing and complexity.

The advantages of his practice model are abundant, and this model generates envy in those of us with larger organizations. A small practice has few employees, and the physical plant is small enough that everyone is in view. The boss' instructions go straight to the employee without an intermediary, and they are there to see if the work is being carried out as directed. The staff is easily focused on one vision. The MD enjoys a long-term, close working relationship with loyal staff. The physician enjoys the pleasure of creating a high-performance team "in their own image." Finally, there is the privilege of paying a few people very well. You can be a generous employer, while saving a lot of money on technical and supervisory staff. Note that the founding principle of simplicity is prerequisite. There are few "moving parts." The optical and surgery center are operated separately, and there is one office location physically optimized for an ophthalmology practice. This is an ideal, simple practice for an MD Administrator.

Case Study 2: MarinEyes and John Campbell, MD

MarinEyes historically started with Dr. Lee's model. It functioned very well from the doctors' perspective for almost 40 years. We'll call those "the good old days." I practiced this way for a number of years. I liked it a lot, it was profitable, and my practice grew. The appointment backlog grew as well. We moved in 1986 to modestly larger quarters. By this time, I had a new partner my age who had no interest in administration. The older gentlemen were all but retired. I hired a tech with experience in office management. We trained a few clinic assistants for limited tasks and things continued to work well. Our surgical practices grew, and we hired an optometrist and more techs in 1987. Additional space became available in our building and we added a few lanes. We were off to a very good start. Growth was fun and life was good.

There came a point, though, where we got stuck. The hospital where we did our surgeries was unwilling to make changes that would permit us to do more than six or seven cases on a surgery day. Our clinic was maxed out and we felt that further reducing clinic time would negatively impact surgery volume. Our backlogs increased (6 to 8 weeks to get OR time, 2 months for an appointment), patient in-office waiting time grew intolerable, and staff performance was, well, "not up to my standards." (See *John Pinto's Little Green Book of Ophthalmology,* Appendix A, on "The Ophthalmic Personality" if you don't know what I'm referring to here.) We couldn't see taking away another day a week to work in the hospital. Space became available across the hall from our office.

• • •

As a historical footnote, the theme of the early 1990s in California medicine was the onslaught of the primary-care driven managed care organization. The common view was that solo practice was dying, and that specialty practices would need to kick up volume in order to cover losses in per-RVU (relative value scale) reimbursement. This would require increased use of space and nonphysician staff to leverage the surgeons' production. ORs needed to be efficient to accommodate the blossoming cataract volumes resulting from the IOL revolution that began in the 80s. I took these visions of change very seriously, in fact somewhat urgently. I was filled with anxiety about being oppressed by managed care.

In 1992, I retained a national consulting firm to advise the practice on how to move forward. We were shown the spreadsheet of the effect on the inexorable reduction in fees vs inflation. We saw the need for leveraged productivity and ancillary income. At this juncture, our practice elected to develop a closely held surgery facility in our own building. The facility was licensed by the state and Medicare certified. Because the surgery facility operated largely as a separate entity, it did not add a lot to the complexity of the medical practice. If anything, it simplified quite a few things for the practice. I retained a very part-time consultant to deal with higher-level compliance issues, etc. It has worked out very well. Just the same, my total administrative responsibilities increased. I now had two corporations to run.

Over the Top

Realizing that the whole package had become too large for me alone to administer, I retained a part-time "consulting administrator." She was only on-site four days a month. Our consultant formed a management team of department heads and attempted to train and coordinate their activities. The plan was to mentor our practice manager with the goal of re-engineering the practice and making her into our administrator. Things got better, but never "good," much less the "great" we sought. Eventually it became apparent that this was a costly and awkward way to operate.

The medical practice continued to add clinical and clerical staff. We opened a small optical. The next attempt at improving administration was to revise the management team (HR, AP/AR, scheduling, tech, optician, and nursing director) to collectively function as administrator. I would be the MP. Things got a little better, but still fell short. I now had two corporations and six direct reports, each with their own supervisees. These managers were people who had come up through the ranks and were each selected for good performance in their basic area, but they were not naturally or trained managers (this is very clear in hindsight, not so at the time).

We absorbed a retiring doctor's practice. We implemented an EHR system, and while we had a clean implementation, a tremendous number of personal and staff hours was required. Increasing numbers of patient visits increased revenue, but the practice manager was no longer able to manage all of the subordinates. Implementation expenses preceded revenue enhancement. Organizational stress grew, and we relied heavily on consulting services again to help us restructure and train management teams, set standards and protocols, and train.

The demands on my time and my aptitude for administration were beyond my limit. Skillful strategic planning, process development and implementation, employee recruitment, and operations management were not my natural skills. I read a lot of books and continued to rely on outside consulting, feeling "I should be able to run things." (Chorus: "I kept hoping that things would quiet down pretty soon.")

Through sheer determination, we made some progress, but as the practice continued to grow, the stress level escalated. I relied extensively on a la carte outside resources (eg, employee development aspect of HR, accounting, IT, strategic planning) to help me. This is more or less the way we have since continued. We recruited a junior associate, acquired practices at various times from three retiring ophthalmologists, and added a second practice location. (Chorus: "I kept hoping that things would quiet down pretty soon.")

Actually, this would have been a great opportunity, a great foundation, for building something better, had I been paying attention. Rather than see the progress and opportunity though, I experienced it as failure. As much praise as the practice and I received, I struggled and felt like I didn't measure up. I worked harder.

Dysfunctional Response to the Need for Change

The practice paid an opportunity cost, and I paid a large personal cost by persisting too long with the physician-as-administrator model. You probably agree after reading this story, but while I was in the midst of it, I really had no perspective. What I lacked in business aptitude and training, I made up with hard work and long hours. I made budgets, planned growth, wrote protocols, and even wrote a computer program to reduce paperwork, transcription, and errors in the surgery scheduling process. When I had a moment, I gave dysfunctional and overdue reviews to employees at all levels. I made more money, and the surgery practice grew; but I felt empty. My home life was very unhappy and so was I. What had begun with every intention of being productive, happy, and generative was rapidly becoming pretty much a bad dream. My income was great but that was little comfort.

In 2005, my same-age associate of 25 years abruptly retired from practice. Fortunately, I had by then a hard-working junior associate as well. We both worked really hard, but the overhead was eating us alive. We began developing a joint management services organization (MSO) with a large practice in a neighboring county. They had an energetic administrator, and this looked like a good way out. This all fell apart when the administrator abruptly resigned under a cloud. Not long after, an ophthalmologist from that practice decided to relocate to our area. He approached us. Ultimately, he joined our practice. The energy, novelty, and new skill set in refractive surgery and additional revenue source gave a new glow to the practice ... for about 2 years. It was 2008, just before the onset of the Great Recession. We were taking home a better-than-average percent of revenue, much better than in the 3 previous years of duress. I was imagining my younger associates making a smooth transition into full ownership of the practice. It would be their problem to deal with. I would simply practice medicine as their employee. I would be H-a-p-p-y. I slacked off a bit in my work. The stock market tanked and I still I felt reasonably secure; I was happy with our rejuvenated practice. I could work part-time and not have to dip into retirement assets. I was starting to have fun again.

Then in early in 2010 it hit: A major staffing/human resources problem surfaced. Conflicts became quite apparent. The practice had grown substantially in complexity. The culture of our established practice was quite different from the accustomed cultural model of our new associate. Silos had developed and camps formed. Shouting and intrigue. I was shocked (though I should have seen it coming) and devastated. I was willing to quit rather than continue that way. Complete burn out.

Moving on From the MD-Administrator Model

I had finally discovered the point where the MD-administrator grows his practice to a level beyond his personal resources to administer. Here, generically, are the signposts we discovered at the end of the road for the physician-as-administrator model.

1. Poor economic performance in a practice that was previously successful.
   a. Rising overhead ratios
   b. Unable to grow revenue in an expanding market
   c. Increasing use of consultants for ongoing operational problems
   d. Poor compliance with third-party mandates
   e. High staff turnover
2. Conflict within the practice, especially between MDs or with managers.
3. You are unhappy: not enough recovery time between working hours. Burnout.
4. The family is unhappy. You're stressed out and irritable, unavailable and distracted.
5. Overwhelmed: too many administrative details come your way to deal with in a timely fashion.
   a. Excessive after-hours work
   b. Ineffective delegation
   c. Poor prioritization

6. You do not know what's going on.
   a. Practice performance measures
   b. Who is productive and who isn't
   c. Staff morale
7. It's 10 years before retirement, and you don't have a viable transition strategy for the practice.
   a. Charismatically driven businesses fail in their succession planning
   b. Many young ophthalmologists have no interest in administration nor in long work hours
   c. Savvy prospective juniors look for the presence of an effective administrator in potential employers
   d. Even more mature junior partners do not want to be as absorbed in administration as their more entrepreneurial senior partner has been. They're afraid of what will happen when he retires.

Many other ophthalmic surgeons would have noticed and taken effective action at the right time to move on to hire an administrator. I am not so gifted, and I have had to learn a lot of things the harder way.

Finally, I "got it." It was 2010, after 30 years in the practice. As I said, I was willing to quit rather than continue this way. Complete burn out. Time for another consultant whose most pointed advice was to ***hire*** an administrator. This sounds so obvious in hindsight!

Personality Trap

I should have hired an administrator 15 years ago. Why didn't I? Without going into detail, I am one of those more extreme "ophthalmic personalities" described in Pinto's books and articles. In retrospect, I was carrying a burden of undiagnosed chronic clinical depression through most of my adult years. I carried a sense of futility, even as I put all my heart into trying to convince myself that I wasn't a failure at my "other job" as the practice's business leader. On a practical level, I was afraid of hiring the wrong person and increasing overhead without supportive revenue. I didn't really know how to go about it. How would I know who to trust? After all, haven't I made many poor choices over the years? A bad selection here could ruin the practice.

I thought I "should" be able to administer if I just had the right team of managers. The smorgasbord of consultants I retained were very happy to continue being helpful. Don't misunderstand: They have done some very fine work and I like them personally. But it's a bit like hiring a stockbroker to be your investment advisor. Better to have a fee-only advisor at the top of the pyramid. For this over-the-top "ophthalmic personality," it took me a very long time to finally admit that I needed a different kind of help.

Have I followed through? Yes. We have scrapped the outgrown physician-as-administrator model and as this book goes to press have our first real business leader in place.

Summary

Smaller practices can do well with an engaged MD-administrator. This is an economical solution to administration of a small, one-location, independent, single-specialty ophthalmology practice. But there are limits.

Pinto says that one objective marker of the upper limit is when total annual revenue reaches $4 million. We certainly over-shot that limit. Symptoms indicating the time for this transition are clear cut: The doctor becomes burned out from excessive hours and stress. Professional goals are not being met because of the time and effort going into business management. The organization suffers from chronic, unrelenting problems in communication, staff turnover, and a lack of statistical benchmarking. Partners, managers, and staff are in conflict. Don't wait as long as I did.

Ophthalmologists like to be in control. Change and delegation can frighten us so much that we live too long with a difficult situation. But when the time comes for the transition to professional management, there is truly an opportunity to have a happier, more productive doctor; happier, better cared-for patients; and a motivated, well-rewarded staff.

CHAPTER 46

Congratulations! (I Think)

Preparing to Become the Next Managing Partner of Our Practice

John C. Shin, MD

Several chapters in this book discuss ideas on how to be an effective MP. The perspective of this chapter is that of a physician who has been chosen to assume the position (corporal pun sort of intended). I admit that this was not a position I was keen for, but came to accept as a new challenge with the encouragement of my partners.

If you are a physician who is looking forward to becoming the MP, then count yourself lucky as having one less issue to slow you down as you prepare yourself for your inauguration. In this chapter, I'd like to share with you a description of my experiences during the transition and the activities my practice and I have undertaken to help prepare me for this challenging new role.

Pinto JB. *Ophthalmic Leadership: A Practical Guide for Physicians, Administrators, and Teams, Second Edition* (pp 273-278).
© 2022 SLACK Incorporated.

I realize that some of you may be in a large, well-established, dominant "legacy" practice that has had several planned turnovers of MPs, with deep management and administrative resources and collective experience to ease the transition. I envy you. This chapter is aimed toward partners in more average two- to five-physician group practices with much less of such resources.

Have We Done This Before?

Not really. For some background and context, I am a partner in a three-physician general ophthalmology and refractive surgery practice located in two offices in Marin County, just north across the Golden Gate Bridge from San Francisco. We each have an equal one-third ownership interest in all components of the practice and currently employ three optometrists and eight technicians. We own a single-specialty ASC in our larger office with eight staff and per diem employees, and have dispensing opticals employing six. Scheduling, billing, and managerial lay staff comprise another 11 employees. We have a fully implemented EHR and an in-house billing system.

Our practice has been in existence since the late 1940s and was the first Bay Area ophthalmic practice north of the Golden Gate. My senior partner John Campbell was hired by the founding partners in 1979. It was John who shepherded the practice into the "modern era" of medical practice and had been the dominant figure in its growth to what it is today. He effectively served as the practice's MP ***and*** administrator and writes about his experiences in these roles in the previous chapter of this book.

I joined the practice in 1998. My other partner Chris Kim joined us after 10 years at another practice.

Several years ago, John announced his decision to retire. Upon hearing this Chris and I had a staring contest, initially wondering if either of us was coveting the position, but quickly realized we were actually in a game of hot potato.

A Man's Got to Know His Limitations

Over time John Campbell, to his credit, had come to realize that even his considerable abilities and energy might not be sufficient to sustain the ongoing success and growth our practice has enjoyed. Given the increasing demands, uncertainties, and complexities of a growing medical practice, and a simple desire (deservedly so) to not work so hard, he had over the years *attempted* to delegate more of his formerly micromanaged tasks to managerial staff, outside consultants, and his partners.

This willingness to let others independently take on increasingly larger tasks was the first critical step in the process of transition from one leader to another, and is an integral part of a senior partner's succession and retirement planning if they are approaching that age. A potentially much more disruptive scenario would be an MP unwilling to let go, forced to do so only after some crisis in the practice. Many practices, especially larger ones, rotate the MP position as a matter of course. For us, the writing had been on the wall for the last few years, but it was only after hearing John's proclamation of his retirement that it became a reality.

A thing that John has known for some time is that delegation's true meaning is the challenge of getting others (including his partners) to actually get things done. As an assigned task languished, a take-charge guy like John would tend to take the task back and do it himself, exacerbating the tendency for the assigned owner of the task to not get future tasks done!

After experiencing this frustration for a while, it became clear that we would need outside help to put in place the organizational, administrative, and managerial systems to allow the delegates to succeed. John's natural internal system, which had served the practice well, now needed to be replaced with a more formalized and ***documented*** system. To be fair, our practice has over the years attempted to create these systems and documents in house with varying success.

After an initial site visit by one of our latest advisors, we were relieved to learn that the bones of the practice were sound, that we had significant unrealized potential, and that we were generally on the right track. The benchmarking and metrics of the practice really appealed to our "normal limits" physician mindset and objectified things that had previously seemed esoteric.

These benchmarks were organized, graphed, and are to be updated every couple of months. Of course, data collection and analysis is not enough. The organizational and governance structure of the practice was formalized. Strategic goals were identified and documented. Tasks, benchmark goals, and problem lists were organized on a simple grid with ownership and timelines. It was made absolutely clear that *everyone* in the practice needs to be involved in the process. Our mission and core values have been posted for all to see. Marching orders were given.

Production and review of detailed protocols has been an ongoing activity for us, so that the hard-won collective knowledge of our successful practice is not lost. We have made an effort to incorporate as much of this into our EHR and information systems to allow easy staff access.

Several months later, midstream in our process to reorganize the company, John explicitly stated his desire to retire within a year. Considering a variety of factors, including my tenure in the practice and Chris staring a hole into his shoes, the decision was made for me to become the MP.

In reality, while I did not relish the idea, I was flattered and, all things considered, I do think I was the logical candidate. The few short months I had remaining until I took the helm certainly didn't feel like a lot of time to me. If you have the luxury, I advise you to start your own preparatory activities as early as possible.

Getting our administrative and benchmarking house in order and designating an office manager was invaluable in reducing my anxiety.

The next thing that was done was to officially announce the changes to the rest of the staff. No backing out now! This caused some squirming in the managerial ranks, but also dislodged some inertia. I've noticed a subtle change in the way the staff approach me with a little more respect, or is it fear? On my part, I've tried to be more receptive to issues that come up and have noticed the managers approaching me with more issues for my opinion.

So What's the Job Exactly?

In a broad stroke, the MP works with the practice administrator or office manager to turn the mandates of the board of directors (the top of the organizational pyramid, in our case the three owner-physicians) into actual performance that keeps the practice on course.

More specific duties may vary from practice to practice, but usually include: presentation to the board of financial/budget data and analysis (monthly), provider and overall practice volume/performance/profitability analysis (monthly), and outreach and marketing activities, all ideally with recommendations.

The MP, with the help of the administrator, frequently checks "action grid" progress, holding lay managers accountable by rewarding and reprimanding accordingly. Frequent meetings with the administrator and management staff are mandatory. The practice's strategic and developmental plan is revised at least annually by the MP and administrator for presentation to the board for approval.

Another critical role now assigned to me as the MP is the management of the medical staff. This includes recruitment, clinical quality control, utilization review, mentoring, conflict resolution, and disciplinary actions. The MP is in a unique position to address these potentially highly charged, uncomfortable matters head on and is expected do so bravely.

Abstracting from Pinto's writings, here are my new marching orders in the form of a monthly checklist:

1. Have two or more formal meetings with the practice administrator and review monthly financial reports, action list, graphs, and forecasts.
2. Do a quick rereading of the practice's strategic plan and ask yourself, "Are we still sticking to the plan, or is it time to revise it?"
3. Attend and participate in the regular senior managers' meetings.
4. Prepare for and conduct the monthly provider's meetings.
5. Review and take action on any open provider discipline or quality assurance matter.
6. Spend a minimum of 2 hours per month (ie, in aggregate ... just a few minutes a day) walking the halls, visiting informally with support staff, asking questions, and praising performance.
7. Do a mental scan of all external relationships (eg, hospitals, referral sources, competitors, payers, vendors) and follow up on written, telephone, or face-to-face action PRN.
8. Hold a breakfast, lunch, or similar meeting with one practice department head per month and with one of the practice's providers (separate or combined meeting as desired).
9. Reading/scanning of one *general* management book. (Pick up several titles during a bookstore visit and get through them in the intervening months). Read/scan a business weekly or monthly such as *The Economist* (ie, subscribe to one or more). Distribute relevant articles to the management staff.

10. As a monthly exercise, ask yourself, "What have I done this month to understand and improve my weakest management skill, be it *gathering information, making decisions, or taking action?*"
    Whew!

Now I'm Really Anxious!

Yup, that's exactly how I felt as I further investigated this MP stuff. So how should someone about to become an MP prepare? First realize that you probably already know more than you think. The simple fact that you have been chosen to be the MP shows that you have either spent a relatively long time at your practice, have demonstrated qualities that have caused your partners to choose you, or both. If you are fortunate, you have had the benefit of observing a capable senior MP to emulate. I have. You must find a mentor or two.

Knowledge is power. So, I'm reading up a storm. I've subscribed to the *Economist* to provide me a more "big picture" perspective and as a foil to the more practice-specific and leadership-themed books I've collected. It also tends to be more fun to read and keeps me up with the news. There are a myriad of books in the other categories. Here's the list I'm currently working through:

- *Buzzmarketing* (Hughes)
- *Coach Anyone About Anything* (Porche)
- *Crucial Confrontations* (Patterson)
- *Delivering Knock Your Socks Off Service* (Performance Research)
- *Finance for Non-Financial Managers* (Tuller)
- *First Among Equals: How to Manage a Group of Professionals* (McKenna)
- *Good to Great* (Collins)
- *On Strategy* (Trout)
- *Patient Satisfaction Pays* (Brown)
- *Pinto's Little Green Book* (Pinto)
- *The 17 Laws of Teamwork* (Maxwell)
- *The 21 Irrefutable Laws of Leadership* (Maxwell)
- *The Efficient Ophthalmologist* (Pinto)
- *The E-Myth Physician* (Gelber)
- *Turnaround* (Pinto)
- *Whale Done* (Blanchard)

As an adjunct to all this reading, I've also attended some of the administrative, management, and leadership seminars held at the ASOA/ASCRS and AAO meetings. If you have an ASC, the OOSS generally holds seminars at the Academy and ASCRS meetings.

I've always thought of myself as relatively illiterate in the nomenclature of finances, so some remediation was definitely in order. I've found a great website called Khan Academy (www.khanacademy.org) and relearned some embarrassingly basic financial concepts (eg, *truly* understanding P&Ls, balance sheets, cash vs accrual accounting, depreciation) that have loosened several mental logjams, helping me to better digest the finance-related books and practice data I've looked at. In addition to finance, it has video didactics on a panoply of topics. Check it out.

I have become a student of the numbers of our industry. They're data, and as a physician we should be able to figure it out. I'm memorizing about 50 financial benchmarks of the practice, which feels like a trip back to medical school memorizing lab norms.

Before he left, John and I had been having biweekly lunch meetings to "talk shop" and strengthen the mentor/student relationship that helped to ease me into my new job. For his part, John was expected to work several hours MORE a week to ensure that the house is as stout as it can be to withstand the storm I may create before his departure.

Get in There!

While my clinical schedule currently still dictates my free time, I've tried to sit in on as many manager's and committee meetings as possible. Our MDs have an evening meeting on a biweekly basis. I've been assigned the duties of clinical director for the ASC and the technical crew.

I think good leadership is hard to define. Some would argue that leadership is something you can't learn. I believe, like most things in life, that one is born with a certain amount of talent for it, and that this talent must be nurtured with constant learning and effort.

I'm certainly not the best ophthalmologist, but I'm good enough to be successful. Since ophthalmologist are born achievers, I have faith that the talents and hard work that have gotten me this far will hold me in good stead as I approach another milestone in my career. From what I've gathered so far, leadership is critically related to will, communication (especially listening), and collaboration. Hopefully, I'll continue to get better at it as time goes on.

I wish you luck. I know I needed it!

CHAPTER 47

Through the Eyes of a Lay CEO Who Has Evolved From Employee to Owner

John Swencki, MBA

I work in a very unique and forward-thinking medical practice in the great state of Florida. For most of my career in health care administration, I've practiced management and leadership as an employee. On more than one occasion, I contemplated how my leadership approach might change if I were ever the owner of a business, as opposed to an employee of a business.

Would the core basis of my leadership and decision-making philosophies change? Could this ultimate alignment of incentives with my physician partners make me a better manager? Or would I somehow become so concerned about the bottom-line income of the practice that my decisions would be biased toward short-term gain rather than long-term investments? Having been offered the opportunity to become an owner in a group practice, I've had what could probably

Pinto JB. *Ophthalmic Leadership: A Practical Guide for Physicians, Administrators, and Teams, Second Edition* (pp 279-286).
© 2022 SLACK Incorporated.

be considered an uncommon experience of leading and managing staff and resources both as an employed CEO and as a nonprovider owner, which (unlike most settings in America) is legal in Florida.

With an ownership stake, you have skin in the game, as the saying goes. Now it's not just the doctors' capital at risk, it's mine as well. And with that figurative and literal transformation in structure, changes in my thought processes have occurred.

I've become bolder. My communication with doctor-owners has become more comfortable and probably more assertive as well. I no longer must toggle between the perspective of the owner and the perspective of the employee. This allows for total focus on the issues with minimal interference in message delivery. Ultimately, as owners of a business, we are working toward the same goal. And that has created a camaraderie that didn't exist before. I believe my ownership has created a bond that fosters more of a peer-to-peer relationship rather than boss-subordinate.

Ownership fosters a greater sense of duty and responsibility upon you than could be achieved as an employee. It's a model that works for our organization and that works for me. Now the question is, can I develop my leadership to the point that it will help instill a sense of virtual ownership in all of the organization's employees?

As a former US Army officer, I was fortunate enough to begin working in the private sector with plenty of training and some real-world experience in how to motivate and manage teams. To be able to fulfill its mission of defending our nation in the time of war, the military must have well trained, educated, and motivated leaders. Because of this requirement, the military places a lot of emphasis on leadership doctrine and development programs. The military's philosophy on leadership and development can easily transfer to the private sector and to your medical practice. I've found success in management by using many of the techniques that I first learned in the military and applying them in the private sector.

Four Factors of Leadership

Army leadership doctrine defines four factors of leadership that are always present under any circumstances. These factors are: communications, the situation, the led, and the leader. These factors always affect the actions you should take, they may also influence when you take those actions and the style of leadership you should apply. Taking into consideration the four factors of leadership can serve as your guide when making decisions, managing resources, and leading the staff required by a modern medical group practice. If you can master these competencies, you will become an effective leader.

Leadership Factor 1: Communications

Communication is the exchange of information, ideas, and data from one person to another. Successful communication occurs when others understand precisely what you are trying to tell them and understand exactly what you want. I suggest that effective communication is the single most important aspect of being a successful leader.

In my experience, the root of most workplace problems, issues, or breakdowns can be traced back to a communication problem of some kind.

This breakdown can range from a lack of communication to miscommunication, misunderstanding of the message, or misinterpretation of the intent of the leader's message. As a young Army lieutenant, I learned a very important lesson about effective communication that has remained with me throughout my career in the private sector.

During one of my first training exercises, my platoon was given the mission of securing a bridge that crossed a small river. In this scenario, the bridge was needed by a larger unit (a company) to transport troops and equipment forward to reinforce another battle-weary unit that was running low on supplies. After receiving our orders, my platoon sergeant and I spent a few hours planning, detailing, and rehearsing each step of our task. We reviewed maps, examined terrain, checked weather forecasts, estimated enemy avenues of approach, reconnoitered the area, calculated risks, and basically covered everything we could think of. I wanted to make this mission a resounding success and set the standard for others to follow.

Once we finalized our plan, we met with each squad leader and assigned each their respective tasks. Each squad was assigned a role that once completed would ensure our bridge was secure and allow the company secure passage across the bridge. Under the management of myself and my platoon sergeant, I was sure that we would secure that bridge and complete the mission in record time. Looking back on this situation now, I realize that we had a very experienced trainer who was keenly observing our efforts.

As soon as I assembled my platoon to begin our mission, the trainer stepped in and said, "Platoon leader and platoon sergeant have been killed by the enemy. Squad leader number one you must now take over." At that point I realized we had made a critical mistake. Although we thoroughly planned each step in our mission neither I nor my sergeant had taken the time to communicate the overall goal of the mission to ***all*** of our troops. Each person knew their individual roles inside and out, but no one (other than I and my sergeant) knew the missions' overall objective of securing the bridge.

Because of that, our mission failed and was over before it even started. I learned a valuable lesson about leadership that day and have tried to utilize it when leading teams in the workplace. That lesson is to communicate the mission (ie, the goal) to each and every member of the team. You must ensure that every employee knows and understands not just their individual role, but the overall goal of the team. I've found that when every member of the team understands the goal it not only helps to assure success, but it allows for and even cultivates a level of independent thought and creative decision making.

This is a critical in a medical practice setting where most of the interaction with our patients is through staff members, not the physician leaders. Managers and staff need to understand the desired goal in order to think on their feet, react appropriately, and make decisions that lead to completion of the mission.

This leads me to another lesson learned about effectual communication. I've concluded that email can be a terrible form of communication when it is used in preference over a face-to-face conversation. Although it is very convenient for the sender, it is hopelessly one-way in nature for the person on the receiving end.

Email strips the message of subtle, but very important, nonverbal ques. The reader has no easy way of discerning which words are being emphasized; there are no facial expressions, no hand and body gestures, etc. A simple question or clarification required by the reader for complete understanding must now be composed, edited, sent, received, and replied too, often with hours or days in between. And possibly most important, is that the synergy created by an actual face-to-face discussion (ie, the brainstorming effect), is nonexistent. The lesson here is to communicate face-to-face, communicate often, and communicate with everyone.

Leadership Factor 2: The Situation

All situations are different and the type of decision making used by the leader should vary based on the situation. Leadership styles that may work in one situation, will not necessarily work in another. Displaying flexibility and being adaptable are key ingredients to success here. There are three distinct approaches to leadership and decision making that can be utilized dependent on the particular situation: directing, participatory, and delegating.

The "directing style" can be utilized in a situation where you need to direct what is to be done, how it is to be done, and when it is to be done. This approach seems to be well suited for a surgeon in the operating room. When using this style of leadership, it is important to follow up and monitor closely to ensure the task is completed exactly as instructed.

The "participatory style" can be used when you want to involve others in the determination of what should be done. This is the technique I like to employ when faced with decisions that may not have a very clear right or wrong path. I use a simple, but very effective, strategy for making these tough and often nebulous decisions. I gather our management team together, explain the situation, review relevant facts, and open the floor for discussion of the issue at hand.

Each member of the group gives their respective thoughts on the situation. Once the discussion winds down, I ask each manager to tell me what their selection would be. I carefully listen to each person's explanation of the thought process that led them to that conclusion. At this point I typically have clarity on the decision I'm going to make. Remember, while using this participatory style the burden of the final decision is still borne by the leader. The advantage of this strategy is that you evaluate the issue through many different lenses, and often this technique will prompt you to scrutinize the issue from many more perspectives than you would on your own.

The "delegating style" should be used when you wish to delegate both the problem-solving and decision-making authority to a subordinate or group of subordinates. This is a great technique to use with managers, when there is a secondary goal of leadership development. By assigning the responsibility of evaluating the situation, developing the solution, and implementing the solution, you are building the foundation for that next generation of managers to rely upon. You will also begin to build a level of trust that will pay dividends in the future.

To increase success using this method you must make absolutely sure that you delegate the "authority" together with the "responsibility." All too often, employees are given the responsibility for something and absolutely no authority to do anything about it. That is a mistake that will only foster frustration among staff members. Also, keep in mind that when using this style, staff will inevitably come up with solutions that you may feel are not the best course of action or even agree with. It is important to not interfere and second guess the decision that has been made. Mistakes are an integral part of learning and often times the best teaching tool available. You should consider all four leadership factors when selecting a style to use for each particular situation.

Leadership Factor 3: The Led (Your Followers)

As a leader, one of your primary responsibilities is to allocate and manipulate resources in a way that generates the most return from those resources. More often than not, those resources are limited in nature. You're probably familiar with the usual resources in a typical medical practice. Some examples would be the facility itself (bricks and mortar), including the waiting room, exam lanes, procedure rooms, and possibly a surgery center. Also included are all testing and diagnostic equipment, supplies, medications, etc.

But, what about the people in the practice?

Human resources (do you see the basis for this term now?) are universally the single largest expense item on your income statement. Your employees are the "led." And those resources—these people—are always the most challenging resource to manage. Leading and managing people is an art that must be mastered over time, with lots of mentoring and mistakes along the way before one becomes proficient at it.

It's not an exact science and typically you must use different approaches for different people. Each individual is different, and leadership styles that are effective with one may not necessarily work with another. You'll find some respond to financial rewards, others respond to praise, some are internally motivated, while others require lots of external direction and handholding. Whatever the case, get to know your people as individuals, learn their strengths and weaknesses, learn what motivates them, and adapt your style as necessary.

Leadership Factor 4: The Leader

To be an effective leader, you must have an honest understanding of yourself. At a minimum, you need to consider who you are, what you know, and what can you do. You need to know what your strengths, weaknesses, limitations, and capabilities are. It is typically the followers who determine if the leader is ultimately successful. And the follower's ***perception*** of the leader may be just as important as the leader's actual abilities running your business.

Always remember that as the leader, you set the example, the tone and the culture of the organization. You are always under a microscope, employees listen intently to each and every word you say. Be careful and do not promise anything you can't deliver. Staff will listen to your words, but it is your actions that demonstrate what is acceptable and what is not.

Never let emotions influence your actions. As the leader, you must instill confidence in your team and give your followers a reason to follow. It is your responsibility. Effective leaders are not afraid to take risks. Effective leaders are not threatened by change; instead, they know that organizations must evolve to thrive. Leaders relish and push for change; they are adaptable and flexible. A leader who demonstrates these traits would never say, "No, we've tried that before and it didn't work." Instead, they would say "Let's try it again, and this time we'll do this part differently and see if we can succeed."

The military's four factors of leadership were the basis or the foundation on which I managed staff and resources prior to having an ownership stake in our practice. And after becoming an owner, I've discovered that the core foundation of my leadership style has not changed. I still rely on the four factors of leadership as I go through each day in the office.

Avoiding Common Management Mistakes

The four factors of leadership can help you manage the operations of your medical practice. Although each practice and situation is different, there are some common traps that leaders should avoid.

When it comes to decision making, I try never to make "hallway decisions." Let's face it, modern day ophthalmologists (and managers) are very busy people. They are routinely expected to see 40 or more patients per day. As practice owners, they must also find time to think both tactically and strategically about their organizations. Lunches and dinners are routinely high-jacked and transformed into business meetings. Family and personal time take a back seat. Time is at a premium. So, there is great temptation to make what I call a hallway decision.

You've probably had it happen before. A supervisor comes to you and explains that Suzy, the new receptionist, is late for her shift and did not call. She wants your permission to terminate her, which you immediately grant. Suzy is terminated. What you don't know is that Suzy did call and explain to your partner that her car would not start and that she was taking the bus and would be 30 minutes late for her shift. What you also didn't know was that your supervisor was clandestinely angry because her boyfriend had spent too much time speaking with Suzy at the holiday party last weekend.

You just made a major decision with only a portion of the information required. If staff members are coming to you in between patients to ask permission for something, it's because they don't feel comfortable with or lack the authority to make the decision themselves. And if that's the case, you won't have all of the information needed to make a well-thought out, sound decision. These questions can range from permission to hire or fire a staff member, approval to purchase a piece of equipment for the practice, or perhaps to change a protocol or procedure.

Whatever the case may be, resist the temptation to make a hallway decision. There is another side to the story, which you have not been briefed on or had time to consider.

You should understand that avoidance of decision is, in itself, a decision. And in fact, no decision is the worst possible decision you can make. It will always be the "wrong" decision. It is also the sign of a weak leader. Leaders must be able to take risks and make the call, even when the correct call may not be apparent.

Watch out for the "law of triviality." (This comes from a book written by C. Northcote Parkinson.) Imagine a board of directors that has two items on the agenda for discussion. The group has 1 hour to decide on these two matters. The first item is to determine a suitable location for construction of a brand-new nuclear reactor. About 5 minutes of discussion ensues when a location is proposed. The vote is taken, and the issue is quickly resolved.

The group then moves on to the second item, determine a suitable location for the new staff bicycle rack. Discussion drags on, everyone in the group has an opinion to express, and hours are consumed debating on the correct placement of the bicycle rack. Why is it that the group spends 5 minutes to decide on an issue that is immensely complex and carries long-term consequences, and yet when it comes to something as simple as a bicycle rack, hours of debate and discussion occur before an agreement can be reached?

According to Parkinson, it's because the time spent on an agenda item will be inversely proportional to the complexity of the issue. Since the construction of a nuclear power plant is multifaceted and very complex, most group members will defer to the expert's analysis and recommendation. However, location of a bicycle rack is an issue that all can understand. Because of each member's desire to contribute and be part of the decision, much more focus and involvement will be spent on an issue that all can understand. These time-wasting situations can be avoided by making simple decisions on your own and saving the complex issues for the group.

Hire experts. A common mistake made by inexperienced managers is to believe that in order to be the best manager possible, they themselves must be the most knowledgeable person in the organization. This couldn't be farther from the truth. The larger the organization is, the more apparent this becomes. How could one person be an expert in accounting, operations, marketing, human resources, clinic, optical, etc?

A strong and effective manager is not threatened by a subordinate that is an expert in their field. In fact, an effective manager will quickly realize that the more competent people they can surround themselves with, the stronger, more profitable the organization becomes. Trust is a big part of this. You must be able to trust your people, be comfortable delegating to them, and stay out of their way.

Medical care has become exponentially complex. Our government and third-party payers are doing their best to make the administration of a medical practice equally complex. As this complexity increases and margins continue to shrink, more pressure will be placed on practices to employ formally trained leaders who apply processes and techniques that create efficiencies that maintain profitability.

• • •

So, did becoming an owner in our medical practice compel me to take my leadership game up to the next level? In retrospect, I would say no, ownership is not a prerequisite for better leadership. In fact, the reverse may be true. If you want to excel as a leader, then practice leadership as if you already have an ownership stake in the organization. What I discovered was that it was my dedication and commitment to the organization that changed.

I still use the four leadership factors as the basis for my management style, but now situations and decisions are viewed through an additional lens of permanency. You don't need to be an owner to take your leadership up a notch. To do that, you simply need to consider the four factors of leadership: yourself, your staff, your situation, and your communication.

CHAPTER 48

Transition Times Two

A New Administrator's Efforts to Reposition and Update a Second-Generation Practice

Hayley Boling, MBA, COE

Stepping in as the new administrator to a second-generation practice has been both a challenging and rewarding experience. A well-established corporate culture, loyal patient base, and untapped potential for growth were among the rewards. That same well-established corporate culture, strong opposition to change and lack of organizational structure were the glaring challenges. I knew that I could make a positive difference for this practice; however, creating a culture of change and adaptability were going to be the key to our ongoing success.

Moving forward with the understanding that change is typically unwelcome and always uncomfortable, I knew that I had my work cut out for me. To prepare myself for the battles that most certainly lied ahead, I reflected on the words of the wise:

Pinto JB. *Ophthalmic Leadership: A Practical Guide for Physicians, Administrators, and Teams, Second Edition* (pp 287-295).
© 2022 SLACK Incorporated.

- *If we don't change, we don't grow*—Gail Sheehy
- *Change brings opportunity*—Nibo Qubein
- *Change in all things is sweet*—Aristotle
- *Things alter for the worse spontaneously, if they be not altered for the better designedly*—Francis Bacon

Upon reflecting on these quotes, I again reminded myself that change is necessary for this practice and essential for success. With this in mind, I began laying a solid foundation for the future generations of our practice.

Strengths, Weaknesses, Opportunities, and Threats Analysis

Prior to implementing any changes, my team and I did a lot of observing and listening ... nearly 8 months' worth, in fact. I figured if we did not have a clear understanding of the way things were, we would not be able to identify what could be better either. With this in mind, I had a number of key staff members complete a SWOT analysis (strengths, weaknesses, opportunities and threats). In learning more about the perspectives of the employees, we were better able to align what needed to happen with what they wanted to happen. Naturally, this established employee buy-in that allowed us the opportunity to identify a few allies early on and secure some support from within.

Bring on the Strengths and Opportunities

The staff had no problem shining light on all the great things it had done in the past. A solid reputation built on 50 years in practice, great people with great hearts, and a willingness to invest in high quality technology and marketing campaigns. There was no doubt about it. A strong brand has definitely led this practice through some glory days! A family atmosphere that encouraged compassion and generosity was instilled from the top down. The best equipment was backed by significant experience and promoted by cutting-edge marketing tactics. This was all great; however, nobody is safe resting on their laurels. Not even a company with little perceived current competition. After all, it is my job to predict the moves of our competitors and properly prepare our practice for the future. To do this, it was time to put on our innovators' hats and align our practice with resources that could not be matched.

To begin, I interviewed each member of the practice and asked them two questions: (1) What is the company mission statement? (2) What are the company core values? Although there were similarities in the answers, not one member of the practice had the same answer as the next. I felt that this was a big opportunity to improve our internal brand image, as I am a big believer in giving people a purpose and helping them realize what they are working for and how they are contributing on a daily basis. To do this, I held an in-service training day with all managers and doctors and we spent time identifying why we do what we do. We discussed what we believe in and what we stand for.

After tossing out words and phrases on a white board, we started drafting our mission statement. The goal was to develop a one- to two-sentence statement that accurately captured the words and ideas we had written down. Once developed, we all learned this statement and felt that it was important that the entire staff learned it as well. Since then, we have proudly displayed our mission statement and three core values in our lobby in 12-inch letters. We did this for three reasons: (1) to remind staff to live by the mission and values of our practice on a daily basis, (2) to inform patients of our mission and values so they feel comfortable and confident in the care they receive, and (3) to declare what we stand for in order for others to hold us accountable. Now when you walk through the halls of our practice and ask an employee our mission statement and core values, they will be able to recite them from memory—a major indication that they truly understand what our organization stands for.

The internal brand image continues to be strengthened by the morale committee that we implemented early on as well. This committee is responsible for employee recognition, theme days, community event participation, etc. The morale committee is light and lively and meets quarterly, at minimum, to discuss and plan the various initiatives and events they want to employ.

The external brand that the practice had built over a 50-year time period was solid; however, we felt that it was time to step out of the box a bit and strengthen our presence through a bold and edgy branding initiative that would definitely increase attention to an already established community pillar. We decided to contract with a local organization that specializes in brand management. We developed standard marketing procedures that defined our brand down to the colors and dimensions of our logo, the mediums preferred, and the alliances that were acceptable to consider. These procedures have allowed us the opportunity to develop unique and dynamic campaigns that will further secure and enhance the company brand as we proceed into the future.

To supplement the marketing and branding initiatives, we felt that focusing on business development was critical to ongoing success as well. Aligning with local organizations and seeking out opportunities to develop a "preferred provider" relationship was a major focus. In these tough economic times, it is not uncommon to see a lack of vision benefits among employers. Offering "preferred provider" relationships with these organizations that do not otherwise offer vision benefits encourages the employees to be proactive in the health and well-being of their eyes. Additionally, they have the opportunity to receive high quality eye care while benefiting from significant discounts and unique opportunities exclusive to that place of employment. Maintaining these types of relationships will not only keep our schedules full, it will also create community alliances that are able to weather the storm of creeping competition.

Technology proves to be an increasingly important aspect of ophthalmology. Whether on the clinical side, management side, or bringing them both together in an EPM/EHR setting, it is time to accept that the future is now. In preparation for this major transition, we invested in an IT department in order to meet goals and ensure we are meeting deadlines for federal incentives. They also tend to equipment malfunctions, development and implementation of the corporate IT strategy, training of new staff members on the EPM/ EHR system, and training of current staff following system upgrades. Investing in an IT department was a necessary opportunity early on and has proven to be a major strength moving forward.

The opportunities and strengths of our practice definitely brought us along the first 50 years, and with the strategic updates we have implemented, I can honestly say that we are positioning ourselves for many more years of success in the future.

Identifying the Weaknesses and Threats

The employees identified consistency issues as a weakness and potential threat for the office. I certainly agreed. To improve these issues, we began working on getting policies and procedures down on paper. Since the practice originated in 1960, handshake agreements and unwritten understandings had governed the decision-making process. Unfortunately, this allowed room for favoritism and inconsistencies to dwell. Being well aware of the problems that this creates, including the possibility of fostering a hostile work environment, we contracted with a human resources company to aid in the development and implementation of an employee handbook, job descriptions, wage grids, performance reviews, company memorandums, and organizational chart.

This was a huge shock to the corporate culture as each and every employee was asked to abide by the same rules and was held to the same expectations. A formal wage grid was developed and implemented to ensure compliance with the Equal Pay Act, equal pay for equal work, in addition to providing justification for bonuses and raises. Furthermore, employees were asked to read the company handbook and assigned job descriptions prior to signing an agreement acknowledging receipt and understanding of company policies and procedures. This allows the practice the opportunity to hold employees accountable for their actions in and out of the workplace in addition to reducing job ambiguity, confusion, and lack of consistency.

In times past, the scariest week of the year for the staff contained the employee performance reviews. I heard stories of previous supervisors critiquing personal appearance, focusing solely on negative behaviors, and stating that a raise would never be an option. This certainly had to change, because I have always viewed review time as an opportunity to connect with staff and look ahead to the future. Rather than a potentially punitive experience, I believed that performance reviews should be used to promote personal and professional advancement. With this, we implemented a process that is to be used as a positive venue to discuss the vision of the company, set goals for growth and development, and identify opportunities for improvement as well as increased satisfaction for both parties. Needless to say, the fear was reduced and a healthy respect for the performance review process remained. The improved method not only enhanced the experience for staff, but it helped reduce inconsistencies overall.

To aid in the delivery and receipt of office communication, and to avoid the fueling of gossip, we have implemented company memos that are distributed to all staff members with the intent of informing them of pressing office information that cannot wait for an all-staff meeting. This system allows all employees to receive reliable information simultaneously, which has significantly reduced office drama spurred on by ill-informed gossipers. This has naturally reduced confusion caused by the spreading of inaccurate information.

Finally, to reduce confusion regarding supervision, and eliminate the urge to run straight to the top, an organizational chart was implemented. This chart clearly displays every employee's name, position within the company, and the appropriate chain of command to follow when faced with an issue. By distributing our organizational chart, confusion and inconsistencies have been reduced.

Although a culture shock most certainly occurred, we were confident in the changes that needed to take place in order to reduce the consistency issues and confusion that had been a long-time culprit to an underlying hostile environment. Compliance is priority to us, and with confusion and consistency falling among the major concerns, there was certainly room for improvement. With everybody in the practice being held to the same standards, our organization became compliant with the human resource laws and took our first giant leap in repositioning and updating our second-generation practice.

Identifying Talent and Strengthening the Management Team

The most difficult part of the last 2 years consisted of the deliberate transition of the management team. Unfortunately, the administrators of the past promoted individuals that held longevity rather than the desired skillsets, resulting in a middle-management team that had been "Peter Principled." Upon realizing that the additional training and coaching, as well as the reassignment of job duties, resulted in little to no performance improvement, it became time to cut our losses. Again, I reminded myself that change was essential for growth, and in order to avoid perpetuating mediocrity among middle management, and the entire practice as a result, focusing on identifying the right people for the job was required. As Jim Collins, author of *Good to Great,* says, "leaders of companies that go from good to great start not with 'where' but with 'who.' They start by getting the right people on the bus, the wrong people off the bus, and the right people in the right seats."

This philosophy changed my perspective as an administrator. Was I really willing to putt along with the wrong people in the wrong seats when the right people were perfectly willing and able to jump on board? After nearly 18 months of this, we took action and released two individuals from their job duties. Of course, the process was difficult for all involved; however, I wish we had made this move months earlier, since we are still cleaning up the messes from employees past.

What did I learn from this experience? That I am no longer willing to compensate for others' poor performance and allow myself and the practice to suffer when there are plenty of qualified individuals that will be able to complete the job duties with diligence, accuracy, and timeliness. Simply put, I now look at the practice much like an apple tree. Without proper pruning, the apple tree will not develop proper shape and form, nor will it bear high quality fruit. In the practice setting, we must prune the people that are not willing or able to give the effort that will bear high-quality results. It's that simple ... but not always that easy.

To aid in this process, we consulted with our human resources company and had documents drafted by an attorney. We held meetings with our staff to ensure understanding and reduce anxiety. We were intentional in our hiring process, and after a few additional modifications, I am confident that we have identified the right people for management, have placed them in the right seats, and we are all on our way to the same destination ... together.

Tracking Our Progress

To ensure the management team communicates regularly and that we are performing our duties diligently, we have monthly meetings to review our goals, performance, ideas, and needs. We are all assigned specific metrics that we track throughout the month and report at the meeting. The results are color coded, green and red, for at-a-glance review. We can instantly focus on those that are red in order to create action items intended to rectify any issues that may be present, which will ultimately help us meet the goals the following month. To track our progress daily and weekly, we conduct dashboard exercises. This gives management the most current performance information possible, allowing us the opportunity to identify potential problem areas and make sound daily decisions. Finally, to measure our results next to other practices, we take part in national benchmarking projects to identify areas that we excel in as well as those areas needing improvement. We believe that tracking our progress is essential, because our goals and performance remain in our sight and not out of mind.

Our compliance committee is another initiative we have implemented that allows us to monitor our performance on the clinical and billing side. Our clinical supervisor currently performs five random chart audits per technician per week. Our billing supervisor does the same. This committee is overseen by one of our doctors and has employees from various departments to aid in employee buy-in process. Our goal is to be able to reduce the number of audits per person once the necessary improvements are a thing of the past. Our audits have proven to be very successful thus far, and management is thrilled that performance improvement is happening on a daily basis rather than waiting until review time.

Management Is Set ... Now What?

Now that the management team had been identified and empowered to lead, it became time to make sure the rest of the staff was on board as well. Upon casting the vision and encouraging the team, it became obvious that there were individuals that were merely loyal to the paycheck and not the mission of the practice. This became apparent when these employees complained about the new accountability and their desire to "keep things as they were" when the necessary checks and balances were put in place. There was not a newly implemented policy or procedure that they did not complain about or completely disregard altogether. These people were more interested in where they fell on the organizational chart, rather than the direction of the company and plan for our future.

With this in mind, we held an all staff meeting and gave everybody the opportunity for an "out." We discussed the type of employees that we were looking for, and if they were unwilling or unable to be that employee, we let them know that this was the time for them to leave. Of course, nobody physically got up and left during that meeting; however, over the next several weeks, the weak links trickled out and found new places of employment. We had no trouble waving good-bye, as we only wanted loyal employees—those that truly believed in and lived by the mission and core values of our organization wholeheartedly. If accountability and an "out" were enough to move them, they certainly were not right for the company in the first place. By observing nature, I have learned that it is important to shake the tree every now and then and allow the rotten fruit to fall. For if we do not … they will cling to the branches and shrivel up and die into mummified fruit, only to hold onto disease and infection and ultimately spread it to new fruit through the twigs and branches (true story!). In management, this means get the bad people out so they do not have the opportunity to spread negativity to others.

Hiring, Orientation, and Continued Employment

We successfully managed to rid our company of some negative people. As a result, it was time to hire a new generation of employee that did not have the "but we always did it this way" mentality. I sat down with my management team and determined the qualities we were looking for. We all felt that working for our organization was quite an honor; therefore, we wanted to make sure that any new hire not only fit into the culture, but truly wanted to make our practice their home. In doing so, we revised our hiring process into four separate phases.

The first phase is a resume screening to determine the qualifications of the individual. The second phase is an initial interview with two members of the management team, who then narrow down the applicant pool to the top third. The third phase is a second interview with me, where I determine fit by asking for real world examples of our core values. Finally, we distribute a comprehensive personality analysis, which consists of 131 questions and takes approximately 45 minutes to complete, to further identify the right person for the job. Yes, this hiring process is extensive, but it allows us the opportunity to make a well-informed decision early on that will naturally reduce employee turnover long term and eliminate the costly mistake required to rehire and retrain.

Upon identifying the "right people for the bus," the revised orientation process begins. One week prior to start date, we send a welcome package to the new hire's home that includes a welcome letter, introductory material to be read prior to the first day, a company t-shirt, and other goodies that express our excitement about their decision to join our team. The training of our new employees is completed in phases and consists of lecture, hands-on training, role playing, daily quizzes, games, incentives/rewards, take home assignments, and skills assessments. We assign mentors to each new hire and have designated individuals available for questions in order to ensure accurate and consistent information is being given.

On day one, the hires understand that certifications are required within 18 months from their date of hire for continued employment. This applies to the following positions and certifications: technicians—COA, opticians—ABOC, receptionists and scribes—OCS. All new employees are required to complete a customer service training to ensure our patients have the best experience possible; this takes place within the first 15 days of employment. Finally, all employees are required to attend monthly continuing education classes to keep skills up to date throughout their employment with the practice. Naturally, our employees end the orientation process with a solid skillset, a firm understanding of our expectations for them, and a desire to grow and develop as an employee.

To further solidify our relationship, all hourly employees are required to sign a nondisclosure agreement. Due to our extensive training process, and solid reputation within the community, competing practices often try to cherry pick our employees. Of course, we would never want to hold back anybody from professional growth and development. However, we felt that it was important to make sure that our employees fully understood that they would be held to strict confidentiality terms and would be unable to contact staff members regarding employment opportunities if they elected to leave our practice in the future. To show appreciation for their loyal service and hard work, we felt that enhancing our employee benefit package would be a well-received perk. We increased health insurance benefits, life insurance benefits, and in-house vision benefits for employees and their family members. By adding these additional perks, our hope is that the employees feel valued and happy to be a part of our team.

For salaried employees, including doctors, an employment contract was put into place. We realize this is likely common practice for most; however, please remember that handshake agreements and unwritten understandings used to rule this practice. To protect the practice as well as the employees, contracts were an essential element to this transition. This process was not comfortable, nor was it well received; however, it was a necessary part in taking another giant leap in repositioning and updating this second-generation practice.

Hard Work Pays Off

I am proud to say that the hard work is finally paying off. We received the Business of the Year award from our local Chamber of Commerce, celebrated our 50th anniversary and the retirement of our founding doctor, have been quoted in *Review of Ophthalmology,* and our current managing member received the Indiana Academy of Ophthalmology Humanitarian Award for his extraordinary commitment to helping others throughout his lifetime.

Additionally, we have started the construction of our new ASC, clinic renovations, and facelift to our refractive suite. This has been a long time coming, and we look forward to the continuity of care that the onsite center will provide to our patients. This also aids in the succession planning of our practice as buy-in opportunities are always attractive options to potential partner docs.

Finally, our alliances remain strong with local organizations and we continue striving to establish and maintain relationships through our community outreach initiatives. We invest in our community and, as a result, our community invests in us. We look forward to an ongoing relationship with our surrounding area as we continue to love the people and the community that we have the absolute honor to serve.

• • •

The past 2 years have been a whirlwind of activity for me as a new administrator. As you can imagine, many of the decisions made were not always popular with the staff. As we all know, it is easy to get stuck in a rut and fall into the "if it's not broken, don't fix it" mentality. Unfortunately, the staff cannot detect the tiny fractures that lie just below the surface—those that have been insidiously developing and increasing with each passing day. It is like stepping out onto a freshly snow-covered pond after the first freeze. It looks safe. It feels secure as you shuffle your feet and proceed toward the center of the pond. Little do you know; however, it is just a matter of time before the tiny cracks break and you fall into the icy water. It was my job to detect these tiny cracks before we found our practice falling. It was my job to identify potential threats and seize ideal opportunities. My job was not to be popular with the staff, nor was it to make friends. I simply set out on a mission to lay a solid foundation for the future of this amazing practice.

I believe that this new culture of change and adaptability has made us better than when we started and will allow us to continue improving with each passing day. These changes were not spontaneous, but designed. I knew that if we did not change, we would not grow. I saw the opportunity lying within the changes I implemented. With this, I can honestly say that this transition was necessary and good—that the changes were, in fact, sweet. Finally, it is important to note that these efforts remain ongoing; however, they have already successfully repositioned and updated this second-generation practice. I look forward to feeling the momentum shift in order for these changes to perpetuate the growth that will sustain our third generation and beyond.

CHAPTER 49

Leadership at a Time of Crisis

William Shields, MD

There's only one thing that's predictable about crisis.
Sooner or later, almost every organization will endure one.
—Rajat Gupta,
former managing director of McKinsey and Co

Note: I first met retinologist Willie Shields a decade before he experienced a carotid dissection and was forced to upend his vibrant practice life. True to type, Willie has always had a hyper-detailed, logical approach to everything he does. This shines through in this chapter, interweaving a personal narrative with graphs and pictures to help convey the author's perspectives. At the very least, this chapter will confirm your suspicions about the way that retinologists see the world. —John B. Pinto

> *The patient is in the ICU, where the room is dark, matching the weather outside—it is the onset of winter. There is a propofol drip, familiar to the patient, but unfamiliar in this setting. Shadows of nursing staff and visitors*

Pinto JB. *Ophthalmic Leadership: A Practical Guide for Physicians, Administrators, and Teams, Second Edition* (pp 297-308).
© 2022 SLACK Incorporated.

move in and out. Consciousness moves in and out. Doctors move in and out. Family slips in and out. And the doctors and family are very worried.

It is not clear what has truly happened, but there is a clouded memory of troubled breathing, intubation, and a rushed passage though many hallways. The tubes smell strongly of plastic. And even through the fog of awareness, it is clear that residual function, and even survival, is discussed by the doctors. And there is a family to care for. And there are patients to see. And there is a business to run.

The events described here are just a small part of the much longer story of my recovery from a personal health crisis. The purpose of this chapter is to discuss approaches to leading during a time of crisis. It is, I think, best to view managing a crisis as something that will eventually be necessary, it is really only a question of when and what. When a crisis occurs, and what it is, will of course impact the decisions made.

With respect to perspective, some background: I am a retina specialist and started as a soloist many years ago. My practice is devoted exclusively to managing retinal disease, and we have been fortunate to grow. Our practice has expanded to multiple offices and doctors. I have functioned in the roles of founder, surgeon, and managing physician. As such, various challenges have surfaced from time to time.

• • •

Crisis is defined in at least one dictionary as "an important or deciding event; the point at which change must come, either for the better or the worse."

Given this definition, it is worth noting that what constitutes an "event" that leads to crisis could be almost anything. I have found it useful to try to classify "crisis" into different categories, much as one might "grade" a clinical disorder. As an example, consider the possibility of staging a crisis, with a model something like this:

The Five "Ms"

Stage	"M"	What	Impacts	Response
1	Minor	Issue easily addressed	One to two people	Fix it
2	Modest	Challenge	One to two departments	Galvanize customary resources
3	Medium	Significant	More than two departments	Invest in outside help, bring in atypical resources
4	Major	Existential threat	Entire company	Major investment of all resources
5	Maximal	Terminal	Entire company	Liquidation

Magnitude: the size of crisis and impact on your organization.

A crisis can be further classified as to its origin, as originating from either inside the practice (internal) or outside the practice (external). If you think of your practice as being like an egg, it can be cracked, in essence, from forces outside or within.

In the model below, a small practice or business that could be represented by a smaller egg is more likely to be disrupted by external forces than a larger practice. This makes sense, because a smaller practice has fewer resources available (eg, staff, capital, expertise, experience). In effect, the smaller the practice, the more likely it is to be extremely negatively impacted by external factors.

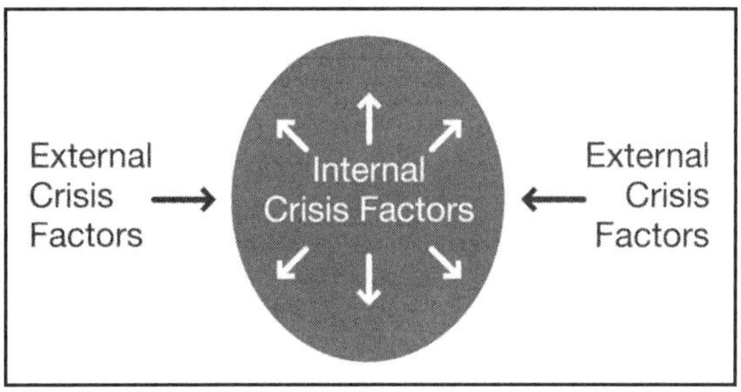

However, a smaller practice may perhaps be less likely to be impacted by internal factors, simply because a smaller practice, having fewer pieces, is more easily monitored by an owner. This brings to mind the old saying: "there is no fertilizer like the farmer's shadow."

Some examples of the two major forms of crisis are tabulated below:

Internal	External
Personal	Environmental (eg, flooding)
Personnel	Governmental/regulatory
Patient	Legal (eg, tort)
Technical/equipment	Economic (eg, recession)
Financial (eg, embezzlement)	Competitors
Partner differences	New technologies that disrupt business models

And sometimes crisis factors lie on a continuum between internal and external poles, such as arson or theft. As an example, a criminal act by thieves (eg, breaking into your office) is, of course, arising externally. The removal of equipment, drugs, charts, and destruction of property could be classified as internal.

Thus, when facing a crisis, we have found it helpful to determine where on a spectrum it lies, and this can be graphically depicted:

Internal______________________________External
Crisis

It is useful to note that in characterizing crises in this way, that tools start to emerge in terms of ultimately responding to the crisis. One helpful tool is assuming an objective viewpoint.

Developing an appropriate, objective viewpoint in looking at a crisis helps to remove emotional bias. Ultimately, doing so allows for decisions and judgments to be made, despite a measure of painful personal cost. The term I use in this context is abstraction: I have found that the more a crisis can be looked at in abstract terms, the easier it can be faced down.

As an example, an external crisis likely has elements within it that may be beyond your personal control. However, because most eye specialists deal with scenarios where millimeters or even microns make a difference in outcomes, eye specialists as a group tend to be very interested in small details and great control. Although it sounds simple, I have found that acknowledging that external factors can be out of my control can actually be a big step in approaching such obstacles.

I believe the major reason I have attempted to classify crises in these ways is to develop an ability to abstract the challenges being confronted. There is a huge advantage to doing this: Being involved too personally can cloud judgment. As they said in the *Godfather* films, "It's not personal, it's just business."Unfortunately, the closer disaster or crisis strikes to you, the more personal it becomes. In my case, the disaster was as internal and personal as it can get. Nonetheless, in my case, making a deliberate effort to think beyond myself and abstract the "what ifs" in considering appropriate responses helped me, and helped my practice, get through a spectacularly difficult time.

One of the tried-and-true methods to "abstract" your way through a crisis is, of course, to get outside help. This is where professionals come in, such as lawyers, accountants, consultants, and the rest who can more objectively assess your position and options. These advisors helped especially by bringing their past, often collaborative experience, to bear.

Advisory support was imperative and enormously helpful. In my own case, it was nice to have a team of professionals, assembled in advance—before my crisis hit. Our team included experts we had worked with for many years. This allowed us to respond more rapidly to the myriad unforeseen consequences that followed. I cannot stress enough how vital it was to be prepared with our team in advance.

As a result, when our practice crisis developed, our team included professional management consulting, financial planning, legal, accounting, banking, insurance, disability, intellectual property, information technology, and real estate professionals. All had knowledge of, or direct working experience, with each other from past projects.

Also extremely important was the experienced management team and the other great retinal specialists in house. And perhaps most importantly of all, the stalwart efforts of my family, friends, and especially my wife. All had been heavily relied upon in the past, and I owe them all a heartfelt debt of gratitude for their spirit and expertise in getting through our crisis.

Finally, not the least in our case, was the support of our community of referral doctors, and even patients. I must acknowledge it is humbling and sobering to realize the support and patience demonstrated by all during a time of profound transition for me.

In responding to a practice crisis with professionals, it may be helpful to note that this is really no different from the role doctors play in their careers. In many respects, doctors may actually have an advantage in dealing with crisis: Because we are trained to enter into crisis points in the lives of individuals on a very common basis (eg, myocardial infarction, cancer, suicidal ideation, retinal detachment). What is less common for doctors is experience with crisis in a business setting. Relying on a mindset of medical practice solving and applying it to business problems can orient a doctor through challenges—as it helped me.

In leading through my crisis, the speed of decision making really helped. Having a team in place allowed for a much faster response to change. The sudden nature of my crisis required that decisions be made quickly and decisively, and often with limited information and a paucity of time for review.

In this setting it would be my advice to any fellow practitioner before a crisis hits to get prepared to make decisions quickly. Give your team and yourself the freedom to make decisions while recognizing that some will not be correct or good decisions. Mistakes will happen, and it must be clear that you, your staff, and advisors will make them. Careening your way through crisis is not a controlled, perfectionistic environment—one has to try to not think like an ophthalmologist.

It was important to delegate some decision making, and important to let my team make mistakes. In my case, business decisions began to flow from my hospital ICU bed. With the assistance of my wife Celia, who functioned as something between a translator, watchdog, and decision-maker in her own right, visitors were engaged, including members of the professional team at the bedside. All functioned admirably, and truly remarkably, given the circumstance at hand.

Aside from assembling your team and being able to delegate, and learning to abstract, I found it helpful to recognize that decisions and responses made naturally require balance. In effect, moves that are made can be considered reactive or proactive, and this can be represented graphically as well:

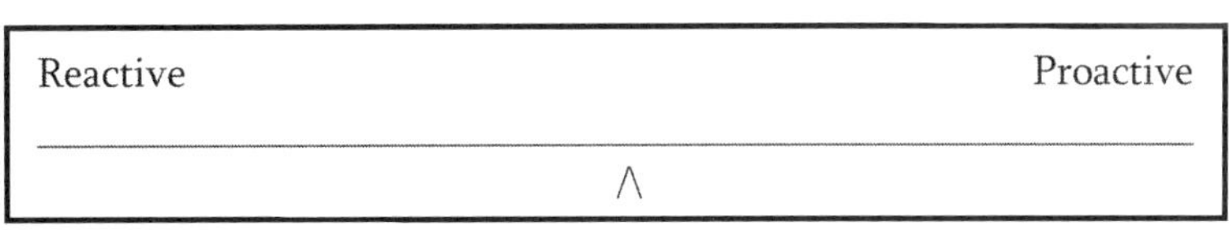

Keep in mind that responding too impulsively or reactively creates imbalance (eg, stuffing cash into the mattress at home). And note, being too proactive can also be destructive, in that planning too far ahead creates imbalance (ie, building home nuclear bomb shelters in the 1950s).

In many ways, developing the perspective of balance while leading through crisis required, in hindsight, what I might call a "zoom" perspective. While abstraction and seeing the big picture in the midst of crisis was important ("zooming out" for the larger view) there was also a need to be detail oriented ("zooming in"). Of course, even before a crisis strike, a balanced perspective is something we all apply. Zooming in and zooming out can also be graphically depicted:

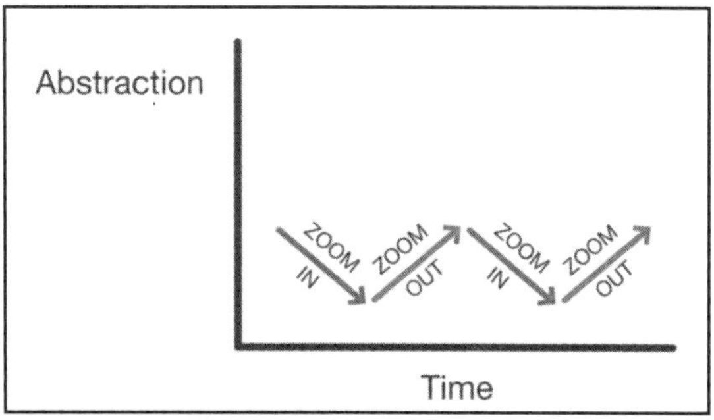

While examining your response to a crisis, remember also that periods of crisis tend to proceed in an evolutionary way, and that often things unfold in ways that are not completely predictable. Managing in this scenario required, in my mind, the true essence of leadership: Managing and guiding the team when the true outcome is uncertain. Looked at in another way, following a proven or established path is like reading a map. While it is nice to have guidelines of what to do; if this were the case, then obviously just about anyone could do it. However, true leadership in crisis requires an ability to find solutions and guide the team—without much of a map.

This concept plays out, of course, in health care more broadly. Those who are leaders in medicine think beyond old maps, in new and innovative ways. While many doctors limit themselves to treating patients out of standard protocols, medicine can only be moved forward by those who think differently and develop new treatment strategies.

While having an open mind is essential to getting through a crisis, so to is a resolute attitude. This brings up the concept of being positive during a crisis. Successful business owners need to be optimists, almost by definition, in risking time, energy, and capital in hopes of better things down the line. Being an optimist as a leader is never more important than during crisis. While it is important to be realistic, your team needs to feel there is light at the end of the tunnel; this can only occur if the leader is positive, even unrealistically so in a pinch.

In an effort to lead in a positive way during crisis, the staff need to believe in you, and this requires that you communicate and are straight with them. When my health crisis arose, we made a serious effort to communicate what was important, without dwelling on obsessive detail. Although my health issues would of course be considered personal, I made the decision early on that I wanted my staff to be engaged in terms of what happened. Once again, balance is important: Releasing too much detail takes time and may obscure the issues, while releasing too little information may encourage destructive speculation and rumor.

Recognizing that the staff were legitimately concerned, and not the least from the standpoint of their own self-interest, we decided to give the managers the freedom to discuss things openly with the staff. We used personal contact more than email, and I held executive level meetings at home as soon as I was able. This was followed by meetings at our main office, with all hands on deck, even when my mobility was restricted.

I think it is also important to keep in mind that in dealing with crisis, it is very hard on your staff. To address this problem, we used some group activities and humor to direct our attention away from the crisis at hand and to blow off some steam. As part of this, we created a project with some scenes with the intent of cobbling together a slide show. In creating this project, the entire office staff, my family, and I were included. Although on a certain level this could have been viewed as a waste of time and energy, the end result was exactly the opposite. Not only did everyone want to participate, but I was surprised to some degree by how much the staff rallied behind it. I have to say I find myself chuckling when I go back and review our efforts at the time.

As we used humor in this context, there is another point to be made. And that is I have a strong opinion that during a crisis it is important to be creative. Not just creative in terms of thinking, but literally creative: In effect countering loss by making something new. In addition to our slide show, we also moved to a new satellite office, began to redecorate, created educational materials, and began to upgrade our computer systems, among other projects.

As a crisis unfolds, it evolves. While many elements cannot be known in advance, I believe some characteristics of crisis evolution, may in fact be predictable. This perhaps can be seen with regards to the impact on the staff, and those around you. The following stages can be observed:

1. All upset
2. Staff support
3. Staff fatigue
4. Outside forces will begin to have an impact on staff
5. Crisis reverberations and oscillations affect staff

The evolution of crisis is such that I think it is helpful to think of a timeline for crisis management. When I think of a crisis, I think of five distinct phases:

1. Precrisis
2. Crisis
3. Aftermath
4. Downstream
5. Epilogue

The flow of events in a crisis can reverberate; that is, a crisis event tends to spawn subsequent issues. It is perhaps typical that as a crisis unfolds, that follow-up crises, or at least challenges, will occur: staff may quit, patients may get upset over delays in service, cash flow is interrupted, etc. We came to call this an "echo crisis."

Closely related to this echo crisis was "crisis creep" ... and the need to pour a steadily increasing amount of resources into fixing the inciting problem. Looking at resources consumed over time during a crisis, this can be portrayed graphically:

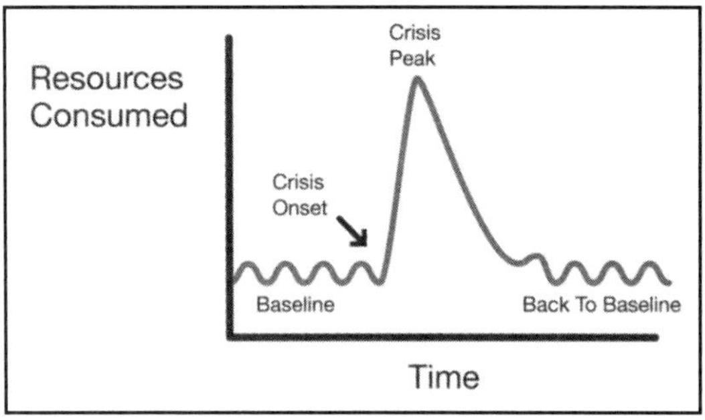

In this model, the magnitude of the crisis is reflected in terms of the amount of resources consumed, measured for example in terms of hours of attention, numbers of staff involved, money expended, or expertise called in. Note that a sharp rise over baseline is typical for a crisis, as well as a relatively slower decay of the curve back to baseline. What is ideal, of course, is a more rapid return to baseline:

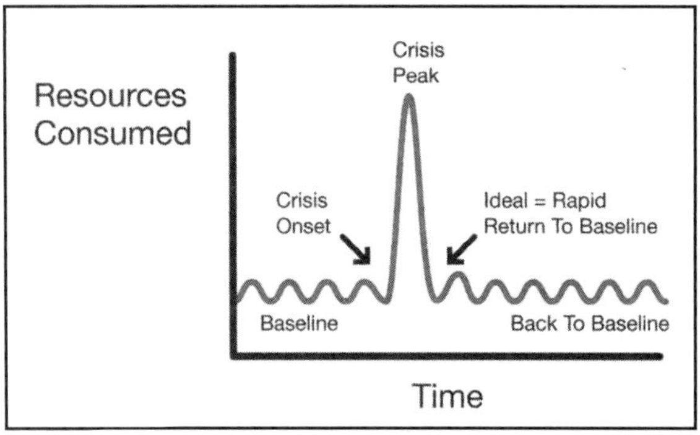

An escalation in resources required to tackle a crisis over time ("crisis creep") can be shown as follows:

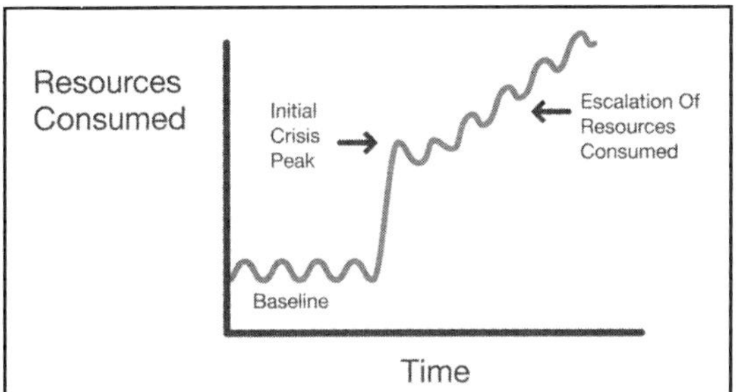

Crisis Creep

Post crisis, a continued heightened increase in resources may be required to continue running the organization, as a crisis necessarily disrupts established patterns of efficiency:

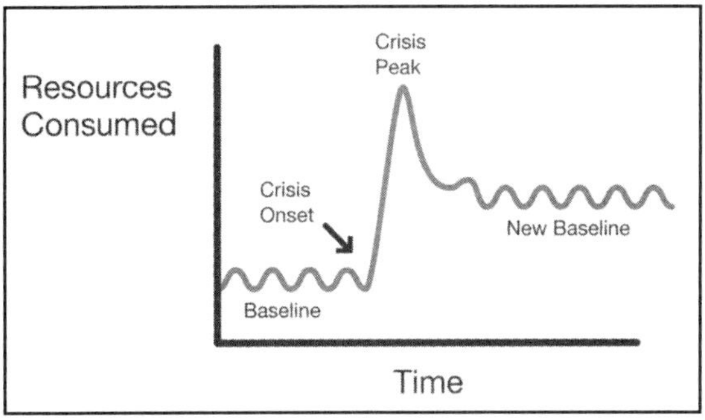

With this graphical model, note that how a crisis evolves can be portrayed in different ways. Subsequent challenges or events, or "echo crises," can be portrayed:

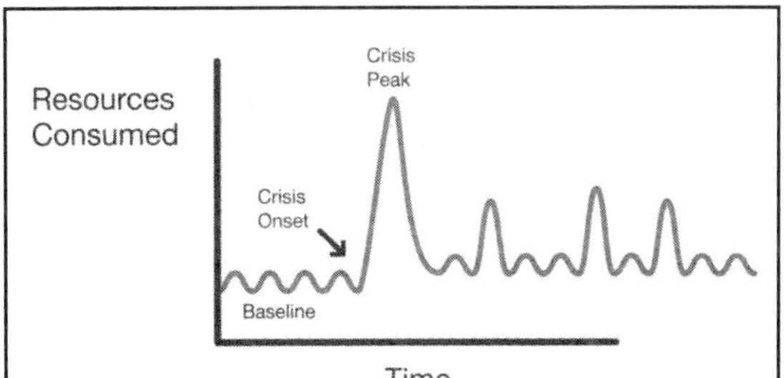

Echo Crisis

Further note that a subsequent echo crisis may have a magnitude larger than the inciting event. This is depicted here, where crisis B is greater than crisis A in terms of energy and resources consumed:

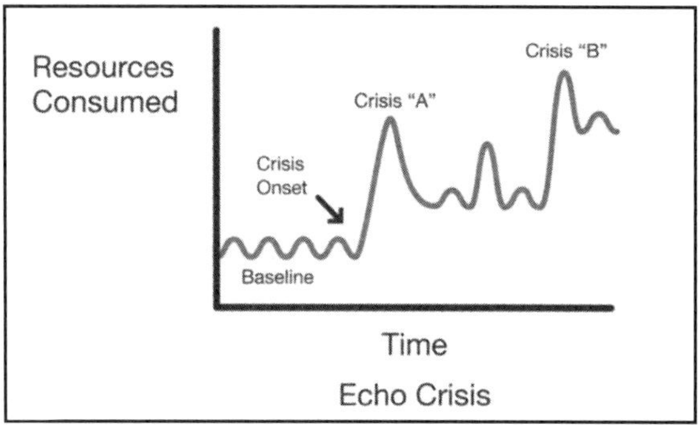

Note also that multiple crises in succession can be difficult to sustain: Simply too much may be expended in terms of resources consumed. This existential event, resulting in sale of the business or liquidation, can be represented as well:

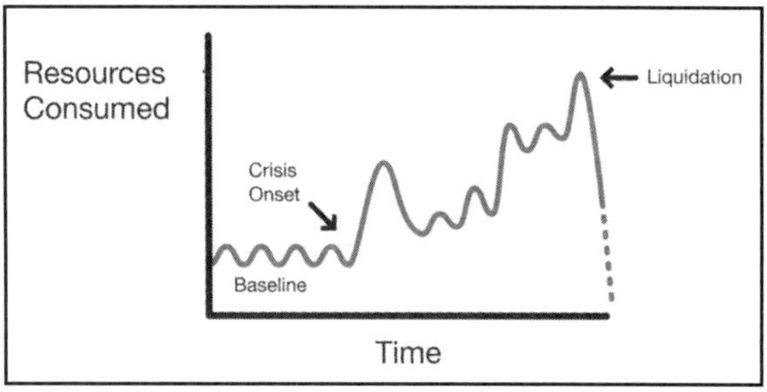

What really matters in terms of the survival or impact on the business, when a crisis is encountered, is the area under the curve … as this reflects the totality of resources consumed:

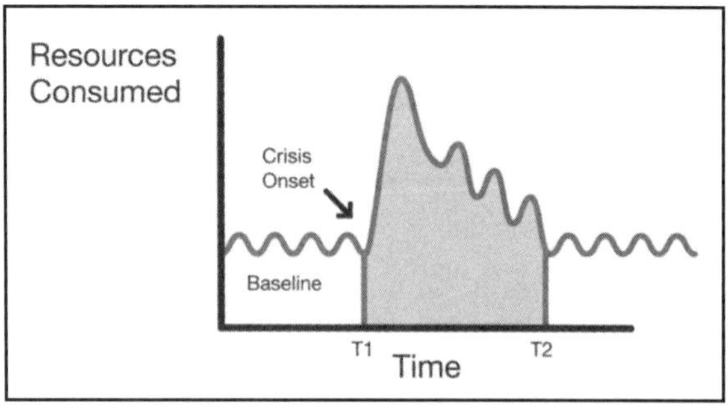

This also can be loosely reflected in equation form as well:

Resources Consumed x Time = Real Crisis Impact

This could perhaps be refined further by subtracting the amount of typical "baseline" resources consumed from the total of resources consumed during a crisis, in an attempt to determine the "extra" resources required to deal with a crisis:

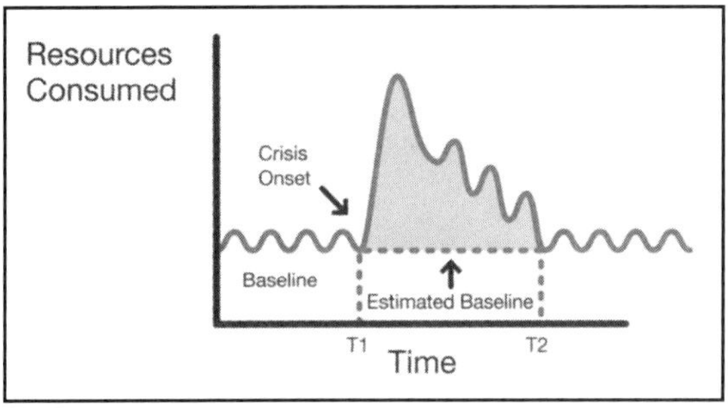

In abstract terms, this model can also reflect the personal impact of a crisis, to some degree, by carrying this to three dimensions:

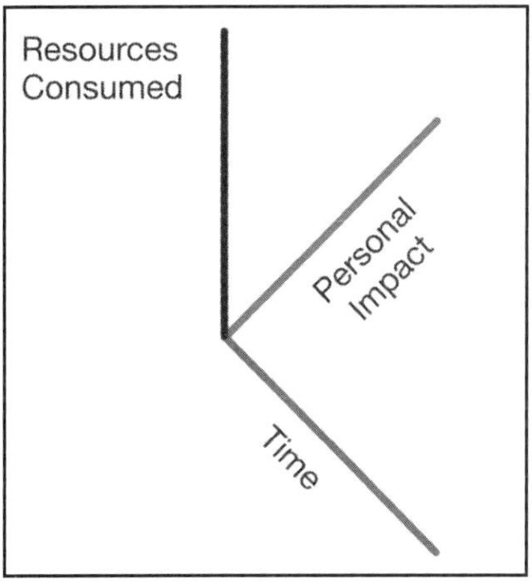

In this model personal impact could be measured in terms of personal hours consumed, spouse hours consumed, the amounts of personal legal or doctor bills, and so on.

How can we gauge that a crisis is nearing its end? In answering this question, one thing that you may observe is the conduct of the staff. Early in a crisis, the staff will likely be highly engaged, open, and flexible. As the crisis ends, look for more quotidian matters to resume their importance.

> *Two years later, the company has changed. The practice has stabilized. There is talk of growth. The practice is different now—more intent on purpose than ever.*
>
> *The phones ring. There are new doctors, and there is new equipment that smells of plastic. Surgery is being carried out, and the team is in place. And there is a family to care for. And there are patients to see. And there is a business to run.*
>
> *And the staff are again grumbling about lunch breaks—and this is a very, very, very good thing.*

Despite—or perhaps because of—the crisis we all faced together, our practice is actually stronger in many ways than it was before my health issues surfaced. That this could be the case during the worst economy since the Great Depression says volumes about the outstanding people within our practice, our patients and colleagues, and the wider community supporting our company.

CHAPTER 50

Critical Care

Health Care Leaders and Political Issues

Priscilla Arnold, MD

Politics is the art of preventing people from taking part in affairs which properly concern them.
—Paul Valery

The art of leadership requires understanding and involvement—not necessarily management—of all aspects critical to the operation of a medical organization. This book discusses those various important concerns of the medical leader, which include maintaining clinical expertise, establishing practice operations, and selecting technology capable of multiple functions. Overall, there is responsibility for a wide spectrum of business functions and personnel management in the office, and for external relationships and marketing. One additional aspect that should be the concern of the effective ophthalmic leader is involvement in the world of politics. While some might question inclusion of such a topic as a more

Pinto JB. *Ophthalmic Leadership: A Practical Guide for Physicians, Administrators, and Teams, Second Edition* (pp 309-313).
© 2022 SLACK Incorporated.

"peripheral" issue, the facts tell a different story. Evaluation of how the political world interfaces with the practice of medicine increases appreciation of the importance of political involvement.

In the United States the practice of medicine is to a great extent controlled through several political systems, both on the state and national level. The authority of these various entities is a jealously guarded power—often a few individuals exert enormous influence over very broad, critical decisions. The wise leader should strive to know about and influence these deliberations, to become a part of the process as much as possible. Unfortunately, experience has shown us exactly the opposite tends to be the case. Consequently, we live and work in a system with only few in ophthalmology having any meaningful input. Hopefully, this chapter will stimulate more to become involved and offer some avenues make a difference.

The first and most powerful interface of the political world with medicine is through ***legislation.*** In the United States, Congress directs the largest health care system in the country. It approves the budget and allocates funding to the CMS, and therefore to all who provide medical services under this agency. Congress establishes regulatory agencies and laws that determine much of the patterns of practice in the United States and oversees the activities of these agencies (more on this later). Much of Congressional decision making, and therefore the point of necessary influence, is done in a few powerful committees. The members who serve on these committees are, in almost every case, nonmedical in background with limited understanding of the actual impact of their decisions in daily practice. They are routinely given volumes of information on multiple topics to act upon, with little expectation of developing any detailed knowledge on the subject.

Because the practice of medicine operates as a business, other legislation impacts it in more general ways. Congress determines federal taxes, establishes wage limits, and promulgates employment laws—all of which have enormous consequences for medicine as for any business entity.

State ***legislative*** bodies have specific authority for scope-of-practice legislation. Sadly, we have seen repeated instances in which medical privileges are given away by vote without clear public need for this expansion, without appreciation of skills and training required, and without understanding of the serious implications for such sweeping changes. It is usual that these actions are the result of successful targeted lobbying efforts of groups standing to gain economically. But such decisions are also the result of ophthalmologists' absence in this arena of serious responsibility. Financial and personal investment is required to achieve a positive outcome, and historically few step up to this plate.

Decisions concerning ***regulation*** also address the practice of medicine. Nationally, the two most important regulatory entities are CMS and the FDA. The wide authority of these agencies include determination of amount and methodology of payment policy, the accreditation and operation of facilities that receive payment, the availability of medication and technology, and the guidelines/restrictions for use. CMS has established increasing mandates for participation, such as specifications for adoption of health information technology. Much attention is now directed toward development of accountable care organization systems. Both of these initiatives may restrict practice options, especially for the smaller, independent offices. Most definitely they establish significant economic and personnel demands on every practice.

On the state level of ***regulation,*** licensure and accreditation of facilities is an important function that responds to active political involvement. Any practice located in a strict certificate-of-need state knows the limitations of these decisions on opportunities to offer less costly, more efficient surgical care. Once again these restrictions are usually in response to strong lobbying efforts and are based on economic interests rather than on reasoned clinical and business evaluation.

The political system in which we practice has important implications for the ***rights*** of both patients and physicians. Decisions of Medicare participation vs nonparticipation result in strict limitations for the physician, and impose lengthy periods of enforcement if the decision is not to participate. The guidelines of these regulations also restrict (through financial penalties) a patient's right to select the physician from whom they wish to receive care. Patients are actually prohibited from using their own resources to seek out what they determine to be the highest quality and best options for their care.

So, clearly it is important for the practice leader to be engaged in this political process—but how? As in every other aspect of any discipline, the process should begin with education. In that regard, the medium of electronic communication has made information and education dramatically more accessible and timely. I am going to mention a few examples in the field of ophthalmology in particular, as that is the topic of our discussion in this book, but a number of other opportunities are available.

In ophthalmology, weekly advocacy e-publications are produced by both ASCRS and the AAO. The format of both of these is very user-friendly, with "headlines" followed by more detailed reports that can be accessed immediately by hot-links. This is a convenient method for understanding the issues of important news in the legislative and regulatory arena. These sites also highlight educational offerings and access to advocacy events. Many state ophthalmology organizations also produce email notification of situations of particular importance, and all of these societies send special alerts on an as-needed basis for "late-breaking" news. Attention to these educational messages can maintain a current base of knowledge and a platform for advocacy involvement.

A growing format for more specific education is by online access programs. These are regularly offered for administrative and clinical staff members of a practice, especially in the areas of compliance and participation in federal programs. Features in print such as *EyeNet, EyeWorld,* and *Administrative Eyecare,* the publication of the American Society of Ophthalmic Administrators (ASOA), spotlight issues of importance in legislation and regulation. Some focused educational offerings are available at every meeting of state and national ophthalmology groups. These special events often feature outstanding experienced presenters, providing excellent opportunities for learning about advocacy and interacting with other concerned individuals.

While it is a positive step to educate oneself concerning political issues, the critical step is to get personally involved. This involvement is most effective on a personal, local level. There simply is no substitute for a relationship developed with a member of the legislative body. Most leadership begins on the state level, and there are many opportunities to make those contacts early. Learning from our most difficult lessons—the state scope of practice battles—successful local personal and financial support usually carries the day. Unfortunately, this trumps any sort of rational argument about the wisdom of decisions in many cases. The opportunity to meet personally with a rising political figure, to explain your professional position, to offer support and to act as a resource for future medically related issues is the most powerful investment an ophthalmic leader can make in terms of advocacy for our profession.

How might one learn the skills needed to make this approach most productive for representing ophthalmology? Both ASCRS and AAO encourage every member to join their grassroots advocacy program and encourage participation in Capitol Hill visits to members of Congress. These events offer on-site training and scheduled visits—perhaps the very best way to learn how to effectively communicate with legislative representatives. They also provide an opportunity to meet and work with others who share advocacy interests. If you happen to be one of the "old hands," the time spent interacting and encouraging young professionals is mutually rewarding. I wonder how many of the readers of this book—obviously a group interested in improving leadership skills—have made a personal visit to a member of Congress or the state legislature to promote ophthalmology?

Another valuable avenue for personal involvement is to serve as an appointed representative for various state and national groups. Our ophthalmology societies have members who serve on several multispecialty organizations. This type of commitment ordinarily requires a volunteer term of several years' service, and has a learning period of policies and procedures. Our profession is always in need of articulate members who are willing to invest time to participate in such activity where the focus is not strictly clinical. This includes representation on groups concerned with advocacy, quality issues, and regulatory activity. Effective leadership in such "political" life is important, and involves interaction with many other dynamic leaders in medicine. In particular, one learns to appreciate the complexity of decisions regarding health care in our country. Ophthalmology needs to be at the table in these deliberations.

One additional benefit is that these personal activities may provide entry into the organizational structure of our professional groups. Those interested in becoming more active within a society's committee structure should consider advocacy as an avenue for productive volunteerism.

One of the easiest ways to personally participate and promote the political concerns of ophthalmology is by financial contribution. As mentioned earlier, there is no secret that fundraising functions as one of the most basic avenues to political access. While we may regret that this is the case, there is no arguing the fact. I would encourage every ophthalmic leader to contribute in two ways. First, ***direct personal contribution*** for individual political figures opens a door for dialogue. A reasonable challenge would be for every practice leader (and every practicing ophthalmologist) to identify and support personally one specific member of their state or federal legislature, and to communicate with that person on a regular basis. It's a safe prediction that the impact of such a commitment would be significant.

The second method of financial contribution is that of ***organized political action committee (PAC) contribution.*** Both of our largest organizations have very active PAC groups that are worthy of support. It doesn't take much experience on the national scene to recognize that having a consistent presence in Washington by organizational staff, making targeted donations to key political leaders, and executing well-planned visits by ophthalmology constituents to Congress deliver our advocacy message in a way not possible by efforts of a single individual. Here is another more ambitious challenge: If each ophthalmic leader made a commitment to pledge a donation, and to make a personal visit to DC at least once every 4 years (not an unreasonable idea), our message could be greatly strengthened. This same presence is also necessary on the state level—so there is plenty of political work to go around!

The challenges issued here probably seem unrealistic to many. But there is one last challenge for all those who just can't seem to accomplish any of the other goals. If you can do no more for our profession, at least go to your computer immediately and register yourself as a grassroots contact with either AAO or ASCRS. It is a very easy step. The ASCRS website is www.ascrs.org, and the AAO's is www.aao.org. You will be sent issue topics with discussion points, and simply asked to contact your members of Congress with the message. (Interestingly, one of these important calls to action came through at the very time this manuscript was being completed!) Read the email alerts from DC weekly and become familiar with the issues. Please do not put off accomplishing this one basic step of political activity. These websites are portals into all the aspects of education and involvement discussed in this chapter.

Currently, our nation's largest health care entity, Medicare, is likely to undergo the most definitive changes since its inception. The reason for this, as we all are aware, is that the financing structure is not sustainable, and things simply ***must*** be changed. The shape of this transition is not yet clear, but whatever "solution" is developed, it will be worked out in the political forum. Surely there can be no better reason to get involved with advocacy for our profession and for our patients. Who knows—you might enjoy it, and you surely could make a difference.

CHAPTER 51

Ten Signs That It May Be Time to Change Administrators

John B. Pinto

It is not necessary to change. Survival is not mandatory.
—W. Edwards Deming

If you don't like something change it;
if you can't change it, change the way you think about it.
—Mary Engelbreit

All changes, even the most longed for, h
ave their melancholy.
—Anatole France

In a variation on the old dating joke, there was once a doctor, let's call him Dr. Jones. He looked high and low to find the perfect practice administrator. He interviewed job applicants who were wicked-smart, but whose ethics were merely wicked. Dr. Jones interviewed candidates who were very hard working, but who simply didn't have the intelligence to run a modern office. He talked to one candidate who was perfect, except they could only work 25 hours a week. And Dr. Jones interviewed ethical, smart applicants who simply didn't have enough experience.

Then, after months of fruitless searching, Dr. Jones finally found her. Lauryn had it all. A PhD in medical economics. Gobs of ophthalmic experience. She lectured on ethics at the local university, and she routinely worked 65-hour weeks, taking off only 1 week a year for vacation.

Pinto JB. *Ophthalmic Leadership: A Practical Guide for Physicians, Administrators, and Teams, Second Edition* (pp 315-318).
© 2022 SLACK Incorporated.

Unfortunately, Lauryn was only willing to work for the perfect doctor. And so it goes.

• • •

Doctor-administrator relationships are not unlike dating and marriage. On most days both parties feel the union is sound enough, the exchange fair enough. A long, rosy future is anticipated on both sides. But on other days, one or both parties want out.

These feelings wax and wane. For many surgeons reading this, a love-hate relationship has existed for years between you and your lay staff leader. You're often saying to yourself: "They are too good to fire, but too (insert adjective of your choice here) to keep on the payroll."

Let's explore 10 over-the-line signals that it may be time to terminate or demote your current office manager, administrator, executive director, or CEO.

1. *Trust has been breached.* This first signal is impossible to quantify. It's a feeling thing. Such feelings can be sparked by one obvious ethical lapse (like letting a personal expense slip onto the company credit card) or an accretion of small items adding up over time. When the "distrust score" is over a given mark—and all of us have different tolerance and forgiveness levels in this area—the manager has to go.
2. *Your practice has outgrown your manager.* Managers and their practices should be closely matched pair. Ideally, as the practice grows in complexity your administrator will grow in competency. Sometimes the practice is static while the administrator blooms (in which case the administrator should be the one to leave to find greener pastures). Just as often, the practice grows at a faster pace than the manager. Unless your administrator is able to keep up, it may be time for a change … this could mean more CE time at the national meetings, coursework, a more engaged physician-leader, or the engagement of outside expertise.
3. *Your practice is stale because your manager is stale.* In an ideal world, the administrator and lead physician are a dynamic duo, keeping the company fresh and acting as a pacer for each other when one or the other gets stale. Your practice is a living organization. To be successful it needs to feed on the ideas and energy of its leaders. If your administrator is burned out or has simply been drained of their creative juices by too many years in the same position, it may be time for a change.
4. *Your manager's numeracy is not up to contemporary requirements.* In days gone by, the acceptable core competencies to run an eye clinic were things like product knowledge, an instinct for managing people, or marketing. Today, the number one competency required is numeric skills (followed closely by clear written and oral communication and raw endurance). If your current manager is, "Like, not really into math," it may be time to exchange them for someone more numerate, or to at least buttress their weakness in this area with an in-house accounting resource.
5. *Practices are merging, and only the strongest manager is needed going forward.* This one is pretty straight forward, and as soon as merger talks commence both managers pretty much know the score. In some cases, the leadership role can be shared, at least through an initial period of operations consolidation. But in most settings a zero-sum choice is obliged, with one winner and one loser. Have the class to make your choice early and help the loser find a new position in the community.

6. *Interpersonal conflicts have risen to the breaking point.* If you live with a teenager (or act like one in your off hours), you probably know all about "life points" … scores you build or shrink based on your success in a video game. Administrators play the same game, only in real life. They start a new job in your practice with 100 points. Then they lose points whenever they argue with you unpleasantly or make a mistake, and gain points with critical accomplishments. Lose too many points, and a manager is pink-slipped … or in many cases should be.
7. *Your present manager is good … but you've discovered someone who is great.* Unlike romantic relationships, a roving eye is good for business and it's perfectly acceptable to trade up every once in a while. Even when you're not looking, you may run across a manager so superior and such a great fit with the needs of your practice that it trumps your loyalty to your present administrator. When this happens, do the right thing. Give your otherwise great outgoing manager significant notice, a generous several package, and abundant support in their job search.
8. *Your manager's life situation no longer allows them to focus on your practice.* Life changes. Your manager may have domestic wobbles, start a family, or start taking care of an older parent or spouse. If they have a new personal challenge to manage this can take away a critical slice of management time and attention they need to commit every week to your company. Their distraction may be permanent or just temporary. Offering a last chance to get back in the game or a leave of absence may be more appropriate in these situations than frank termination.
9. *Your practice is faltering, you don't know why, and your administrator isn't struggling by your side to turn things around.* Ideally, you're in this together. If your practice is on the skids and you feel like you are more engaged with the turnaround than your manager, talk about it. If on most days you still feel like the only sled dog pulling in the harness, it may be a signal to find another manager.
10. *Practice revenue is shrinking, and economics no longer warrant a higher-level executive.* This is rare today, but we may see more of this in the future. In the typical practice, the "brains" of the outfit (your office manager along with various outside accountants, attorneys, and other professional advisors) will cost about 2% to 10% of practice collections. In a typical $1 million practice, that might be $60,000 for an office manager, $15,000 in annual accounting fees, another $20,000 for miscellaneous other advisors, or about 9.5% in all. The percentile figure skews lower in larger practices due to economies of scale. A $10 million practice might have a $150,000 administrator, $35,000 in accounting fees, and another $60,000 in professional fees, for a total of about 2.5% of cash flow. If you have a high-priced administrator and your top-line collections are shrinking, it may be necessary to downsize the cost of your "brains" to fit new circumstances. In the future we may see a trend in smaller practices long observed in optometry, where an engaged physician-owner takes over running day-to-day operations. Experience shows this is not ideal, but it can work fine for selected providers in selected settings, and in practices up to about $4 million in annual collections.

These are 10 reasonable reasons to consider terminating your administrator. There is at least an equally long list of reasons to ***not*** terminate, and I've seen all of these in the eye care boardrooms of America over the last 33 years. They include:

- One-time errors and omissions. Remember that although you may hold yourself to standards of near perfection as a provider, the rest of the world is human. One or two crummy management decisions a month is par for the course.
- Firing as a direct result of scrupulous honesty about bad news. You want to create an environment where you administrator doesn't fear for their job every time they bring you the truth.
- Failure to recognize that no manager has a 100% complete skill set. Strong financial managers may need outside help for marketing or IT or human resource expertise.
- Letting things build up in silence ... failure to confront your manager in the moment when they disappoint you. You should give your administrator ongoing feedback—plus and minus—about their performance so that over time they'll do more of what you like and less of what you dislike.
- Failure to provide progressive discipline. Rather than lowering the boom abruptly in response to poor performance on the part of any staffer, corrective action should be taken in stages ... verbal warnings ... written warnings ... formal retraining ... wage reductions and the like.
- Judging your manager's job performance based on their affability or lack thereof. There are plenty of communicative incompetents in every industry who should be weeded out. There are also a lot of relatively dry, dour—but administratively brilliant—business leaders out there in the world of ophthalmology. As a practice owner, it pays to know the difference, and not sack an otherwise committed executive just because they don't smile and ask you to lunch every day.

Section V

Doctors Leading Doctors

CHAPTER 52

Managing Partner
The Dirtiest Job in Eye Care Today

John B. Pinto

A wild television series, *Dirty Jobs,* was launched a few years back as part of the continuing wave of popular reality TV shows. In this show, oil rig roustabouts, hog farmers, and sanitation system repairmen (among others) are profiled on the job in a largely successful effort to gross out the audience. The show's ratings were through the roof, as might be expected given the state of popular culture.

But this show missed a huge opportunity. To draw higher ratings, the producers should tape a segment called, *Managing Partner: The Dirtiest Job in Eye Care.* They would find a lot of pretty awful material:

Pinto JB. *Ophthalmic Leadership: A Practical Guide for Physicians, Administrators, and Teams, Second Edition* (pp 321-325).
© 2022 SLACK Incorporated.

- Partners who support the lead doctor publicly, but undercut him at every turn.
- Lead doctors who spend hundreds of uncompensated hours annually with nary a thank you from the board.
- MPs who start their tenures with high hopes that their contributions will make all the difference ... only to learn that this "difference" is not so much practice-based as it is personal in exhaustion, frustration, and a new appreciation for the challenge of working in groups.

Although I have scores of similar examples, here's one anecdote that says it all. Several years ago I sat in on a board meeting for a very profitable $26-million practice in the east. On an evening with a very full agenda, the partners spent 45 minutes arguing whether the new MP's monthly honorarium—compensating him for about 10 hours a week of blood, sweat, and tears—should be $1500 or $2000. As you can imagine, the new practice leader started out feeling like he had less than the board's full confidence.

So it goes for an unfortunate majority of MPs. It's always been lonely at the top.

As a neutral observer in such dealings, I've developed a few practical recommendations that may help whether you're the MP, a member of the board, or an administrator caught in the crossfire.

The prime directive—aside from picking the right leader in the first place—is that the MP's scope of authority and position description must be formally articulated in writing. Without this document, even the best-intended lead partner will either overreach or underreach their reasonable boundaries. Here is some sample language about your duties:

- Up to 12 hours per week as an average time commitment
- Financial acumen sufficient to monitor progress toward agreed-upon profit targets
- The ability to communicate directly
- The ability (and widely held credibility) to actively mentor fellow doctors, and to not avoid uncomfortable confrontation
- Sufficient discipline to stick to board-agreed directives, and not succumb to "mission drift" or self-serving projects
- Willingness to be the doctor's disciplinarian, intervening when fellow providers are underperforming or misbehaving
- Willingness to ride to the defense of a partner or associate who is being unfairly picked on
- Helps to prepare and periodically revise the practice's strategic plan, leads the board approval process for each subsequent edition
- When other partners temporarily lose faith in the practice's plan, shows a willingness to carry the torch
- Ongoing work to coach individual doctors, helping them reach their profit and volume goals, brisk intervention when patient volumes or revenues lag
- Serves as a member of the practice's management committee (a group composed of selected senior staff) that manages day-to-day operations
- Chairman of the practice's board of directors

- Maintains ongoing, senior-level contacts with the practice's sources of referrals and with third-party payers in the region
- Is involved with all provider and senior staff recruitment
- Conducts risk management, utilization, and quality assurance reviews, or delegates these chores to fellow providers ... in consultation with the board, has the ability to suspend or revise any clinical practices believed to be inappropriate
- Works to resolve provider-to-provider conflicts in such areas as scope-of-practice issues, patient assignment, compensation methodology, etc
- Responsible for applying a progressive discipline system to misbehaving partners and associate doctors, ranging from informal peer-to-peer counseling to termination

Compensation for an MP is influenced by many factors. If all the partners within a practice take the role in equal rotation, then the position can be noncompensated. In most practices, however, the MP duties are not equally shared. Compensation, in this case, should definitely be paid.

What's the proper amount? In the best of circumstances, the stipend ends up being little more than a token honorarium, roughly proportional to the size and success of the group. In a two- to five-doctor practice, a payment of $18,000 to $36,000 per year is typical. As you can see from this, a partner working 10 hours per week on the practice's behalf is only going to earn about $50 per hour ... far less than they would seeing patients. In larger practices, where more time is required and the lead-partner's stipend is divided among more owners, the MP may receive more than $50,000 per year.

In a small number of settings, MPs receive a bonus based on practice collections or profits. However, this is uncommon and doesn't seem to influence performance. If anything, a struggle can erupt because the MP then tries to boost his bonus by overworking his colleagues.

Tenure in this leadership role should be 2 years or longer. An annual rotation—often chosen out of a misplaced desire to assure perfect fairness by giving everyone a shot at the job—results in doctors stepping down only as they are starting to learn the nuances of the position.

Succession in this role from one partner to the next should be handled with great sensitivity. Rather than a simple majority approval, it's preferable to nearly follow the rules for a Papal election—where nothing less than full consensus must be achieved.

In my experience, any practice with two or more owners should designate a formal leader, even if at this smaller scale all policies and decisions are typically derived through the complete consensus of the owners. Line staff in the trenches especially benefit when the organization chart makes it clear that they report to their immediate supervisor (eg, head tech, billing supervisor), who in turn reports to the administrator, who then works most closely with the MP to execute the board's mandate.

Here are some coaching points and success factors we've learned through the years from long-term lead partners who not only enjoy the durable support of their peers, but who have an absolute ball doing the job.

- *Stay informed.* One of the best compensations of being the leader is the status of informational privilege that it confers. Knowing the way the wind is blowing both inside and outside of the organization is critical to both your success and satisfaction in a leadership role.
- *Delegate avidly.* You can't do it all. In the busiest years, you can't even touch half of the opportunities personally. You should be personally engaged ***only*** with those areas and projects that are the most interesting to you and crucial to the company. Remember that the best way in any group setting to stimulate involvement is to give people a job to do.
- *Set firm boundaries at the outset.* For example, when you send an email out requesting feedback, set a deadline and follow up early in your tenure with stragglers. Do not let your partners get in the habit of blowing off meetings or failing to follow up with your reasonable requests.
- *Make everyone responsible for success or failure.* Unless you're a practice dictator—in which case it's really all on you—your organization is going to rise or fall based on everyone's contributions.
- *Find the right balance between dictatorship (which on the toughest days sounds pretty attractive), guile, and collegiality.* Sometimes it's appropriate to be in touch with your "inner-Machiavelli," and play one side against another for the benefit of the organization.
- *Hold your management accountable for their agreed projects in terms of content, quality, and timeliness.* Be clear about the specific outcomes you expect from them.
- *There are going to be lots of times when you have to give speeches to the board, management team, or total staff.* If you're not a natural orator, or tend to stray off your core message, speak from written notes.
- *Arrange a time every few weeks to meet over a casual lunch with a few staff.* These informal sessions will not only give you a glimpse of life in the trenches, but your staff will see you as more approachable and will seek you out with their future concerns. This feedback is invaluable as a leader.
- *Be honest.* Long-term success is only possible if you are authentic, approachable, and ultimately vulnerable in your dealings with others. If you are at wit's end with your board, your administrator, or an outside party, say so, and let the chips fall where they may.

Being the first among equals in your practice is not a position from which you ***command*** … it's a position from which you ***lead.*** There's a difference. A military commander's directives are followed without question. A corporate executive can fire his entire cast of subordinates. But a leader—particularly in a medical setting with a slew of smart peers hanging around—starts with a clean slate every day and has to defend every new initiative. If you're not ready for the frustrations and gaps in control incumbent in this reality, don't step forward and volunteer for the position.

Very few MPs are ever abruptly fired. Actually, their tenure is usually quite long—which may be a better measure of the lack of willing substitute candidates than a vote of confidence in most of the settings that I visit.

However, this does not mean that most practice owners are overjoyed about your performance as an MP. Their greatest concerns commonly center around fair dealing. The fastest way to lose your board's support is to appear to be spinning opportunities in your own direction at the expense of the rest of the partners. Instead, the most successful MPs often have to vote actively against their own interests to be viewed as impartial.

Doing this job requires a perpetual "Goldilocks" sense of balance. Get too involved with the details, and your board and administrator will accuse you of micromanaging. Become too aloof, and you'll be accused of abandoning the team. How should you determine the right tipping point? That's simple. Ask everyone you work with how you're doing with this balancing act, and follow the advice that you're given.

Any way you look at it, being the MP of your group practice is a dirty, thankless, long-suffering, underrewarded, overstressed, and certainly undercompensated job. Every new lead surgeon's get-started kit should include a thick skin, an abundant sense of humor, and a hazmat suit. It's a tough, dirty job. Welcome to the head of the table, chief.

CHAPTER 53

How to Be a Better Physician Supervisor and Break in Your Practice's New Doctor

John B. Pinto

You would think that after some 25 years of schooling, every newly-graduated ophthalmologist would be fully ready—ripe, even—to competently report for employment in your practice. But this is far from being the case. In one client practice after another, I'm astounded by the degree of "finishing school" still needed in many cases.

Who is responsible for this gap? The doctor's parents? Their training program? Employing practices? The young physicians, themselves? Everyone is probably co-responsible. However, let's move beyond the question, "Who's responsible?" to the more practical question of, "Who can make it better, and how?"

Pinto JB. *Ophthalmic Leadership: A Practical Guide for Physicians, Administrators, and Teams, Second Edition* (pp 327-330).
© 2022 SLACK Incorporated.

Here's a 12-point list to help ease you over the first year of your associate's tenure with your practice, starting with choosing the right doctor in the first place.

1. *Screen all prospective doctors for their level of maturity, "coachability," work ethic, and lack of "entitlement issues."* Some arrested development is to be expected of any 30-something doctor who is only now getting out into the real world. But is your final candidate willing to let their ego down and take direction? One of the best predictors of this is prior, successful work or play as a member of a team. As a broad generality, doctors with a life history of team sports (football and volleyball being better than singles tennis) or of group activities (eg, clubs or scouting) are more moldable to work in a group. A strong predictor of your candidate's work ethic in your practice is how early they took their first job. You may want to jump on candidates who cut lawns or babysat at 12 … and pass on candidates who would draw their first real paycheck from your back account.
2. *Get the employment contract right.* As many details should be worked out in advance as possible. A generation ago, it was common for partner-track associate deals to be sealed with a handshake, with no finite provision for what the partnership transaction was going to be. Many years later, it's now clear that this is not the best approach. You should outline your performance expectations. Do not take anything for granted. Spell out hours, duties (both clinical and business), call responsibilities, and promotional chores. An intelligent associate doctor employment contract today still doesn't guarantee partnership, but it spells out the steps that will ensue if partnership is mutually desired. Really smart contracts outline how partnership buy-in, compensation, and governance will work in the years ahead.
3. *Get to know your new doctor.* When young, associate doctors complain to me about their employer (my client) everything usually revolves around communication gaps. Listen to your associate surgeons actively and often. All doctors (both partner and nonpartner) in even the smallest group practices should meet at least once every month, ideally over a social meal, to work out the kinks in their professional relationship. Along the way, get to know what career drivers are the most important to your new associate. Is it financial success or quality care? Case volumes or clinical or outcomes? Your understanding of your associate's priorities will underpin your approach to managing their work in the months ahead.
4. *Remember that it's called a "residency," not "cotillion."* Assume that your new *Dr. Young and Wonderful* knows nothing about the nuances of social interactions with staff, colleagues, or referring doctors. The most astute professional practices in law and accountancy discovered many years ago that their new associates were not quite ready to interact with the professional world. As a result, they set up formal training sessions, including such practical lessons as which fork to use for the salad course. No less attention to detail is called for in your practice. Make sure your young associates are ready for prime time before you send them out into the world to win referral support. Rather than allowing them to fly solo with the first few meetings with referring doctors, join them at get-acquainted lunches and end each such meeting with a constructive (but not overbearing) postmortem.

5. *At the risk of being somewhat paternalistic, be sure to orient your young doctors to the most common career-builders and career-killers.* Here are some talking points:
   a. If you have not yet done so, grow up. Take yourself seriously and professionally. Dress and speak and act the part.
   b. No matter the temptations, do not socialize with lay staff. It's lots of fun to flirt with techs at the Friday night bowling party. But it's best for your career to find your own crowd outside of the office.
   c. Lose the nine-to-five attitude. Arrive at least 30 minutes before your first patient and stay at least 30 minutes after you've wound up the last encounter to help tidy up the office and get ready for the next day.
   d. During down time, when patients thin out, don't waste your employer's time reading journals or surfing the internet. Spend your time wisely on activities that further the interests of the practice (remember, if you make partner it will be ***your*** practice one day). The time you spend is your employer's … use it to their benefit, not your own.
   e. You are not quite yet a "medical deity." Before you get there, show a little humility. Remember your "yes, sirs" and "yes, ma'ams" along the way.
6. *Score some early wins.* Don't let months pass before helping your young doctor be successful. Discuss two or three measurable goals, write these down, and work together to achieve them. Examples include:
   a. Achieving a clinic volume of six patients or more per hour
   b. Yielding optical sales of $25 or more from the average patient visit
   c. Generating at least one surgical case for every 30 patient visits
   d. Meeting face-to-face with at least 10 potential referral sources per week
   e. Mastering the details of coding and charting so that periodic audits reveal a diminishing number of errors
7. *Track progress graphically over time.* It can get pretty frustrating in the first few quarters as an associate twiddling your thumbs and waiting for the next patient to arrive on a slow day. It helps immensely to see the broader trends. And there's no better way to do this than by graphing by week or by month the number of patient visits, cases, average revenue yield per patient visit, and other metrics.
8. *Nearly everyone needs and wants a boss.* As the doctor or administrator supervising a young associate doctor, do not assume that they want a hands-off approach from you. Set and continuously reaffirm expectations. Unless your supervisory style is overbearing, your associate will appreciate honest feedback over the rough spots … and relish praise for progress. Show abundant support and celebrate even the small wins (like your young doctor seeing the 1000th patient of their career in your office). Remember that it's quite lonely being a new associate. In my experience, the average doctor-supervisor orbits their charges much less closely than they should.

9. *Offer more than just blunt complaints.* Instead, you should offer abundant praise for everything that's going well and occasional redirection when problems surface. If your associate doctor requires more than just the occasional course correction, this may be a signal that it's time to consider stronger medicine: A formal probationary period or frank termination.
10. *Take responsibility.* As the administrator or managing partner of your group, do not blame practice problems on your associate doctors. Let's say your practice volume is faltering, and your associates have a lot of extra time on their hands. Who's been minding the store? Who determined that more doctors were needed? Who hired them? Who has supervised their work? Who has been responsible for a marketing program to keep them fully employed?
11. *Get close to your young doctor's allies.* Chances are good that as the administrator or lead doctor of your practice you're not the most important person in you associate doctor's life. Work to get close to those who are. These people include spouses, techs, and even sales reps who have insinuated themselves with your young employee surgeons.
12. *Finally, have fun.* One of the greatest joys of owning or managing a professional practice can be bringing up the next generation of providers. Like parenting, this process can involve sleepless nights and lots of mistakes along the way.

CHAPTER 54

What Does Your Associate Doctor *Really* Want?

John B. Pinto

Among the many great mysteries of the ophthalmic world, one of the most enduring is summarized in the question, "What does my associate doctor want, anyway?!?" A significant portion of my phone calls and emails revolve around this topic. What's left after you feel you've given the moon, the sun, and the stars—and your employee doctor is still not happy? There's no easy answer, especially when an overly tight senior doctor is the employer of an overly grabby junior doctor. Here's a brief digest of the most common complaints I hear from junior associates, along with a few ideas to help their employers and practice managers.

Broadly, associate doctors, whether permanently tabbed as associates or on a partner track, want respect. They (at least usually) understand that they are not first in the practice pecking order. But they do want lay support staff to be

Pinto JB. *Ophthalmic Leadership: A Practical Guide for Physicians, Administrators, and Teams, Second Edition* (pp 331-333).
© 2022 SLACK Incorporated.

responsive to reasonable requests. They want to hear their employer say during a staff meeting, "Now I want you all you all to realize that in the eyes of our patients and the eyes of our staff, Dr. Smith is my colleague and equal in this practice." Some associate physicians (and optometrists as well) undermine their own authority by trying to be one of the gang or being a little too familiar. "Call me Dr. Dave. Or just Dave is fine. And what time is staff happy hour on Friday?"

As an owner, foster a group spirit and talk about the "team." Be an "us" practice, not a "me" practice in all communication: at staff meetings, in speaking with patients, and in marketing materials. It's in marketing coverage that some of the rawest conflicts arise, not only interpersonally, but in a very practical business sense. If your practice advertises, we know that using one doctor's name as the name of the practice, like "Michaelson Eye Center," works better than a generic name like "Western Eye Center." And we also have learned that using one doctor spokesperson as the public guarantor of quality works better than a parade of different faces. If your practice can overcome the ego strains, stick to one person in the ads. If the associates insist on their 15 minutes of fame, use a group shot and use the fact that you take a team approach as one factor distinguishing your service.

The best quality associates want to get involved with decision making and with special projects they can call their own. Allow associates to sit in on nonsensitive portions of your practice's partner meetings. Give them a voice, even if they do not have a vote. There's no need to discard an associate because they do not volunteer for extra duties like coming eagerly to these meetings, but it may be a signal that they are not partner material. By allowing a young doctor to participate in the group's discussions on strategy and spending philosophy today, you'll be helping a partner-in-training make better decisions for *you* in the future.

Doctors who have not yet made partner, along with younger partners, are often exquisitely sensitive about how new patients are assigned in the practice, especially if the compensation methodology leans toward top-line production. There should be a written protocol for scheduling new patients, and the front desk or appointment clerks should be checked periodically so that the very human tendency to please the senior partner by feeding them patients is not biasing the system.

Most associates (and partners, too) detest being clinically pigeon-holed, and kept from areas of practice that they enjoy. There are numerous conflicts arising today as the senior doctors in some setting are carving out LASIK surgery for themselves. (Just watch—the tide will turn as procedure fees settle down to earth and it becomes most profitable once again to provide general eye care and cataract surgery!) As a general principle, unless an associate has been hired with the expressed agreement that they will stick to defined practice areas, it works best if every doctor is permitted to provide whatever care they are trained to perform well.

Even the most junior doctors will commonly—and understandably—complain if they are forced to report solely to a lay manager in the practice or answer to a clinician or paraprofessional they deem to be of lower status. I ordinarily construct client organization charts with dual reporting lines so that doctors report to a medical director or an MP for clinical affairs and to the practice administrator for business matters.

It's not unusual for doctors—even pure, permanent employees—to react adversely when the partner-doctors are using staff and other practice resources for personal purposes. I'm speaking here of the common practice of a senior doctor sending someone out for personal errands or over to their home for child care or housekeeping duties. It's clearly your right as an owner to deploy staff as you see fit, subject only to your accountant's comfort with this, but try to not rub these perks in your associate's face. If you are in solo practice (where such line-blurring between personal and business expenses are most common), be sure to install a charge-back protocol for quasi-business expenses when your associate becomes a partner.

Partner-track associates obviously want an equity stake in the practice. But owners and associates are rarely on the same page regarding a fair percentage. Owners can be too parsimonious, offering just 5% or 10%, even if their associate is now doing nearly half of the work. I find even more often that it's the associates who are overreaching. It's not unusual for me during a consulting assignment in this area to speak with an associate who perhaps generates just 20% of the practice's revenue, but expects to be granted a full 50% equity position. If you're an associate surgeon reading this article, put yourself in your employer's shoes. They are likely either going to want to retain a 51% majority control, or at the very least have legal documents obliging a supermajority vote (which they control by contract even with a minority position). Precise fairness to both sides calls for an equity position for all partner providers pro rata to their revenue or profit contributions, subject only to the preferences of a founding or MP, whose word—legally and morally—should be law.

Believe it or not, associate doctors want clear boundaries. A common complaint I hear from associates we're about to terminate is, "I never knew I was expected to do that … why didn't somebody tell me?" Every new associate should be given a written summary of your minimum performance expectations. This list may reasonably be quite different for partner-track associates, who should *cheerfully and skillfully* take on extra work in such areas as staff training, community outreach, and quality assurance review.

Whether you're an associate or an owner—or a manager stuck in between when these two parties get into conflict—it may help to hand out copies of this short chapter to help stimulate a discussion and reach a resolution.

CHAPTER 55

Deciding If Your Associate Provider Is Ready for Ownership

John B. Pinto

Quick decisions are unsafe decisions.
—Sophocles

All our final decisions are made in a state of mind that is not going to last.
—Marcel Proust

In most professional firms besides medicine, the pool of applicants materially exceeds the number of job openings. There can be scores of great applicants for a low-level associate position in a law, architectural, or accounting firm. And 5 years later (commonly years of 60-hour weeks), one's elevation to partnership is by no means secure.

This is quite unlike medicine in general, and ophthalmology in particular, where the number of open positions is growing faster than the number of available candidates, and the demand for care is rising sharply with the invasion of baby boomer seniors.

Pinto JB. *Ophthalmic Leadership: A Practical Guide for Physicians, Administrators, and Teams, Second Edition* (pp 335-337).
© 2022 SLACK Incorporated.

As a result of this, some practices are lowering their guards—and their standards—admitting partner-track associates who are unlikely to ever be partner-worthy and offering partnerships to doctors who are destined to be a poor fit.

Compatibility Screening

If you have a partner-track associate heading for partnership, or even if you're only starting to interview for a new doctor, here are 12 simple screens for compatibility.

1. *Sufficient passage of time.* The prepartner associate period is typically as little as a year or as long as 5 years. The average figure in ophthalmology is 2 or 3 years. Does that figure sound familiar? It's about the same time that couples date before they seriously consider marriage. The similarities are apt. For at least the first year, everyone in both settings is on best behavior. But eventually, the true personality of both marital and business partnership candidates shines through (or fades to black). Beyond giving both sides time to see whether there's a fit, waiting at least a couple of years has a practical advantage—before this, it's unlikely that the new doctor has developed sufficient revenue productivity to be able to afford to start paying for a buy-in.
2. *General affability.* Pathologically unpleasant individuals—even the smartest ones—are usually screened out well before they complete an ophthalmology residency. Still, eye surgeons come in a wide array of flavors, from cuddly and affable to individuals who are described thusly by everyone in their world: "Well, Dr. Andrews is not the kind of guy you go to for a good time, but he will give you a great surgical result." If affability counts in your practice (and it should), hold out for Dr. Cuddly.
3. *Clinical and judgment skills.* These are two separate skills, and both should be obliged in your candidate partner. Clinical skills are essential, obviously. But great didactic knowledge without the judgment to apply it properly will lead to disaster on the clinic floor. And in the courtroom.
4. *Surgical skills.* Over the last 31 years as an advisor to ophthalmologists, I've often asked the question, "How do you know a great surgeon is a great surgeon?" The answer that typically comes back is the same as Justice Potter Stewart's 1964 Supreme Court dictum on pornography: "I know it when I see it." And so will you, if you're judging your young colleague's fitness for partnership. Watch carefully.
5. *Compatible work ethic.* At any one time, I'm working with a large number of 60-something ophthalmologists who lament the lower work ethic of their 30-something colleagues. If you are a workaholic surgeon, it's not likely that you are going to be happy with the average new graduate's idea of a full work week. You either need to accept that their work–life balance is going to work for you, or keep looking for the uncommon young individual today who puts their career ahead of all other life domains.
6. *Staff interaction.* One of the best partnership screens is to stay keyed into what your staff think about Dr. New becoming a partner. If their thumbs are still up in the air after a couple of years, yours should be too. And vice versa. If your candidate partner is humble and self-effacing, willing to drop what they are doing to

help out the crew, and someone who makes them proud to work as support staff in your practice, you're anointing the right candidate.

7. *Patient relationships.* Even the sweetest doctor will tote up a few patient complaints each year, especially when they are being compared to the "old man" who founded the practice. A few complaints a month should set off alarms. A few complaints a week should lead to termination. Let your patients vote your associate in or out of partnership.
8. *Utilization and volumetric productivity.* It's helpful to pull the last year's Current Procedural Terminology (CPT) report on a candidate partner and check their utilization statistics against the average for the practice. If the existing partners have a 40% YAG rate and the junior doctor is at 15%, some comparisons around the table may be in order. The same goes for the utilization rates of special testing, assertiveness in charging for refractions, and the overall revenue yield per patient visit. Laggards should be coaxed to higher performance before they become partners. Outliers who overtreat should be counseled and if needed, removed.
9. *A well-adjusted ethical compass.* Most choir-boy, Eagle Scout ophthalmologists do not have the belly for what's become of modern medical economics, where being sufficiently assertive in coding and case selection is unfortunately the obligation to also make payroll and get your rent check in on time. That said, aggressiveness has to be tempered by an underlying sense of what is defensible and absolutely in each patient's individual interest. It's a fine line and getting finer all the time. As the practice owner, you call the line. Make sure your partner-to-be is on the right side of it.
10. *Financial productivity.* I'm often called with a question along the lines of: "I'm the founder of a two-doctor practice. Dr. Maybe has been on staff as an associate for 3 years. His collections were $620,000 last year. Mine were $1.9 million. Is it time to bring him on as a partner?" The answer is a definite "maybe." If he passes the other screening dimensions discussed here, he could be a good fit. But since Dr. Maybe is only generating 25% of total practice collections, equal partnership may be less appropriate than a minority share of the company … or a delay in granting partnership until the two doctors are a little closer to being economic peers.
11. *Business instincts and behaviors.* When you nominate a new partner, you are not just advancing a clinical peer up the ranks … you are drafting a new board member. Each new addition to the table should ideally improve the net skill, judgment, and commitment of the board to your company. Rethink your decision if the new owner candidate is overly timid, disruptive, or absolutely disengaged from all business affairs (yet unwilling to trust and delegate business authority to others like you who are interested).
12. *Giver vs taker mentality.* As the old man used to say: There are only two kinds of people, givers and takers. Two willing givers make the best partnership. A taker can partner well with a longsuffering giver. The most toxic practice environment is a cohort of takers. Measure your candidate in black and white terms … this is not a matter of degrees. They are a giver or they are a taker. Do they volunteer for extra call? Cheerfully take on special projects? Or do they push work and worry that they should personally bear off to others? Partnering with a taker, even the most productive one, sets up the rest of your career for misery.

CHAPTER 56

What Is a Partnership, Really? What Kind Do You Have?

John B. Pinto

In an average year, I spend hundreds of hours constructing, deconstructing, and patching up doctor-to-doctor partnerships. At the surface, there are scores of hot-button issues that make partnerships so difficult to make and keep happy. But at deeper levels, there is perhaps just one core attribute, the degree of partner equality.

Not that *unequality* is bad. Extremely strong business partnerships (and for that matter, other kinds of partnerships like marriage) exist where both sides agree who is going to lead and who is going to follow. But the most extraordinary environments for surgeons to work in are often those where equality prevails.

Pinto JB. *Ophthalmic Leadership: A Practical Guide for Physicians, Administrators, and Teams, Second Edition* (pp 339-342).
© 2022 SLACK Incorporated.

What is a partner, really? Here's a dictionary definition that's suitable for most competitive ophthalmic environments: "A partner is one of two or more people who play together in a game against an opposing side." A drier, more legalistic definition is, "A partner is someone involved in a close, cooperating relationship with others, regulated by mutual rights and responsibilities, to further a common enterprise."

All English lessons and legal jargon aside, ophthalmic partnerships fall into two very broad and profoundly different categories.

Unequal Partnerships

Surprise! This is the most common form of partnership, in eye care and elsewhere. Even if partners are legally and economically equal, they are rarely equal in actuality. An examination of the typical ophthalmology practice reveals a rank order of leaders and followers. The hierarchy is most commonly along lines of either tenure (who came first?), economic production (who collects the most?), or natural leadership (who by raw personality is granted the most authority?). In these kinds of partnerships, decisions and resource allocations are lopsided. The senior doctors get the choice midweek, morning hours in the practice's surgery center— the junior doctors get Friday afternoons. The seniors get their pick of the best technicians—the juniors by default run the tech training program. The seniors are excused from call sharing, the juniors are excused from a sound night's sleep. Not a bad arrangement ... if you're a senior. So long as everyone gets to rise through the ranks and agrees to this approach ahead of time, unequal partnerships can work just fine.

Equal Partnerships

In these rare partnerships, doctors most often (but not always) have equal shares in the practice and all of it's subsidiaries such as optical shops, buildings, and surgery facilities. Both younger and older doctor partners have an essentially equal voice in management—more decisions are made by consensus rather than formal vote. Perhaps the most important contribution to harmony is that everyone in an equal partnership setting gets an equal share of resources. Marketing dollars are split equally among the various subspecialists. Everyone gets to rotate through the most productive satellite offices. Every doctor gets a turn at being the MP. Perhaps most importantly, all partners rise or fall with the total success of the total organization.

• • •

Here's a recent example from a client setting. A large Midwest practice was exploring the admission of a new partner, a well-respected local surgeon who would be merging his smaller solo practice into the larger organization. For the first several hours of our merger conference, the five partners of the larger practice were adamant that the soloist, if he joined, would have to be 100% at risk. His compensation methodology was going to be different from everyone else for the first year or 2, in a way that I saw was going to potentially result in the new partner's income rising while the old doctor's income fell—or vice versa. I suggested that for the first several years the partners might index their split of available profits to their current incomes. If the profits rose 10% after the merger, every doctor would get a 10% pay raise. All boats would float together. It's interesting to note that as soon as the doctors in the larger group understood the inherent fairness of their incomes rising and falling together based on the success of the entire team, they went on during the rest of our conference to equalize everything else: access to the best techs, sharing of the evening and weekend hours, and responsibility for covering distant satellite offices. I have a high level of confidence that this merger is going to go very well, indeed.

What Kind Is Yours?

When two or more doctors draw themselves together, the kind of partnership they choose—equal or unequal—has huge implications for everyone around them. In an equal partnership, the practice administrator is less likely to take sides. In equal partnerships, even junior staff realize that it will be hard to play one doctor off the other. I suspect that even patients get a sense that all doctors are interchangeable, and are more willing to see whichever doctor is most available. I think the reverse is also true. If there's clearly a dominant, "head" doctor, patients gravitate to that one provider, especially for their surgical care. This can amplify rivalries that naturally occur in unequal partnerships.

It's more likely for truly mutual, equal partnerships to form naturally when two young, equally novice doctors start a practice together. Equality is far less common when a young surgeon joins an established doctor 10 years or more ahead in their career. In these situations, the young surgeon, even after a successful associateship, will likely remain in the senior doctor's shadow until the older doctor retires, although there can be hope for greater equality with the passage of time. It's been my observation that with age and success, senior ophthalmologists become somewhat less controlling and more acquiescent to true partner equality. Of course, this usually happens just about the time when the younger generation is wanting to take over and control the practice themselves, which is why most unequal partnerships stay that way. Perhaps this article will stimulate an internal discussion within your group practice on how authority and control is shared.

A discussion of partnership models wouldn't be complete without reviewing how young surgeons make it through the ranks from employed associate to partner. I've always been critical of the all-or-nothing approach most commonly taken in private practice medical employment, where junior doctors are often moved after 2 or 3 years, in one leap, from "associate" to "full partner." This works against basic human nature and the experience of most large institutions (eg, military, educational, religious, trade union, business, political). These institutions move their members from novice to expert in small, incremental stages. Perhaps the most intelligent approach to granting partnership in an ophthalmic practice is to grant similar, incremental shares—"merit badges," if you will—so that junior doctors feel a sense of steady progression in their early years.

Whether partners are equal or unequal, the biggest factor for success and harmony is mutual agreement about the development path of the practice. Partnerships are hardest to maintain when there are no large goals held in common—and yet, few group ophthalmology practices have anything like a written business plan. The angriest doctors I counsel are those with partners who don't share their goals; or far worse, hold them back from accomplishing their dreams. In extreme cases, these toxic pairings can lead to the polar opposite of my favorite saying about partners and partnership: "A partner is someone with whom you can accomplish things that you can't accomplish alone."

Finally, some doctors do not really play well in groups, and should probably not be part of a partnership, just as some people should probably not be married. It may take you several years of struggle (or several practice divorces) to learn this about yourself. Fortunately for such doctors, the environment today is allowing eye surgeons who would like to remain solo to do so, with open access to managed care patients, more and more underserved rural pockets of the country needing doctors, and practice costs that have at least temporarily stabilized.

CHAPTER 57

Eight Rules for Getting Along With Your Practice Partner

John B. Pinto

Benjamin Franklin once famously said: "Keep your eyes wide open before marriage, and half shut afterwards." He could have just as readily been giving advice to partnering eye surgeons, who today have a disharmony and divorce rate that nearly matches that of the ordinary kind of matrimony.

Even in the most congenial practices I visit, significant time has to be spent getting at least one or two strained relationships back on track. Through the years I've developed a simple how-to list of recommendations that may help you reverse partner discord, or even better, stay out of trouble in the first place.

Pinto JB. *Ophthalmic Leadership: A Practical Guide for Physicians, Administrators, and Teams, Second Edition* (pp 343-346).
© 2022 SLACK Incorporated.

Partnership Rules

1. Don't compare your "deal" (eg, your hours, wage, call schedule, case mix, burden of scutt work) with your partners and get burned up because Joe gets more cataracts than you get, or Mary makes more than you do, or the practice's senior partner is now off call rotation. Instead, it's a lot easier on your nerves to compare your present situation as a partner with what life would be like as a soloist. I often counsel junior partners who are steamed because they don't have the same high surgical loads or incomes as the senior doctors, "Wait. If you have the right talent your turn will come. Imagine you were off on your own … how many fewer cases would you be doing then? How much more overhead would you have to cover all alone? Who would you talk to about difficult cases?"
2. Accept the fact that all partnerships are flawed because all people are flawed. Even the coziest partnerships have a 5% grief and regret factor. There's no one in this business that I know who's holding hands with their partners singing hymns around the campfire. Indeed, being an affable partner is something that many eye surgeons have to struggle with for their entire career, it's their "adapted" personality, not their natural state. The ophthalmic personality is not often given to playing well in groups. On top of all that, ophthalmology is now an increasingly disciplined business. Resources are tapering. Profit margins are shrinking. There are more excuses to pick a fight. You need to redouble efforts to admit your own flaws and accept the flaws in your partners.
3. Fighting and conflict, to a point, is good. But you need to understand and respect your partner's willingness to confront and his natural conflict resolution pace. If you're the kind of person who blows off immediate steam at the first provocation, but settles down quickly, you can get into trouble having a partner who quietly, gradually reaches his boiling point. If your style is to talk everything out in the open and your partner is more obtuse, you're both going to be frustrated. Discuss your differences and then respect them. This is more easily said than done, obviously. If you're running into chronic strife over differences like these, it may help to have all of the partners (and the administrator and department heads if appropriate) tested with one of the common personality inventories, and then be oriented as a group on the results by a trained professional. It's worth the time commitment—you may just be a few hours away from making your work environment a lot more pleasant.
4. When there's strife, as difficult as it may be, look in the mirror first and ask yourself, "Is it me? Am I causing this?" Ask for and defer to the opinion of a few trusted coaches. I try to take this particular pearl to heart at home and turn to my 9-year-old son Graham to learn if I'm being, in his words, a "butthead" on some issue. In your practice life, you may feel close enough to your administrator or chief tech or semi-retired senior partner to take them aside and find out if you're being a butthead, too. If so, not to worry; it's a big, big club with lots of fellow eye surgeons (and management consultants) as members.

5. Don't use the administrator or other lay staff as the referee for doctor-to-doctor conflict resolution. If you're an office manager and your doctors are in a fight, your first instinct may be to dive in and break up the rumble. You should resist this in most cases. As any police officer can tell you, some of the most dangerous calls they go out on are seemingly minor domestic quarrels. Like an officer responding to a domestic dispute, you should remember that partner-to-partner conflicts can be dangerous for first-responder administrators to get in the middle of. Even if you succeed in lowering tensions, at least one of the partners will likely perceive you're taking sides against them; their resentment will be durable, and you can lose the ability to lead in other areas of the practice in the future. It's far more appropriate for the MP or an outside party to rescue difficult situations. MPs can be rotated out. An outside vendor can be dismissed and replaced with two phone calls. But losing a valued administrator can set your practice back for years.
6. There's no such thing as a 50-50 partnership. Perfect equality is as much a myth as Santa Claus, another idealistic archetype that serves a valuable social purpose to keep naive believers temporarily in line. Somebody in your practice is the smartest. Somebody is the least smart. Somebody is the best with financial details. Somebody is the most skilled surgeon. And chances are, nobody is the best at everything. The *TEAM* acronym, "Together Everyone Achieves More," only works if you harness everyone's unique strengths and simultaneously acknowledge that not everyone is going to get a perfectly fair, perfectly even deal. This year you might make less, but your partner finally gets lanes 2 and 3 equipped just the way they want them. Next year, you can get your LASIK marketing program tuned up, while your partner takes a mild pay cut for you in turn. To be a happy partner, your favorite expression has to become, "I can live with that." Not every partner problem has a solution. Living with a modicum of small inequalities is obligatory.
7. Don't be shy to call 911. You need to know when partner discord has lasted longer or plunged deeper than is healthy. There are all kinds of outside parties you can draw on, depending on what's at issue. A purely financial argument might be best solved by your accountant. An ethical issue can be addressed by a professional ethicist. Interpersonal frictions may yield to an industrial psychologist. Practice management consultants typically provide help with multidisciplinary issues, as when both practice governance and financial integrity have fallen off.
8. Practice divorce is an acceptable, if regrettable and expensive, solution. As I've lectured and written elsewhere, business partnerships are a kind of unconsummated, childless marriage. The relationship glue is your common vision of what you can create together, your stepwise progress, and your fear that practicing outside of partnership will be worse than what you have now. But sometimes even this glue is not strong enough to bond unsuitable partners. If it's at long last time for a practice divorce, make the break as cleanly and as fairly as possible, *but do so only after heroic efforts to work things out and to understand precisely why things failed.* Just like the ordinary kind of marriage, your failure to thrive in the current practice marriage will often lead to successive botches.

• • •

I hope that with the ideas here, you and your partners will be able to stop well short of divorce. With any luck it may be as easy as ceasing to look so hard for what's wrong and focus instead on what's right about your partnership. Accentuate the positives. As Ben Franklin might have said, were he an ophthalmologist, "Enter a partnership with crystalline vision and thereafter work hard to develop a progressive case of macular degeneration."

CHAPTER 58

Twenty Rules for Group Practice Harmony

John B. Pinto

If you're an ophthalmologist, odds are high that you work well with other people—or at least need to learn how to do so. That's because two-thirds of America's ophthalmologists in private practice today work in a group practice setting, either in a single- or multispecialty group.

I'm often called in to restore doctor-to-doctor relationships in practices where the providers are no longer harmonious. Here's a checklist to improve harmony in your own setting.

Pinto JB. *Ophthalmic Leadership: A Practical Guide for Physicians, Administrators, and Teams, Second Edition* (pp 347-350).
© 2022 SLACK Incorporated.

1. *Have a written business plan.* Until the owners of a practice are clear about their goals, it's easier to have partner relationships go adrift. Your goals can be abstracted into a terse punch list or elaborated into a major document. Either way, you'll have a reference for prioritizing near-term actions and acquiring the resources you need to get ahead.
2. *Employ a strong administrator.* Although no lay manager can—or should—act as a referee between arguing practice owners, the best management executives can help you keep your practice humming along well enough that there are fewer reasons for discord.
3. *Select the right physician-leader.* The best practices are led by one strong lay manager and one strong physician. Too frequently, the latter is an unpaid, figurehead position only. Your group practice's MP should be elected for 2 or more years, and receive a stipend that is equal to about 5% to 10% of their total professional compensation.
4. *Always have a new physician-leader in the wings.* Unless your term of office exceeds 3 years, nominate the next MP in the "batter's box" who will be stepping up in a few years. It takes at least a year or 2 to get ready to lead. Selecting the next leader is easier in a large practice with a deeper bench of prospects.
5. *Run formal, fact-based board meetings.* It's common as practices grow to maintain the old informalities of their mom-and-pop stage. Reread *Robert's Rules* and follow them. Your meetings will be faster, fairer, and more effective. Make decisions based on facts more than feelings.
6. *Support the board's decisions. Always.* Does this happen in your practice? You make a decision by majority vote. Then one or more of the dissenters go out the next day and tell their staff, "I know we voted for 'X', but I'm going to do 'Y' instead—the board is wrong." Nothing will undermine overall practice morale faster than an owner who can't respect majority decisions.
7. *Pick the right doctors to join your practice.* No matter how much you interview, how much you check references, or how closely you observe their surgery tapes, only about 50% of the time will you hire the right doctor to join your practice. The other half of the time "Dr. Wonderful" will end up being the wrong fit. Work hard and you'll be 55% correct.
8. *Remove the wrong doctors quickly.* When you pick the wrong doctor to join your practice, make your mistake as quickly as possible and find a new home for your mismatched associate. In hindsight, most hires that don't work out are visibly wrong within the first 120 days.
9. *Oblige every owner to understand the business.* There was once a time when all you needed to know as a practice owner was the location of the key to the back office door. Not any longer, especially if you're in a complex group practice. Small errors in judgment or a lack of proper financial oversight can now balloon into a significant business killer. Rather than having just one or two doctors in a group understand the business, it's helpful to teach every owner—and every partner-track associate—the basics of business.

10. *Ensure that every owner has a personal financial plan.* In the typical five-doctor client practice it's almost certain that one of the partners is mismanaging their personal financial life. This is usually due to either a lack of spending or savings discipline, that is usually linked to the absence of a personal financial planner or involved accountant. If one of your partners is making poor personal money moves, this will adversely impact their judgment in the boardroom.
11. *If you need a second subspecialist, protect the first one.* Imagine you have one overworked retinal specialist in your group. You know you need a second subspecialist. But if you add Doctor #2, you're going to hurt #1's income for a year or more. What should you do? The easy and fair solution is to build a floor under Doctor #1's income, so that for a period of 12 to 36 months after hiring, #1's income is preserved at (let's say) 80% of their historic levels. Since ***everyone*** gains over time with the addition of a new doctor, it's only fair that ***everyone*** should take the same financial hit transiently.
12. *Control your practice's access to patients and share them fairly.* It's easy to control capacity—just hire a new worker or equip a new exam room. It's a lot more difficult to control the *volume* of the practice. Marketing, contracting, and customer service must work just right to bring you the correct mix and number of new patients. Meanwhile, make sure that the patients you do serve are shared fairly among all practice providers to preserve harmony.
13. *Let doctors do their own thing....to a point.* It's best to not unduly limit a provider's scope. For example, every appropriately trained surgeon should be able to perform cataract surgery or provide LASIK, rather than only allowing the senior doctors to get the "good" work. But don't be shy about requiring lower-quality surgeons, despite their abundant other attributes, to give up operating.
14. *Coach individual providers actively.* If you're the administrator or MP of a group practice, it's easy to focus so hard on the big picture that you forget that your practice is really composed of a lot of individual careers. These careers should each be coaxed along, at the same time that you're managing and coaching the entire team.
15. *Be clear about provider productivity expectations.* Most practice overhead is fixed. If partners or associates drop off in their productivity, practice overhead goes to waste and profitability can plummet. As part of their individual contracts with the practice, providers should have specific volume and revenue production expectations.
16. *Make the practice as profitable as possible.* As a wise old man once said, "If you think it's not about the money, then it's probably about the money." Money, as crass as it may sound, is a wonderful solvent for partner-to-partner squabbles. I've noted that partner discord is rising sharply just as profitability is declining in recent years. Do all that you reasonably can to optimize profits.
17. *Share practice profits fairly.* There is no perfect compensation methodology in a group practice. That said, you need to continuously adjust and fine tune the compensation model over time to at least assure that every partner is equally *unhappy* with the math.

18. *Treat partner-track associates well.* Many practices are set up to treat prepartner associates as second-class citizens. Instead, provide your partners-to-be with abundant access to performance data, a voice (if not yet a vote) in management, and a robust education in the intricacies of practice ownership.
19. *Hold plentiful group meetings between management and owners.* At least once a quarter—monthly is better—there should be a time when all of a practice's owners and all management staff gather to jointly identify and solve problems. Do not leave your administrator obliged to act as postmen, passing messages back and forth between the board and the managers.
20. *Play together outside of the office.* The happiest group practices are those owned by those who not only respect their partners as surgeons and clinicians, but who truly enjoy each other's company. If your practice is less "kumbaya" than you would like, try to engineer better relationships with an annual board retreat, quarterly partner social dinners, or sporting tickets shared around the group.

• • •

The Greek philosopher Plutarch wrote (2 millennia ago) that to understand and treat in medicine one has to first examine disease. In the same manner, to understand and nourish harmony in your group practice, it's important—even if occasionally unpleasant—to face up to areas where you and your colleagues are discordant.

CHAPTER 59

Tips for Running a More Effective Practice Retreat

John B. Pinto

The Portuguese have a lovely, melodic, aching word that even when spoken poorly with an English accent sounds exactly like it means on the streets of Lisbon. "Saudade" refers to a special kind of nostalgia for a past happiness that one perhaps never really possessed.

Saudade is as good a word as I can muster for the feelings of a vast number of eye surgeons today, who gaze wistfully and with no small measure of depression, at the past and feel that the best business years for their practices are behind them. They often look only at the fees they once received, instead of examining the balanced ledger of benefits present in modern practice and appreciating the happiness and success that can still be found.

Pinto JB. *Ophthalmic Leadership: A Practical Guide for Physicians, Administrators, and Teams, Second Edition* (pp 351-353).
© 2022 SLACK Incorporated.

Such surgeons need professional renewal. And one of the best, formal tools for business and professional renewal is a practice retreat.

What is a retreat? A retreat can be anything from a half day of private contemplation about the future of your career, to an orchestrated, moderated, week-long, all-hands event at a faraway destination resort. Most practices stake out the middle ground: 1 to 3 days, fairly close to home, held over a weekend to minimize lost production.

In my experience, more doctors and administrators consider and reject holding a practice retreat, than ever go forward with this valuable business tool. This happens for a number of reasons. Concerns about cost and time top the list. Indifference is a close second: If you're already burned out or confused about where you should take the practice, it's hard to muster the enthusiasm for a pow-wow. Some practices are not really sure if or how they should organize a retreat session. Small practices think that corporate retreats are only for the big dogs. Big practices think they've become too large and cumbersome to have retreat-style meetings, or they choke on the necessarily higher cost of getting 15 or 20 principles together for a multiday event.

Here are some helpful pearls gained from moderating a few hundred of these sessions through the years.

1. Who should attend? It all depends on the goals of the retreat and the openness of your practice. Increasingly, lay managers are being let into the board room to help the owners make decisions. So having a doctors/managers retreat is the most common approach. On the other hand, if the goal of the session is to refine a succession plan for two senior partners, the only participants at the retreat may be the administrator, a financial analyst, and the principals.
2. Although it requires more time and cost, it really does take 2 nights and 2½ days to foster the desired sense of being cloistered and part of a close group, especially when you are coming from behind in the area of team development. Four or 5 days are even better, but impractical in most cases.
3. The most common and workable format for a 3-day session is to start on a Friday evening with a social dinner followed by a couple of light, warm-up working hours. In the morning, start early, work through lunch on Saturday, and then adjourn at 1:30 PM or so to let everyone participate in one or more social or sports activities. Even if only half of the group enjoys golf, tennis, fishing or whatever your venue offers, there's lots of growth, education, and comic relief that emerges if you can pair "experts" and "amateurs" as teams for a little friendly competition. Hold another short business meeting after a purely social dinner on Saturday … and find a bit more time on Sunday morning, adjourning at noon on that last day. This format, with about 15 network hours over 2 leisurely days is a much more successful formula in my experience than burning the team out on a death march through 12-hour days.
4. It is certainly very helpful to take over a meeting facility, rather than being lost on a larger property. I've found that with enough advance planning you can rent an entire bed and breakfast property for a lot less cost and a lot more intimate environment than staying at a plastic 2500-room resort. We've also used everything from rustic doctor's vacation cabins, to swank, mid-town Chicago and Manhattan hotels. In the latter case, "group recreation" more often focuses on fine dining or a

night at the theater, than quail hunting from Jeeps or standing around a Georgia piney-woods bonfire smoking cigars and swilling genuine moonshine. (Both are true stories that will have to wait for a future memoir.)

5. You don't have to get on a plane to hold an effective retreat, although some boards treat themselves to an exotic destination every year. Often as not, there's a wonderful and unique setting within an hour's drive of your practice.
6. Try to build your retreat around a defined theme (eg, teamwork, profit enhancement, crisis resolution, or the development of a long-term strategic plan) and be sure to write out and review at the outset as a group exercise the specific goals of the session. Try to avoid the easy trap of saying, "Well, we've got a couple of days ... let's cram in everything."
7. If you have a mixed retreat of MDs and ODs—owners and nonowners and lay managers— and your intent is to not keep everyone together at all times, arrange formal breakout sessions so that during "work time," everyone is working. Try to avoid the embarrassment of having to announce, "We're going to talk about super-secret stuff now, so will all the nonowners please leave the room?"
8. Book the retreat well in advance so that every needed participant can arrange their personal affairs to be completely free. Every participant should stay for their full allotted time and should not have to be distracted by being on call if at all possible.
9. Depending on your preferences, I sometimes find that a doctors-plus-spouses retreat is a nice format. Not only can it increase the social cohesion of the group, but holding a brief joint session for 30 to 60 minutes toward the end of the proceedings, so the spouses can hear a synopsis of how the company is doing, is always appreciated. Obviously, this doesn't work very well if some of the spouses don't get along or if any of the partners are uncomfortable with this level of mixing it up.
10. During the retreat, assign one moderator or chairperson. This person isn't there to lecture or hog the proceedings, but to assure that the group stays on task, and that everyone gives their input. The choice of an internal moderator (eg, the practice administrator or MP) vs an outside facilitator is subject to commonsense judgment: Do you need outside expertise, or does your group have all the experts it needs in-house? Can you afford to bring in an outside facilitator? Will the facilitator actually "facilitate," or will the presence of an outsider inhibit open discussion?
11. If your retreat is effective, you'll not only be discussing topics, you'll be making dozens of decisions. Someone has to be responsible for taking notes and memorializing the agreed action. This scribe can be the moderator or a drafted participant for smaller meetings. For larger, more formal events, consider bringing a recording secretary. Avoid audio or video recording the session. This will inhibit open discussion and the free flow of opinion that is so vital in these meetings.
12. After the retreat be sure to distribute a written summary of the issues discussed and the decisions reached. Consider distributing a questionnaire to all participants while the retreat is still fresh in their minds: Did the event meet or exceed the stated goals? What was done well? What improvements should be made with future events? When and where should the next retreat be held?

CHAPTER 60

From Chaos to Order

Improving Practice Board Meetings

John B. Pinto

Every high school physics class, when the syllabus comes to the concept of "entropy," should be taken on a field trip to the nearest ophthalmology practice to observe a typical board meeting.

Dr. Where-Is-He? arrives 20 minutes late. Dr. Bored spends the entire time going though their mail and signing off charts. Dr. Gotta-Go leaves half-way through the proceedings to see a patient who could have been scheduled later. Dr. Eager Beaver introduces seven perfectly acceptable ideas, except that they have absolutely nothing to do with running a medical practice. The long-suffering administrator counts the minutes but dares not bring order to this random chaos for fear of being chastised.

Pinto JB. *Ophthalmic Leadership: A Practical Guide for Physicians, Administrators, and Teams, Second Edition* (pp 355-358).
© 2022 SLACK Incorporated.

It's been about 40 years since my last physics class, but I still get to go on the board room field trips regularly as a consultant to practices throughout the country. From these, I've abstracted a primer on how to conduct your practice's board meetings more effectively. Here's a 21-point list.

1. Advance preparation is key. Board members should receive a package of materials at least 3 days in the advance of the meeting and have clear instructions from the board chairperson on expectations. These expectations can be laid out in a cover letter describing the key theme of the meeting.
2. If you are the chair of your practice board, it's likely that you're either an administrator or the MP of the group—you're not the king of the world. All the same, both you and your board members should take the mantle of your office seriously. Do not be shy to set high expectations going into the meeting: "In the next week, I would like each of you to (a) talk to your techs about their feelings on the uniform changes, (b) read the chapter I distributed on budgeting, and (c) study last year's financial statements for at least three potential cost savings." You'll garner more respect if you are clear and reasonable in your requests, and if you thank board members abundantly for their efforts.
3. Set the tone for each meeting. If practice performance has been excellent, and it's time to celebrate, then introduce a little levity. Hand out personalized trophies to each board member or bring in a singing telegram. If you're in the midst of a real crisis, assert your leadership and start the meeting with a short speech outlining your optimism that the challenge will be overcome.
4. Work from a written agenda … and if you have the habit of running out of time at every meeting, set time limits for each item.
5. Although it should be obvious, make sure that in making up each board meeting agenda you are devoting prime time to priority topics. Put the most important matters at the top of the agenda.
6. If your group tends to ramble, a little spoon feeding may be in order. Prepare issue/decision sheets. These are simple, one-page documents where you have synopsized the open issue, the relevant facts, and either your firm recommendation (in the form of a formal motion) or a punch list of potential options.
7. You should insist on wide participation by all attendees, and not run the board meeting as a policy speech or classroom lesson. When you report on quarterly practice performance or progress with a project, go around the room asking for comments. When you reach an impasse, table the discussion for another time or send the issue to committee for their recommendations.
8. Despite any personal feelings or excitement in the heat of battle, respect the chair's authority to direct the discussion.
9. The chair must be fearless in defending his obligation and perogative—granted under the authority of the board—to direct the meeting. Any chair who finds himself not being respected by those in attendance at board meetings should wrest back control of the proceedings or offer their resignation.
10. Every board member should ideally be in attendance at every meeting, create a stiff fine system for those who miss more than two meetings in a row.

11. There should be no side-bar discussions; only one person speaks at a time, and only when acknowledged by the chair.
12. Once a vote is cast, the decision is final (subject of course to re-votes based on new information). It is highly destructive to the operational integrity of the practice for dissenting board members to subsequently turn to lay staff and in effect say, "Well, I know that's the new policy, but I'm not doing it." People who can't live with group decisions should not work in groups.
13. Remember your fiduciary responsibility as an owner … board members need to vote wisely for the betterment of the *practice,* not their personal interests.
14. As chair, know the patience and tolerance levels of your board members. Some members may be inexhaustible, and willing to sit through a 5-hour meeting. Others may fidget after 50 minutes. Take formal breaks and mid-meeting stretches to keep the blood flowing.
15. Make sure your room is chilly and ventilated enough to keep members alert. Serve caffeinated beverages and light snacks. Expect that sessions over a filling dinner will tend to be somewhat less effective (though great for periodic morale boosting).
16. Be disciplined. Start and end on time. Be intolerant of late arrivers, chronic interrupters, distracters, and early leave-takers.
17. If you have new participants, have nametags for everyone.
18. Bring middle managers and line staff in to report periodically on issues in their area.
19. One of the biggest errors I see at client board meetings is this: Doctors will bring up an important issue, discuss it robustly—but probably for longer than is necessary—and then the conversation trails off without any resolution. Remember that it is the chair's job to open, direct the flow of discussion, and drive toward resolution with each item on the agenda. Consider this stepwise process to help you get closure on each issue raised:
    a. *Framing:* The person introducing the subject should frame it up in a simple sentence or two: "Our lease rates in the Morristown office are scheduled to rise sharply. We have an opportunity to accept this, lease alternate space, or consider building a new office."
    b. *Facts:* Present the facts and data related to the issue … this might include a timeline, budget figures, contingencies, legal impediments, etc.
    c. *Comments and discussion:* Allow time for comment around the table, but do not allow this to go on indefinitely or for the discussion points to get off-track from the core issue.
    d. *Make a motion, table the item for the next meeting, or send to committee:* One of the more important arts of chairpersonship is that you firmly move your board members from discussion to resolution. This shifting of gears can come from you as a directive or as a question: "Does anyone else here think we should send this difficult issue out to a committee of staff members so they can come back with a possible solution?"

e. *Second:* If a motion has been made (eg, "I move that we direct Carla to get bids to change the décor of the Waterville office"), ask for a second. This saves time and inhibits renegade board members who might otherwise float items that others are really not interested in.
f. *Secondary discussion:* Once a motion has been made and seconded, allow a few minutes for subsequent discussion … "I agree that the Evanstown needs to be freshened up, but I don't think we need an expensive makeover … I think all we have to do is lay down new carpet and paint the waiting room."
g. *Motion refinement:* This secondary discussion will often lead to improvements in the original proposal. Make sure you are creating an "accountable motion," that is, designating an action item where completion can be measured. "We will try to reduce no-show rates," is not an accountable motion. "We will put Barbara in charge of a program to reduce our current 10% no-show rates to industry standards of 5% or less," is accountable.
h. *Vote:* Most votes in a practice setting are held openly. With some especially difficult decisions, it can be useful to have a secret ballot. Know and follow your practice's established rules for balloting, quorums, proxies, majority voting, and super-majority requirements. It can sometimes be helpful, if you're stuck on an issue or only half way through an elaborate matter, to hold a straw poll … "As an indication of interest only, who here by a show of hands would like to omit the last three items from today's agenda so we can devote more time to the matter at hand?"
i. *Assign:* Once a binding vote has been made, make sure the minutes reflect ***who*** is responsible for the action item and ***when*** the item is due.

20. If you must run over, do so with the open acceptance of the group. Thirty minutes before the scheduled end of the session, say, "It's clear that this important topic could take us into overtime this morning. Is everyone ok with staying an extra 15 minutes so we can get closure on adding the new doctor?"
21. Invite feedback on your performance as board chairperson. This can be sought formally through questionnaires or informally in the lounge: "Mike, what do you think I should do to keep the meetings flowing better?" Some effective chairmen will close each meeting with a rapid-fire roundtable question: "What could we have done to make this an even better meeting?"

CHAPTER 61

The Neanderthal Doctor

Habits to Lose on Your Way to a Better Practice

John B. Pinto

According to a *New York Times* report, scientists have found genetic evidence that may explain the boorish behavior of a thankfully small minority of eye doctors. It seems that until about 30,000 years ago, our Homo Sapiens ancestors interbred with our more brutish genetic cousins, the Neanderthals. Perhaps a few of their less desirable ancestral traits are embedded within a few of us to this day.

Of course, every eye surgeon has those occasional tough days when you can easily get in touch with your inner cave man or cave woman. This is perfectly understandable when the new ASC staff is all thumbs, or the billing department reports a longstanding "oopsie" in collecting your old accounts. But such days should be the exception.

Pinto JB. *Ophthalmic Leadership: A Practical Guide for Physicians, Administrators, and Teams, Second Edition* (pp 359-362).
© 2022 SLACK Incorporated.

After more than 40 years consulting with a wide array of clinicians and medical research specialists, I can report from the field that ophthalmologists are happily among the best of the breed when it comes to behavior on the job. However, there are those few surgeons I've met through the years whose behaviors and personality quirks can only be attributed to an overactive Neanderthal gene kicking up.

Chances are good that you have run into one or more of these doctors in your career as a surgeon or as an ophthalmic administrator. Perhaps you can recognize a hint of some of these behaviors in yourself. Let's explore the most common varieties of loutishness, along with tips to cultivate a more genteel and better-bred personality.

The Fault-Finding "Dr. Gotcha"

This is the most common caveman holdover in my experience. Eye surgeons, like every learned professional, are selected and trained in our society to be hypercritical, to find faults and fix them. Few patients would prefer their doctors to be relaxed and casual in the face of serious disease. We like our doctors to be intense, precise, standard-setting, and intolerant of error. But what makes for an especially great ophthalmologist can also make for an insufferable human being to work around.

Here are a few practical ideas for cultivating the opposite behavior if this is a problem for you or someone you work with.

The key is simply this: Wake up and stop being critical, which at this point is probably a completely unconscious behavior. For example, in a situation where you would usually be critical of a technician's performance, reference their otherwise great work and hold this up as your expected standard. "Becky, you are ordinarily the very best of our staff when it comes to taking histories ... but you seemed to be in a rush with Mr. Jones. Could you please get back to being 'perfect' for us?" (For more on this, read the excellent book on developing positive supervision skills, *Whale Done,* by Blanchard.)

Hand out sincere compliments. If this is hard for you to remember, keep a written list of every coworker (lay and doctor) in your pocket. Make it a game to not get through the work week without checking off every name after having provided some kind of positive reinforcement or compliment.

Enlist a trusted member of your staff to provide feedback on how you're doing. This may be a long-time tech or a manager who knows you well. Tell them you are working on being more positive and less negative, and sit down with them briefly every week for frank feedback.

The Pot-Stirring "Dr. Can You Believe It?!?"

This is a behavior related to the "gotcha" doctor. For the pot-stirring doctor, disaster is always around the corner—and he wants you to know about it. "Just you wait. That new marketing program is going to be a bust." "The new fee cuts are going to put us out of business." "Andrea is never going to learn her job." "EMR is not going to work in our practice." Enough of this, and even the most positive staff members will begin to see the world—and their careers—in a pretty gray light.

How to solve this? Again, it's a matter of consciousness. The pot-stirring doctor is probably unaware of their behavior—or at least unaware of the damage they cause to group morale. Someone influential in the practice, typically the administrator or MP, must take the offending doctor aside. In my experience, when sufficient seriousness is applied during the intervention, such doctors are surprised that they are affecting morale and are quite willing to change. In tough cases, an intervention by the full board is appropriate.

Make sure you have one or more other owners providing a balancing influence to the negative partner. Over time, lay staff will begin to tune out the pot-stirring partner. In the most extreme cases, the board may need to censure or even remove the offending doctor, even if they are otherwise highly productive.

The Board-Ignoring "Dr. My Way"

Surgeons love control, and being controlling serves them well in the OR and clinic. But the business of medicine obliges compromise and collaboration—and not a lot of personal control, ultimately, unless you practice alone as a soloist. In group practices you come together as a board of owners, set policies, vote on tactics, and then leave the board room. That's when the real work and maturity begins as an owner, because even when the majority vote goes against you, you have to publicly support the board's decision.

MPs and practice presidents should be empowered to take care of this problem, which is especially common in smaller (or newer) groups where behavioral boundaries have not yet been established formally. As practices grow and encounter new, scale-related problems, it's important to set down formal rules and consequences. I commonly drop into larger practices with $10 million and more in annual revenue that, despite their size, only have a few soft behavioral guidelines and no material consequences for unruly doctors.

You can also short-circuit the damage of "Dr. My Way" by following up major board policy votes with a memo to all hands in the practice affirming the group's decision.

The Finger-Pointing "Dr. Defensive" Who Says, "It's Not Me!"

It's hard to work around people who are incapable of accepting constructive criticism. Play back in your mind your response the last few times that patients, staff, colleagues—or for that matter a member of your own family—was critical of you in some way. It's a mark of both your inner security and your maturity if you typically respond by listening actively (instead of framing a defensive comment), accepting the comment at face value, and exploring the criticism in detail.

By being defensive in the past, it's likely that the people you work with are now inhibited in telling you about your issues. If that's the case, go to your coworkers, acknowledge your defensiveness, and ask for their feedback on how you can improve. Your confession, alone, can erase years of perceived affront.

The Patient-Hostile "Dr. Meanie"

This trait is rarely revealed early in an eye surgeon's career, but rather comes forth in middle age in those surgeons who no longer have the energy or internal control to hold in an underlying dislike for patients that has probably always existed to some degree. Doctors who are even a little mean to patients are often even more unpleasant with support staff, friends, and family members. And they can be very hard on themselves.

Most practices are able to avoid hiring unhappy young doctors who don't really like working with patients. It's more common to observe a self-controlled doctor whose ingrained dislike for people is only coming forward and being unmasked in mid-career. We all seem to become more like ourselves as we age, and mean people tend to get meaner over time. Boards facing a difficult member of their professional staff are well-advised to intervene early and vigorously in such cases.

These behaviors and personality traits are obviously compounded in some individuals—the doctor who is both pot-stirring *and* defensive, or both mean *and* a poor team member. It takes a saintly and impracticably rare array of traits and talents to be Dr. Perfect. But with a bit of energy and openness to feedback, you can effectivly suppress the most debilitating of your latent Neanderthal genes.

CHAPTER 62

Leading Your Team Past the Inevitable Conflicts of Practice Life

John B. Pinto

Whenever you're in conflict with someone, there is one factor that can make the difference between damaging your relationship and deepening it. That factor is attitude.
—William James

Courage is what it takes to stand up and speak. Courage is also what it takes to sit down and listen.
—Winston Churchill

When leading others, even in the most genteel of practices, two simple truths apply that you need to master. First, conflicts will always occur, even among the kindest, best-intentioned individuals in a work group. And second, the excellence of your leadership is not measured by how few conflicts arise on your watch, but by how quickly and effectively these conflicts are reduced and resolved … by *you.*

Practice conflicts have always been prominent when leading in this people-intensive arena. These conflicts issue from a host of innate personalities found in those who gravitate to medicine. The adverse behaviors flowing from these personalities are now being magnified in an environment of progressively tighter finances and sharply clearer threats to business survival.

Pinto JB. *Ophthalmic Leadership: A Practical Guide for Physicians, Administrators, and Teams, Second Edition* (pp 363-366).
© 2022 SLACK Incorporated.

However, in most clinic settings, conflict is not diffuse and generalized. We can often point to one "PITA" who is an enduring wellspring of conflict. I'm not referring to the Mediterranean flat bread here, but the acronym for a "Pain In The Rump." It's likely that some one person in your practice is your major annoyance and distraction to your leadership responsibilities. This can be a provider, a lay staff member, or increasingly, if you work in a health system or multispecialty clinic, an institutional colleague or overseer.

We are all periodically a PITA, even the angels among us. Durable PITAs are the greater challenge. The adverse impact of workplace PITAs is magnified by leaders who fail to lay down strong rules, or have allowed settings where roles are unclear and there are unintended signals sent to your office PITA that it's OK to buck authority and make others miserable.

In the same way that parents are responsible for calming family conflicts issuing from their children, it is the responsibility of the more senior practice leaders—owners and managers—to resolve conflicts occurring at lower levels. Just as an effective physician reveals a disease and applies the appropriate treatment briskly, the effective practice leader finds and fixes conflict without delay. Everyone involved in a conflict needs to be called into the room at the earliest possible moment. But unlike disease managers, business managers can be conflict avoidant and uncertain about how to start the discussion.

In heated settings it can help to draw a conflict diagram to stimulate a group dialog and to better understand who "owns" a conflict. Write down the involved parties—this may be a cohort of doctors or the members of a single department. Array the names at the corners of a triangle (for three people), the corners of a square (for four people), and so forth. Then draw lines between each party and label each line based on your loosely judged objective paired scores for their present level of conflict between each person on a "1" (low) to "10" (high) level.

In the simple diagram shown below, Dave, Mike and Mary are three eye surgeons, partners in their group practice. Mike and Mary have a very low level of conflict—a "2" as marked on the diagram. Dave and Mike have a high level of conflict, at an "8." Dave and Mary have an even stronger level of conflict, a "9."

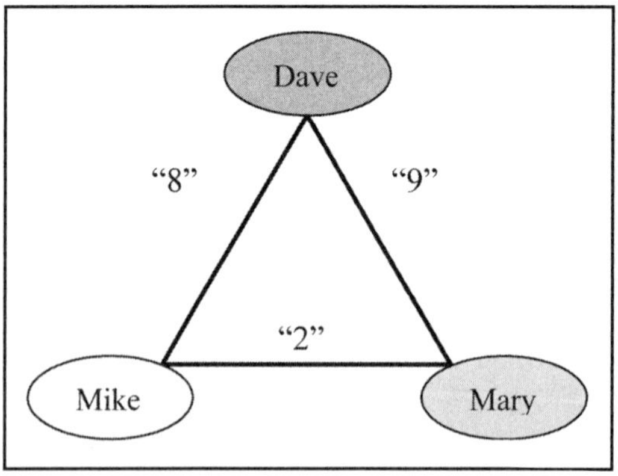

It's a good hunch in this setting that Dave could be the source of the conflict. A diagram like this is especially useful when you have more than three parties and are trying to communicate with your practice's PITA why you believe that they could be chiefly responsible for the difficulty.

• • •

Here are a few insights on conflict resolution abstracted from the writings by Richard Darlington, an eclectic British-Italian trade union negotiator … framed in an ophthalmic context (http://www.rogerdarlington.co.uk/conflict.html).

1. *Be calm.* Conflict usually engenders strong emotions, even anger; but in such a state you are unlikely to be rational or in the mood for compromise. If two conflicting doctors are highly charged emotionally, take a time out and return to resolution efforts at another time.
2. *Show respect.* However much you disagree with a staff member or provider, try to attack the argument not the person. This approach can break down when dealing with individuals who are themselves disrespectful of the discussion process. In such situations, group pressure or removal of the offending party from a group discussion are the common resorts used by effective leaders.
3. *Be magnanimous.* In truth, most conflict is over matters of little substance and often it is mostly pride or status that is at stake. Consider conceding the point to your opponent, just as an effective martial arts practitioner steps aside rather than absorb a blow.
4. *Discuss or debate.* So often, conflict is created or maintained because there is no real discussion or debate. We make assumptions about the other person's point of view and willingness to compromise that might be quite wrong. In addition to discussing an issue verbally, diagram it on a white board or yellow pad.
5. *Be rational.* Much conflict is not about substance but perception. Try to clear through the perception to discover and agree on how things really are. Ophthalmology is a fact-laden enterprise … the management of an ophthalmic practice should be similarly factual and rational. Use benchmarks, industry standards, and the documentation of the best demonstrated practices to agree on what's true, before trying to hammer out disagreements.
6. *Acknowledge emotions.* Facts alone, however rational, cannot resolve much conflict because how people perceive those facts is colored by their emotions. It's no good denying those emotions, so make an effort to see the situation the way the other person does and to acknowledge their emotions before endeavoring to move beyond them. Use phrases such as *"Please allow me to explain why this is so important to me."*
7. *Change the wording.* It's amazing how often we disagree about words and how a change of words can change how people view a situation. Instead of criticizing a young associate for his low surgical volumes, invite him to set future growth goals backed up by new outreach efforts.

8. *Change the environment.* It's no coincidence that some of the toughest political negotiations of all times, for instance those aimed at Middle East peace, often take place in locations like the Camp David presidential retreat. Don't hold tough board meetings in the staff lounge. Reserve a private dining room at everyone's favorite restaurant or borrow your attorney's board room.
9. *Consider sequencing.* Much conflict is created and aggravated by lack of trust. Building trust takes time and proof of goodwill. Consider introducing an agreement in stages with progression toward the ultimate goal.
10. *Seek mediation.* This is a process whereby a neutral third party consults with those involved in a conflict to see if the problem can be presented in a way that facilitates a resolution. The mediator may simply listen and ask questions, or he may suggest other ways of looking at the problem or possible solutions.
11. *If absolutely necessary, apply your authority.* Conflict can sometimes only be resolved by one party imposing their authority as the administrator or MP. Such a "settlement" will cause resentment in the party at the receiving end, but sometimes this is the only way to resolve a conflict and move on.
12. *If all else fails, wait.* Most problems change over time. Either the problem solves itself because circumstances change, or one's attitude about the problem changes as the heat dies down and other practice matters assume more prominence.

APPENDIX A

Administrator/Practice Manager Score Card

Here's a self-test you can take to measure selected aspects of your management ability. This list of attributes is by no means complete, and no manager could be expected to have high scores on all of these attributes.

Score each item on this 20-point list based on the following scale:

5 = I have a very large measure of this attribute, no more is needed for success.

4 = I have nearly enough of this attribute, but could use just a little more.

3 = I barely have enough of this attribute to get along effectively as a manager.

2 = I have a little less of this attribute than I feel I need and should work on this area.

1 = I profoundly lack this attribute.

Pinto JB. *Ophthalmic Leadership: A Practical Guide for Physicians, Administrators, and Teams, Second Edition* (pp 367-368).
© 2022 SLACK Incorporated.

____ 1. *Direct job knowledge.* I could step in and perform the work that I supervise.
____ 2. *Delegation.* I'm good at knowing when and who to go to with a project.
____ 3. *Action oriented.* I plow through my tasks and don't procrastinate.
____ 4. *Grace under pressure.* I am able to be calm and clear in the face of confusion.
____ 5. *Accountability.* I complete on time the jobs I promise on behalf of my department.
____ 6. *Communication.* I am a better than average communicator, I listen especially well.
____ 7. *Discipline.* I work every day to uphold the operational standards of the practice.
____ 8. *Tough love.* When it's called for, I am tough with the people I manage.
____ 9. *Fairness.* I am inordinately tough, but combine this with being extremely fair.
____ 10. *Openness.* I am open to new ideas from my people, and encourage their suggestions.
____ 11. *Forgiveness.* I never hold a grudge with my staff for an error they make.
____ 12. *Adaptability.* I love change and embrace every opportunity to alter our protocols to improve.
____ 13. *Organization.* I am able to work well with lots of loose projects in the air at the same time.
____ 14. *Guardianship.* I see myself as a protector of the organization, the patients, the staff, and the doctors.
____ 15. *Mentoring.* I have lots of patience and a real knack for passing along my knowledge.
____ 16. *Team playing.* I balance being a leader of my own departmental team, with being a member myself of our larger team called the "practice."
____ 17. *Sacrifice.* I am open to early and late hours, open to criticism, and open to the adverse consequences of making the occasional poor management decision.
____ 18. *Maturity and respect.* I publicly respect the decisions of the doctors and administrator, even when I may privately disagree.
____ 19. *Humility.* I readily admit my mistakes and work to correct them.
____ 20. *Personal energy reserves.* I consistently have abundant energy to get me through the week.

Total Score: ________

Add up your score. With 20 different attributes, and with up to five points each, there's a maximum score of 100. There is no objective scale that compares you to others, but this summary score can be a valuable personal baseline of your "fitness," and can help point out areas to improve.

APPENDIX B

Physician Leadership Score Card

Here's a self-test you can take to measure selected aspects of your leadership ability. This list of attributes is by no means complete, and no physician-leader under the rank of "saint" could be expected to have high scores on all of these attributes.

Score each item on this 50-point list based on the following scale:

5 = I have a very large measure of this attribute, no more is needed for success.

4 = I have nearly enough of this attribute, but could use just a little more.

3 = I barely have enough of this attribute to get along effectively as a leader.

2 = I have a little less of this attribute than I feel I need and should work on this area.

1 = I profoundly lack this attribute.

Pinto JB. *Ophthalmic Leadership: A Practical Guide for Physicians, Administrators, and Teams, Second Edition* (pp 369-372).
© 2022 SLACK Incorporated.

_____ 1. I am disciplined. I complete on time the duties and projects I promise my staff, patients, and family.

_____ 2. I don't procrastinate. I push ahead and get even the more unpleasant things done.

_____ 3. I am a better than average communicator. I listen especially well.

_____ 4. I am inordinately tough, but combine this with being extremely fair.

_____ 5. I am open to new ideas from my people and encourage their suggestions.

_____ 6. I never hold a grudge with my staff for an error they make … I get over it, and life goes on.

_____ 7. I love change and embrace every opportunity to alter our protocols to improve.

_____ 8. I have the focus to be able to work well with lots of loose projects in the air at the same time.

_____ 9. I see myself as a protector of the organization, the patients, the staff, and the doctors.

_____ 10. People are attracted to work with me because I am much more often a giver than a taker.

_____ 11. I am a great mentor. I have lots of patience and a real knack for passing along my knowledge.

_____ 12. I am a team player. I balance being a leader with being a member myself of our larger team called the "practice." As such, when appropriate, I subordinate my needs to the needs of the team.

_____ 13. I know when it's time to lead by gentle consensus, and when it's better to put my foot down and simply be directive.

_____ 14. I readily admit my mistakes to others and I work to correct them.

_____ 15. I consistently have abundant energy, more than enough to get me through the week.

_____ 16. When we get stuck on making a decision, I am good at getting us back on track.

_____ 17. Knowing that medicine is extremely stressful, I monitor my moods and affect closely and am excellent at knowing when I need to apply stress management tactics.

_____ 18. I am good at setting myself to reasonable workloads and delegate or defer everything else.

_____ 19. I have written down a manageable list of measurable, core goals for our practice and reinforce these often with all staff.

_____ 20. I avoid "mission drift" … don't pile on new, conflicting goals. And I avoid adding new goals until we've accomplished or formally abandoned old ones.

_____ 21. I work hard to gather the facts, and I let these *facts manage the practice.*

_____ 22. I review financial trend reports and volume performance graphs at least monthly.

_____ 23. I keep a close eye on what is happening in our regional market and what my colleagues and competitors are doing.

_____ 24. I avoid personal conflicts of interest and lead for the benefit of everyone in the practice.

_____ 25. I am more than a figurehead leader. I am realistic about the time it takes to do the job right, and I put real time resources into this part of my job as a clinic owner.

_____ 26. To avoid misunderstandings at home about the demands of my work duties, I have secured my spouse's durable acquiescence to my demanding professional life.

_____ 27. In meetings, I speak little and listen much.

_____ 28. I rarely vacillate or change my mind, but when I do, I explain my reasoning clearly to others.

_____ 29. When I anticipate any resistance to a new idea or initiative, I touch base with senior staff individually before I ever bring things up at a group meeting.

_____ 30. I can answer at least the following questions about each of the doctors I manage:

a. Where they went to school and trained
b. The names of their spouse and children
c. Where their clinical interests lie
d. What their financial and volume performance goals are for this year

_____ 31. I can answer the following questions about the senior managers of our practice:

a. The names of their spouse and children
b. Where their future career interests lie
c. What their greatest strengths and weaknesses are

_____ 32. I know every one of our staff members by name, and I know their position in our practice.

_____ 33. I never break confidences. When told something privately, I don't divulge my sources, even indirectly.

_____ 34. I don't make promises unless I know I can keep them.

_____ 35. I know from experience that it's better to promise a "6" and deliver an "8" than the other way around.

_____ 36. I struggle daily to be the most informed person in our practice … on many days I succeed.

_____ 37. I am not afraid to motivate doctors and managers with an occasional sense of crisis. I use industry news, community gossip, and adverse financial trends to break through staff and doctor lassitude.

_____ 38. I have created a strong advisory board. The practice's consultants, attorneys, accountants, and bankers co-report to me and the administrator when appropriate.

_____ 39. I trust my guts. I only make really important decisions after a few minutes of quiet reflection on the simple question: "Is this the right course?"

_____ 40. I am humble. I consistently remember that "wins" belong to the team, while "losses" are mine alone.

_____ 41. People know there is no job I would be unwilling to roll up my sleeves and do in this practice.

_____ 42. People around here have ample evidence that I enjoy my work. Even on the days I'm not enjoying, I keep up a brave face.

_____ 43. I walk the talk. When I'm preaching practice cost containment, I simultaneously forego family expenditures. If productivity is lagging, I am the first doctor who schedules extra patients in a day ... and then arrives an hour early to see them.

_____ 44. I never use my disproportionately great position and resources to bully others.

_____ 45. When I have to reprimand or terminate someone, I strive to preserve their dignity.

_____ 46. I arrive in the office earlier than is necessary for patient care to give myself time to touch base.

_____ 47. I meet at least weekly with our administrator, even if briefly, and formally review progress. I allow these meetings to take up as much time as my administrator reasonably needs to cover the company's business.

_____ 48. I meet at least quarterly (and individually) with each doctor in our practice ... I know the specifics of where they want to head in their careers ... and they know that I know.

_____ 49. I have real empathy for the feelings of other people.

_____ 50. I tell the truth, even when honesty results in temporarily hurt feelings.

Total Score:__________

Add up your score. With 50 different attributes, and with up to five points each, there's a maximum score of 250. There is no objective scale that compares you to others, but this summary score can be a valuable personal baseline of your "fitness" to lead and can help point out areas to improve. Consider focusing on two or three selected items at a time for improvement.

APPENDIX C

Measuring Your Practice's Level of Teamwork

Every practice agrees with the concept that taking a team approach is a core requirement for providing great patient care. Most administrators work very hard in a day-to-day task sense to foster teamwork. But very few practice teams call a time out in the game to agree on just what constitutes superior teamwork and to nail down missing elements.

Pinto JB. *Ophthalmic Leadership: A Practical Guide for Physicians, Administrators, and Teams, Second Edition* (pp 373-377).
© 2022 SLACK Incorporated.

Part One

Here's a self-assessment you can hand out individually or even complete as a group exercise to measure selected aspects of your group's teamwork. This list of attributes of great teamwork is by no means complete, and no practice could be expected to have high scores in all of these areas.

Score each item on this 40-point list based on the following scale:

5 = I strongly agree with this statement.

4 = I agree with this statement.

3 = I am neutral ... I neither agree nor disagree with this statement.

2 = I disagree with this statement.

1 = I strongly disagree with this statement.

____ 1. Everyone on our practice team understands the historical context of our organization and where we've come from.

____ 2. We have a written plan so everyone knows where we are heading in the future; group goals are clear.

____ 3. We understand the rules of the game and how to keep score. We play to win, and celebrate our wins, both large and small.

____ 4. We communicate well with each other, and we are especially good at listening.

____ 5. We all understand the roles ("positions") that everyone plays on the team.

____ 6. As "players" on the same team, we show respect and appreciation for each other, up and down the ranks.

____ 7. Managers in our practice personally demonstrate good teamwork to the rest of the team.

____ 8. The doctors personally demonstrate good teamwork to the rest of the team.

____ 9. We have fun and enjoy playing "the game" together as a group.

____ 10. We reward staff at every level for their ideas, performance, skills, motivation of others, flexibility, willingness to trying and risk failure, sharing, small improvement, etc.

____ 11. We set standards and expectations for teamwork that are appropriate ... with especially high standards for senior lay staff and partner doctors.

____ 12. We are constantly developing a better group understanding of what the customer wants ... and making service improvements in this context.

____ 13. We hold a common mission to serve and delight all of the fans in the stands: patients and their family members, payers, referring docs, employees and their dependent family members, etc.

____ 14. We organize enough social interaction among the lay staff and doctors to develop great relationships with each other.

_____ 15. We educate ***everyone*** on the basics of ***every*** job, not only so we'll be able to cross-cover job functions, but so that we can have greater empathy for our colleagues' work environment

_____ 16. We have developed specific performance expectations and standards, and hold each other to these; we have created an environment where we each feel accountable to the team.

_____ 17. We understand the minimum standards of customer service, and work to exceed these.

_____ 18. We have boosted our investment in information technology to improve communication and productivity, and to reduce the frustration that comes with using outdated tools.

_____ 19. Each member of the team is open to the input and reciprocal coaching of their colleagues. Our doctors are open to receiving and following through on the coaching efforts of their managers. Our managers are open to receiving and following the coaching efforts of the doctors.

_____ 20. We have a "playbook" (eg, personnel manual, operations manual, care pathways).

_____ 21. We get the team "psyched up," and elevate every teammate's reasonable expectations and enthusiasm about winning.

_____ 22. To watch us in action for 30 minutes, you would think we look more like a synchronized group than a collection of individuals running off in different directions.

_____ 23. We maintain a tempo that everyone can reasonably keep up with.

_____ 24. We seek a steady increase in both the individual and the combined talents of the team; we work hard to improve weak links and give them a fair chance to improve.

_____ 25. We deal with each other with empathy; we don't make fun of weak links in the team, but help them.

_____ 26. When a weak link on the team can't be improved, we are not hesitant to remove them.

_____ 27. We don't withhold difficult information or "triangulate" (ie, when Mike complains to Ann about Mary).

_____ 28. We support decisive leadership and insist that our leaders lead.

_____ 29. We foster effective and appropriate "followership," the ability of team members to rally around the leader, and respect their position always, even if from time to time we harbor concerns about the individual leader involved.

_____ 30. We are time-sensitive, and do not dawdle once a course of action has been ordered.

_____ 31. We sacrifice for, and compromise with, each other.

_____ 32. We remember there is no "I" in "TEAM" and that "TEAM" stands for "Together Everyone Achieves More."

_____ 33. We each take responsibility … others can count on us.

_____ 34. We balance authority with responsibility and give our managers the authority they need to carry out their duties.

_____ 35. We take in all viewpoints and don't discount even the most outlandish ideas.

_____ 36. We are energetic and have great stamina.

_____ 37. We make everyone on the team feels important.

_____ 38. We play carefully, to avoid harming ourselves, others, or the company.

_____ 39. When any of us get our feelings hurt, we work through it and still stay in the game; we do not withdraw or quit playing.

_____ 40. Everyone plays ... nobody sits on the bench for very long.

Total Score:__________

Add up your score. With 40 different attributes, and with up to five points each, there's a maximum score of 200. There is no objective scale that compares you to others, but this summary score can be a valuable internal baseline of your teamwork and can help point out areas to improve. It might be interesting to repeat this scoring instrument again in a year.

Part Two

In addition to specific attributes of teamwork that you've measured above, it might be interesting to know what you think the level of teamwork that's going on in various segments of the practice.

On a scale of 1 to 10, with 1 being low and 10 being high, rate the following:

1. I feel that ***my*** personal level of teamwork is _____.
2. The current level of teamwork for the ***doctors*** is _____.
3. The current level of teamwork in the ***technical department*** is_____.
4. The current level of teamwork in the ***reception/patient accounts department*** is _____.
5. The current level of teamwork in the ***optical*** department is _____.
6. The current level of teamwork in the ***surgery*** center is _____.
7. The current level of teamwork in the ***marketing*** department is _____.
8. The current level of teamwork for our ***overall*** practice is _____ and I believe we should be striving for an ***overall*** practice teamwork level of_____.

What do you observe from this second part of the self-assessment? Which areas of the practice have higher or lower levels of teamwork? Do you think it's easier to improve overall teamwork when doctor teamwork is high, but teamwork in other areas is faltering ... or the reverse, when the lay staff are great at teamwork, but doctor teamwork is poor?

Part Three

As a final—ideally group—exercise, select two or three weak aspects of your practice's teamwork that are suggested by your responses to the questions in this appendix. For each of these weak areas, write down specific goals and tactics to achieve them.

Here's an example:

> No one on our team except the administrator and our partner doctors understand how we're doing as a practice. These "insiders" get the financial and volume performance data, but everyone else on the team has to guess if it's been a good or poor quarter compared to last year. To improve this, we're going to prepare a quarterly score card for the practice, containing five key benchmarks for this year vs last. These benchmarks will be: total patient visits, total surgical cases, a lay staff efficiency ratio consisting of total payroll hours divided by total patient visits, a doctor efficiency ratio consisting of patient visits per clinic hour worked, and the percentile increase or decrease in our collections. We will share this score card with every member of our staff at our quarterly all-hands meetings. Whenever our quarterly score card shows progress, we'll think up some creative way to celebrate our improvement as a group.

APPENDIX D

Does Your Practice Have "Supervisory Deficit Syndrome"?

Eye surgeons, being famously independent by nature, rarely project on themselves (much less the rest of their work world) the need for appropriate levels of supervision. As a result, chances are your practice may look more like it's being run by a substitute teacher than a drill sergeant. Most surgeons, although they would prefer the latter, disciplined approach, typically ask, *"Can't we simply hire the right people around here, so they can do their jobs with little or no supervision?"*

This statement belies the false but keen hope that people don't have to be confronted and challenged to do their very best. The truth is that we all do our best job with a degree of supervision and oversight—even eye surgeons with the best work habits and ability to self-supervise.

Pinto JB. *Ophthalmic Leadership: A Practical Guide for Physicians, Administrators, and Teams, Second Edition* (pp 379-383).
© 2022 SLACK Incorporated.

Quiz

How would you describe oversight and supervision in your own practice? Drum tight or a bit loose? Here's a quick and easy quiz to determine where you and your supervisors set the bar for the rest of the team. When you've finished and added up your score, I hope you'll have new insights about the supervisory tone you set. Obviously, it's more important to use insights from this little test to stimulate a conversation in your practice, than to feel great or miserable about the objective score you achieve.

Direct Job Knowledge

One of the most important attributes of a great overseer is that they know how to do—and do well—the task or job they are supervising. (That's why it's so galling when doctors have their treatment protocols called into question by a third-party payer's review nurse, instead of a fellow physician in the same specialty.) Which one of these three choices best describes the supervisors in your practice?

____ 1. Our supervisors could seamlessly step into any of the job functions that they supervise and do the job as well or better than any staff member. ***(5 points)***

____ 2. Most of our supervisors know at least a little bit about the jobs they oversee and could do them if forced to, but not all that well. ***(3 points)***

____ 3. None of our supervisors could do the tasks they oversee ... they are new to the job or have never taken the time to learn the specific skills they supervise. ***(1 point)***

Written Operational Controls

Even the smallest practice is a vastly complex and changing business "engine." Some few practices have written down a comprehensive "owner's manual," but most still operate based on a verbal culture, relying on the collective memories and experiences of the existing staff. When one staff member leaves, so does their institutional memory for how to get things done. Which of these fit for you?

____ 1. We have essentially blueprinted operations here. We've broken down every practice position into dozens of specific tasks (ie, "refracting" or "submitting Medicare claims") and there's a written guideline for every task. We revise these documents often to make sure they're still the best approach to every segment of operations. Anyone can suggest a new "best" way to do something. In addition, for each department of the practice we have daily and weekly checklists that help remind us to take care of all the details. ***(5 points)***

____ 2. We have some outdated position descriptions written down and a few old, written protocols are in the files, but we really don't take a disciplined approach to operations documentation. As a result, our supervisors tell us what they *feel* we should do, rather than what everyone *knows* to be the best, institutional approach. ***(3 points)***

_____ 3. We take a seat of the pants approach here, with little if anything handled in writing. As a result, staff training and subsequent supervision is hit-and-miss. We're constantly discovering that once- agreed protocols have been dropped or changed without any management oversight. ***(1 point)***

Communication

World-class practices take communication seriously, putting liberal resources into formal meetings, impromptu brainstorming sessions, and abundant bulletins. Which choice here best fits your practice?

_____ 1. In our practice we strike a nice balance between written and verbal communication, and between too many and too few meetings. We meet together for an upbeat, all-hands group session at least every month or 2, and we take enough time so that everyone has a turn to contribute. Each department meets at least every few weeks for training and problem solving. Between meetings, we get lots of memos and procedure updates. Everyone feels they have an open channel here, not only to their direct supervisors, but—if necessary—all the way up the chain of command. Everyone knows our practice's basic plans for the future. ***(5 points)***

_____ 2. We hold large and small staff meetings a few times a year, but only when a big problem comes up or the doctors feel they have something they need to announce. We also get a few memos each year about office policies. The rest of the time we're pretty much kept in the dark. ***(3 points)***

_____ 3. We only find out what's happening in our practice through the grapevine ... if that. There are no open forums here to discuss prospective policy changes or to even find out about new policies. ***(1 point)***

New Staff Selection and Orientation

Great supervisors put their greatest talents to work in recruiting and selecting new staff members ... they know that if they get that part of their job right, subsequent training and supervision will be far easier. Which of these is the best description of your practice?

_____ 1. Because we promote our jobs widely and enjoy a reputation as a great place to work, we always have a large pool of applicants for every new job posting. This increases our odds of finding people who not only have the energy and talent to do the job, but who will fit in with our philosophy of patient care. For most hires, everyone in the practice gets to interview the final candidates. Not only is this a great way of weeding out poor choices, it helps to ensure that everyone will get along after the hire has been made. Also, we put a real effort into orienting new staff members on the special features of our practice. Even the most experienced new staff are matched with a "practice buddy" for several months and really learn about the history and culture of this practice. Far more than 50% of our new staff work out long term. ***(5 points)***

____ 2. We wish we could do better at picking new staff, but we've never been right more than about half of the time. It's hard to find good candidates in our market, and because we're chronically understaffed we often settle for "B" players and cross our fingers. Orientation lasts for the first week at best, then it's sink or swim in our practice. ***(3 points)***

____ 3. We're so busy with patient care chores that we tend to hire the first applicant who comes along and just throw them into the practice without much advance training. It sometimes works out, but much more often than not our new hires don't make it past probation, and we have to start all over again. ***(1 point)***

Loyalty to the Practice and Job Accountability

The best supervisors, without being sycophants, are strong advocates of the practice's and the owner's interests. They are guardians, and see themselves as protectors of the overall organization, its patients, staff, and doctors. In this role these best managers feel profoundly accountable for getting the job done. Which of these describes your supervisors?

____ 1. Our supervisors could just as well be elite commandos. They consistently place their duty to the practice above their own personal interests. ***(5 points)***

____ 2. Supervisors here are by no means neglectful of their duties, but they're not all that committed, either. If they see something that really, really needs to be done or reported, they'll certainly come forward ... but not at personal costs. ***(3 points)***

____ 3. Our supervisors are rather lax in the "guardianship" department. They don't really seem to care about the destiny of the company, and don't evidence much concern about setbacks to the practice. They behave in a way that furthers their own self-interests. ***(1 point)***

Are Your Supervisors Fair?

The most effective supervisors I meet around the country are most commonly viewed by their subordinates as "tough but fair." This latter quality is hard to quantify ... like "tough," "fair" is something you know when you see it. Which describes your practice?

____ 1. Anyone in a new supervisory position with our practice is oriented to the importance of fairness in dealing with staff. They're taught not to play favorites when delegating tasks or assigning vacation time. They equalize workloads, not only within the department, but in the overall organization. They quickly learn that staff confidences must be scrupulously protected at all times. ***(5 points)***

____ 2. Our supervisors try hard to be even-handed, but in an effort to be popular or well-liked are often lenient, which leads to the perception—if not the reality—that they don't treat everyone equally. ***(3 points)***

____ 3. Supervisors in our practice could hardly be considered "fair." They groom their friends on the staff for advancement and pick on people they don't like, often just for personal reasons. This leads to our staff taking sides, which is splitting our practice down the middle and lowering morale. ***(1 point)***

Enthusiasm and Personal Energy Reserves

At the risk of trivializing a serious, grown-up role, supervisors are the front-line cheerleaders of your practice team. Try to remember back to your last live high school football or basketball game. The cheerleading squad's "rah-rah's" are passionate and heart-felt. What's more, in a typical game, the average cheerleader probably burns more calories than the average linebacker—and as every manager in your practice knows, it takes a lot of energy to be a successful supervisor. Which of these describes your practice's supervisors, energy-wise?

____ 1. Our supervisors are upbeat and consistently have an abundance of energy to get through the week. Even on the tough days, they not only shoulder through their own jobs, but manage to chip in to help others and share their time and encouragement with everyone around them. ***(5 points)***

____ 2. We could probably use a little more "spirit" here on the team. We start the week off with a roar, but end with a whimper. ***(3 points)***

____ 3. If our practice was a sports team, we'd probably lose every game. Our supervisors are lackluster ... they barely drag through the work week doing their own jobs, much less have any excess energy to provide encouragement to others. ***(1 point)***

• • •

Now add up your total score, and see where you seem to fit in the ranges below. The maximum score is 35, the minimum 7.

30 to 35 points: Congratulations! Whether by luck or plan, you have mastered one of the most difficult, subtle—and important—arts of business ownership.

22 to 29 points: A close runner-up! And now at least you know a few concrete areas to work on.

Under 22 points: Sorry. It's time to get on with broad improvements in one of the most fundamental areas of practice management and leadership.

Financial Disclosures

Dr. Amir Arbisser has no financial or proprietary interest in the materials presented herein.

Dr. Paul N. Arnold has no financial or proprietary interest in the materials presented herein.

Dr. Priscilla Arnold has no financial or proprietary interest in the materials presented herein.

Hayley Boling has no financial or proprietary interest in the materials presented herein.

Dr. John Campbell has not disclosed any relevant financial relationships.

Keith Casebolt has not disclosed any relevant financial relationships.

Linda Cook has no financial or proprietary interest in the materials presented herein.

Jeff Grant has no financial or proprietary interest in the materials presented herein.

Dr. Adrienne Graves has no financial or proprietary interest in the materials presented herein.

Dr. Paul S. Imperia has not disclosed any relevant financial relationships.

Dr. Erik F. Kruger has no financial or proprietary interest in the materials presented herein.

Jaci M. Lindstrom has no financial or proprietary interest in the materials presented herein.

Dr. Richard L. Lindstrom has not disclosed any relevant financial relationships.

Dr. Marsha Link has no financial or proprietary interest in the materials presented herein.

John B. Pinto is an ophthalmology practice management consultant in his firm, John Pinto & Associates, Inc.

Dr. Craig N. Piso has no financial or proprietary interest in the materials presented herein.

Alan E. Reider has no financial or proprietary interest in the materials presented herein.

Amelia Rogoff has not disclosed any relevant financial relationships.

Dr. William Shields has no financial or proprietary interest in the materials presented herein.

Dr. John C. Shin is the partner/owner of Marin Ophthalmic Consultants and Marin Ophthalmic Surgery Center.

Jane T. Shuman has no financial or proprietary interest in the materials presented herein.

Allison Weber Shuren has not disclosed any relevant financial relationships.

Candace (Candy) S. Simerson has no financial or proprietary interest in the materials presented herein.

Lauren Simon has no financial or proprietary interest in the materials presented herein.

John Swencki has no financial or proprietary interest in the materials presented herein.

Corinne Z. Wohl is an ophthalmology practice management consultant in her firm, C. Wohl & Associates, Inc.

Index